TREATING TRAUMATIC STRESS
IN CHILDREN AND ADOLESCENTS

Treating Traumatic Stress in Children and Adolescents

How to Foster Resilience through Attachment, Self-Regulation, and Competency

MARGARET E. BLAUSTEIN
KRISTINE M. KINNIBURGH

THE GUILFORD PRESS
New York   London

© 2010 The Guilford Press
A Division of Guilford Publications, Inc.
72 Spring Street, New York, NY 10012
www.guilford.com

Printed in Canada

This book is printed on acid-free paper.

Last digit is print number: 9 8 7 6 5 4 3 2 1

Library of Congress Cataloging-in-Publication Data

Blaustein, Margaret.
    Treating traumatic stress in children and adolescents : how to foster resilience through attachment, self-regulation, and competency / Margaret E. Blaustein, Kristine M. Kinniburgh.
        p. ; cm.
    Includes bibliographical references and index.
    ISBN 978-1-60623-625-3 (pbk.: alk. paper)
    1. Post-traumatic stress disorder in adolescence—Treatment.   2. Post-traumatic stress disorder in children—Treatment.   I. Kinniburgh, Kristine M.   II. Title.
    [DNLM: 1. Stress Disorders, Traumatic—therapy.   2. Adolescent.   3. Child.
4. Psychoanalytic Theory.   5. Resilience, Psychological.   WM 172 B645t 2010]
    RJ506.P55B53 2010
    618.92′8521—dc22
                                                                2009044009

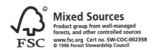

For D. and H.—
for all you have taught us, all you've become,
and all you are yet to be

About the Authors

Margaret E. Blaustein, PhD, is a practicing clinical psychologist whose career has focused on the understanding and treatment of complex childhood trauma and its sequelae. With an emphasis on the importance of understanding the child-, family-, and provider-in-context, her study has focused on identification and translation of key principles of intervention across treatment settings, building from the foundational theories of childhood development, attachment, and traumatic stress. With Kristine Kinniburgh, Dr. Blaustein is codeveloper of the Attachment, Self-Regulation, and Competency treatment framework. She has provided extensive training and consultation to providers and consumers within the United States, Canada, and Europe. She is currently the Director of Training and Education at The Trauma Center at Justice Resource Institute in Brookline, Massachusetts, and is actively involved in local, regional, and national collaborative groups dedicated to the empathic, respectful, and effective provision of services to this population.

Kristine M. Kinniburgh, LICSW, is the former Director of Child and Adolescent Services at The Trauma Center at Justice Resource Institute in Brookline, Massachusetts. She is currently a practicing clinical social worker and organizational consultant, working with agencies to integrate trauma-informed and trauma-specific practices into all facets of service delivery. Over the past 15 years Ms. Kinniburgh has dedicated her practice to work with children and families affected by trauma in a range of settings including outpatient clinics, schools, residential programs and hospitals. Her clinical experience, broad in scope, inspired her to explore and subsequently identify core components of trauma-informed intervention that can be implemented in the array of treatment settings serving this population. Ms. Kinniburgh is the originator and codeveloper of the Attachment, Self-Regulation, and Competency treatment framework and is currently training and consulting on this framework with agencies across the United States and abroad.

Preface

It is a rare privilege to have the opportunity to share with others everything you have ever learned about a field of study. In the pages that follow, you will be introduced to most of what we know about the understanding and treatment of complex trauma in childhood. We feel extremely lucky to have entered into our clinical careers at a time when knowledge about traumatic stress in childhood was ever-expanding, when societal awareness was growing, and when the opportunities for study, collaboration, training, and intervention were continuously unfolding.

Approaches and methods for treatment of traumatic stress in childhood are many, and though there is more consensus than in the past, a great deal of disparity remains within the field as to the "appropriate" treatment modalities for this population. Given the complexity of the topic, it is not surprising that this is so—"trauma" is not singular, those who experience it are not identical, and the contexts and cultures within which each of us lives are as varied as the blades of grass in a field. We believe it is fair to say that no two individuals, no two families, and no two communities will ever have the exact same experience, whether traumatic or otherwise. Because of this complexity—in population, in subjective experience, and in outcome—it makes sense that certain approaches will have excellent results with one child but variable results with another. It is difficult for us to believe that any single treatment method would work with every child, in every family or setting, in every context, every time.

The Attachment, Self-Regulation, and Competency (ARC) treatment framework was developed in large part because of the awareness of that complexity. It is a components-based framework designed not to replace any of the excellent treatment methods that are currently available but rather to organize, encompass, and facilitate their use. Although this text is lengthy, the framework is, in many ways, quite simple: It consists of 10 "building blocks," or key treatment targets. Nine of these fall within the three primary domains of attachment, self-regulation, and competency, with the tenth, trauma experience integration, as an overarching target integrating and building upon all other skills addressed within this framework. Within each block we identify key treatment goals and their theoretical rationale, primary "skills" or areas of focus, potential methods of intervention, developmental and cultural considerations, and applications across contexts. We describe each of these building blocks in detail in Chapters 4 through 13, grounded in the real-world work that shaped our own understanding of treatment. In the first three chapters we describe the theoretical foundations on which this framework is built, and ways to consider its implementation.

This framework is designed to be applicable across settings. Our hope is that this book has value for the range of individuals and systems working with children and families affected by trauma, including (but certainly not limited to) clinicians in outpatient, home-based, and milieu settings; program administrators; educators; child welfare workers; milieu counselors and line staff; and biological, foster, and adoptive caregivers. The framework is meant to be adapted; we have had the great privilege of working with many different agencies and programs that have incorporated the framework into their work, and no two of them have ever applied the concepts in the same way. Because our own learning has been greatly influenced by the work of others, we include examples of applications that have arisen from the creative implementation of our collaborators.

Our approach to treatment is grounded in a deep belief in the ultimate strength of children, families, and systems. We believe strongly that the "symptoms" displayed by children and adolescents most often represent their generally successful attempts to adapt to their worlds, and that the impact of trauma must be understood in the context within which it occurred. Our lens is not one of pathology, but rather of developmental adaptation, and our ultimate goal for treatment is to build positive developmental pathways and competencies that can support present and future resilience. It has been a great pleasure for us to bear witness to the unfolding of resilience in many children, families, and systems over the years, and to learn from all of them. It is our sincere hope that this book offers back what we have learned in a way that continues to ripple.

Acknowledgments

The development of the Attachment, Self-Regulation, and Competence (ARC) treatment framework, and ultimately of this book, has been a process of the heart extending over the past 7 years, and has been influenced by the contributions, support, and wisdom of many different people.

We have the great pleasure of working as part of a strong, vibrant clinical team at the Trauma Center at Justice Resource Institute (TC-JRI) in Brookline, Massachusetts. We are extremely appreciative of the support, collegiality, and contributions of our peers over the past number of years. Although we would love to thank everyone by name, we know that we would invariably leave out a name or two. So we thank all of our colleagues as a group and pull out a few "in particulars." First, our thanks to the Center's founder, Bessel van der Kolk, and members of the senior management team—Alexandra Cook, Richard Jacobs, Joseph Spinazzola, and Marla Zucker—for their encouragement and administrative support, and for their leadership in creating and sustaining a center that strives for excellence and innovation in the very real work of helping those who have been affected by trauma. Our gratitude also to the members of our small internal ARC team for all of their support, creativity, and downright excellent on-the-ground work over the past several years: Leticia Buonanno, Marissa Gold, Michelle Harris, Kristina Konnath, Eva Lambidoni, Kelly Pratt, Jessica Shore, and Dan Williams. To everyone else at TC-JRI—staff, supervisors, and faculty—it has been a sincere honor and a great pleasure to work with all of you, and to learn from your wisdom and dedication.

In 2005 our Center had the great privilege of joining the Justice Resource Institute (JRI), an impressive nonprofit agency that strives for social justice and that has as its mission providing services to the least served populations among us. Among other partnerships, a number of JRI programs collaborated with our team in developing applications of the ARC framework in the range of residential settings serving highly trauma-affected youth. Our thanks to the following individuals from Glenhaven Academy, Cohannet Academy, the Butler Center, and the Susan Wayne Center for Excellence for their support and creativity in the development of ARC applications: Laurie Brown, Rick Granahan, Ligia Hammiel, Bryan Lary, Beth Anne Lundberg, Candy Malina, Tracy Moore, Mike Morrill, Leah Newton, Molly Ober Fechter-Leggett, Abby Perham, Christine Robitaille, Alicia Straus, Karen Vincent, and members of the Cohannet "Trauma Team."

The ARC framework had its earliest roots in a model developed in collaboration with Alexandra Cook and Michele Henderson, and we appreciate their contributions to its initial conceptualization. Our thinking about the nuances of culture was greatly enhanced by rich discussion with and feedback from Beau Stubblefield-Tave of the Cultural Imperative. Our thanks to Dawna Gabowitz, Erika Lally, and Jodie Wigren for providing feedback on earlier drafts of this book; to Wendy D'Andrea for her assistance with tracking down references; and again to Erika for sharing two of her drawings for use in our handouts. Our thanks to Janina Fisher for her generosity in allowing inclusion of one of her activities.

Our work applying the ARC framework within our own community was supported in part by the National Child Traumatic Stress Network (NCTSN), funded by the Substance Abuse and Mental Health Services Administration, and we have very much appreciated the opportunity the NCTSN has given us both to team with systems locally, as well as to collaborate with excellent colleagues from around the country who stretch our minds and expand our understanding of this work. Our particular thanks to the members of the Complex Trauma Workgroup, with whom we have felt honored to work and from whom we have learned much.

Outside of the NCTSN, we have had the great pleasure of collaborating with numerous agencies both within and outside of the United States. Our thanks to all of them for their hard work, creativity, and dedication to the children and families they serve. We have learned a great deal from all of you. In particular, we'd like to express our thanks to Anchorage Community Mental Health Services, Bethany Christian Services, La Rabida Children's Hospital, and the Lower Naugatuck Valley Parent–Child Resource Center for their lengthy collaborations with us.

Taking the step to turn our ideas into a book was a big one, and we are extremely grateful to The Guilford Press and Executive Editor Kitty Moore for believing in this project and being so positive, despite our multiple deadline changes, and to our colleague Glenn Saxe for encouraging us to take our ideas to the next level.

For both of us, our families have provided a foundation and a life lesson in the invaluable influence of support, love, humor, wisdom, and "hanging in" through the tough times. **From MB**—my thanks and love to my parents, Donna and Arnold Blaustein, for . . . well, everything, but among many other things, for the ways you have shown me, in everything you do, the immense capacity of human beings to make it through and transcend the inevitable curve balls that life throws our way, and to do so with grace, compassion, and humor; to Rich, Keri, Josh, Megan, and Nicole—I feel so lucky to have you all in my life, and to receive the ongoing reminder of what health, love, and joy look like in a family; and to Vera Rosenbaum, my thanks for the unconditional love and the many, many life lessons. **From KK**—my thanks and love to Todd for being my partner in everything, for your quiet strength and unfaltering patience, and above all for offering consistent love and support throughout this journey; to my parents, Maureen and Bjorn Jentoft, for instilling in me the belief that I could be anything, do anything, and overcome anything that life should throw my way and for guiding and supporting me in all of my endeavors; to my sister, Wendy, thank you for being my friend and for reminding me about the importance of fun and laughter; and to my daughter, Lexi, for an experience like no other, for the pleasure of watching you learn, grow, and change, and for the gift of pure joy that you have given me every day since you came into my life.

Finally, our deepest thanks go to all of the children, adolescents, and families with whom we have worked. There is nothing we do in our work, and nothing in this book, that we didn't first learn from one of you.

Contents

Introduction

Ryan, age 10, is a generally likable kid, in turns, charming and funny. For the most part, he gets along with adults, particularly in one-on-one conversation, and his peers can count on him to be the "class clown." Despite this, Ryan has no really close friends. He vanishes after school and never gets together with other students on the weekend. He is in the fifth grade, and although he receives some school supports, he spends most of his time in a mainstream classroom. Ryan isn't doing very well in school; he participates in class when he's interested, but can become easily frustrated when uncertain of himself. He never turns in homework. He struggles with authority and confrontation, and when pressed too hard by a teacher, will either shut down or explode. He's gotten to know the guidance counselor as a result of his frequent detentions, and despite the problem behaviors, she finds him endearing and earnest. She notices that Ryan is watchful: In between moments of charm and laughter, Ryan is generally quiet and observes everything going on around him. He is often jumpy and has a hard time concentrating, and as a result was diagnosed with attention-deficit/hyperactivity disorder (ADHD) by his pediatrician at the age of 6. Although he is taking prescribed medication, Ryan continues to have difficulty paying attention in class.

Ryan likes to take the bus to his grandparents' home after school. They struggle with many medical problems and are impacted by cognitive limitations, but they provide a steady source of love and affection. When he is unable to go to their house, he returns home, where he spends most of his time in his room. He likes to lose himself in the world of video games. At night, he climbs into his top bunk and surrounds himself with stuffed animals. The animals make him feel safe: Although part of him knows that it's silly, part of him believes the layers of animals in his bed provide protection from anything dangerous. For extra security, he keeps a plastic wiffle-ball bat tucked under his covers. Although he would probably never use it, it makes him feel just a little bit safer. Sleep always takes a while to come, and Ryan sometimes lays in the dark for hours before finally falling asleep.

Every child has layers of possibilities: developmental pathways waiting to unfold. Every path a child takes in the course of development leads to new pathways and new possibilities. Although these paths are not infinite, it is almost impossible to predict at birth the direction a child's life may take. Our lives are influenced by the intersection of many factors: our biology, temperament, experiences, and relationships; the resources we bring into the world, and the resources that surround us; the layers of challenge we face, and the buffers that protect us—or not—from these challenges.

All of us learn to adapt to our worlds. It is one of the marvels of nature: We learn to respond to the environment that surrounds us, in a way that helps us survive. For many of us, our lives provide a "good-enough" balance of strengths and challenges, resources and stressors. A safe-enough system surrounded us in childhood. We built the foundations for establishing relationships and grew these with our parents, our teachers, our peers, and our larger world. We learned to recognize our strengths and limitations. We faced stress, learned from it (or not), continued to grow, learned new skills, and evolved our adaptations to meet new demands.

We absorbed information and ideas—about ourselves, others, and the world, from the context surrounding us, both in its presence and in its absence. In a noisy home filled with exuberance and love, perhaps we learned to cherish silence but tolerate chaos. As the child of quiet, structured parents, we may have learned to rely on organization but to enjoy the spontaneity of the world of our peers. As the oldest child of a hard-working single mother, we learned responsibility and work ethic, but secretly treasured the moments of unadulterated fun and escape.

Few of our lives were idyllic; it is rare, in this world, to never face stress or challenge—even, at times, overwhelming stress. Research suggests that as many as one in four of us will face significant adversity in childhood, a stress so overwhelming that it taxes our available resources (Centers for Disease Control and Prevention [CDC], 2005). Yet the capacity for human resilience is remarkable. We witness it every day: the ability of individuals, of families, of communities, of entire societies, to cope with, metabolize, and to overcome or transform even the most overwhelming of experiences.

But what happens to the children from the not-quite-good-enough environments—the children who face not one, but two, or three, or four, or seven layers of adversity? How is development impacted for those children who encounter more challenges than buffers?

Ryan is 13 now. He has had increasing difficulty in school. He barely passed sixth grade, and by early in seventh grade was tagged as a "problem student" by his teachers. He has struggled with the increased chaos of the middle school schedule, and after numerous temper outbursts and perceived aggression, several of his teachers refused to have him return to class. Whenever confronted by the vice principal about his behavior, Ryan's facial expression appears flat, and his body appears rigid. Although he snaps at some of his teachers, he withdraws and appears frozen when confronted by this larger authority. Because of his increasing classroom troubles, he now spends much of his time in a resource room. He continues to function better in a one-to-one setting, so his behavior with the special education teacher is improved from that in his classroom, but he appears bored and restless. He has been tested and has high average intelligence with no real sign of a learning disability other than some difficulties with concentration. The resource teacher notices that Ryan appears drawn and pale, with dark circles under his eyes. He is increasingly jumpy and hates the noise in the hallways when classes are changing, often asking if he can put on headphones.

There are many "Ryans" in this world. There are children who, like Ryan, are tagged as "problems" in the school setting. There are others who show up with frequent health complaints in the offices of primary care physicians, or who are referred to mental health centers for treatment of oppositional behavior, attention problems, or mood disorders. Most likely to be referred are those who cause trouble for others: that is, those whom we identify as having some sort of behavioral problem. Just as many children, however, "fly under the radar": They are quiet, or watchful; they learn to follow the cues of the adults around them and to shift accordingly. They exert tight controls on their behavior and show up in the system much later, with depression, eating disorders, substance abuse, or self-injury. Many children, like Ryan, show some of both—alternatively controlled and explosive, they struggle to maintain equilibrium.

Like all of us, Ryan has learned to adapt to his environment. What we label as "pathology," Ryan's brain labels "survival." What we *observe* is the surface behavior: the temper, the academic trouble, the trouble concentrating, and the rigid controls. Underneath it all, though, is a marvel at work: the brain doing its best to ensure survival by sacrificing some tasks for the sake of others.

WHAT IS DEVELOPMENTAL TRAUMA?

Ryan grew up with two parents who themselves spent significant time in the mental health and child welfare systems. His father was placed in residential care by the time he was 10 years old due to severe mood swings and behavioral trouble; the diagnosis of bipolar disorder wasn't made until much later in his life. Abandoned by her parents, his mother grew up in foster care, group homes, and residential programs. Ryan's parents met as adolescents and married in their late teens. Ryan, their oldest child, was born when his mother was age 21. Three more siblings have followed. His parents lead chaotic lives. His father is more frequently unemployed than working; a mechanic, he is often fired for losing his temper on the job. His mother works part time as a waitress. Both parents drink regularly and smoke marijuana; his father occasionally uses cocaine. Ryan is aware that he was a "mistake," an accidental birth. Although his mother is affectionate toward his younger sisters, and his father will occasionally play with his baby brother, their behavior toward Ryan is generally unpredictable. There are infrequent moments of connection, but more often, Ryan is ignored or criticized.

Ryan's father has a temper. Although his mother often yells back, Ryan knows that she is afraid of him. Ryan has seen his father slap and punch his mother on many occasions. During the worst incident, when he was age 8, Ryan tried to get in the middle of the fight, grabbing a baseball bat and threatening his father. On that occasion, the police were called by neighbors, and Ryan, his mother, and his siblings spent 4 months in a domestic violence shelter before his parents reunited. Ryan's father turns his anger on the children, as well, and although he is afraid of his father, Ryan will send his younger siblings upstairs when he senses the escalation and take the brunt of his father's rage. Whenever possible, though, Ryan tries to keep from being noticed; he has started to teach his younger brother how to pick up on signs to stay away from Dad.

On rare occasions, Ryan's father shows interest in him. Although Ryan always feels torn, he secretly treasures these moments and wishes there were more of them. When he wants to be, Ryan's father is charming and fun; he knows how to make things exciting, and Ryan loves when his father takes him fishing or down to the local mechanics' shop where his father's friends work. These occasions don't come very often, though, and Ryan has learned to see his father as two very different people: the "good" parent and the "bad." He tries not to let himself feel too much and often feels like he is watching his own life from afar.

There are, unfortunately, many overwhelming experiences children may face. In its definition of posttraumatic stress disorder (PTSD), the *Diagnostic and Statistical Manual of Mental Disorders*, 4th edition, text revision (DSM-IV-TR) has classified traumatic experiences as those events that involve experiencing or observing actual or threatened death, physical injury, or threat to physical integrity (American Psychiatric Association, 2000) and that result in feelings of terror, horror, or helplessness. This definition is limited, however, and many rubrics, including experts examining a newer diagnosis of developmental trauma disorder (van der Kolk, 2005), expand this definition to include other overwhelming experiences of childhood, often occurring within the attachment relationship, such as neglect, psychological maltreatment, attachment separations, and impaired caregiving systems. It is widely agreed that there are qualitative distinctions in outcomes among those children who experience more acute and particularly noninterpersonal traumas, such as motor vehicle accidents and natural disasters, versus those who experience chronic, interpersonal stress (Cook et al., 2005).

It is without question that trauma has the potential to have a significant impact on individual outcome. In a national epidemiological study involving nearly 17,000 adults, the CDC established unequivocally that exposure to adversity in childhood increases the risk for myriad adult health risks and negative outcomes, including depression, substance use, cigarette smoking, and obesity, and social risks such as teen pregnancy and paternity as well as experiencing or perpetrating domestic violence in adulthood (Anda et al., 1999, 2006; Felitti et al., 1998). Although only 5–13% of individuals exposed to a traumatic event will develop PTSD (Breslau, 2001), among those with this diagnosis, the incidence of comorbidity may reach as high as 80% (Solomon & Davidson, 1997). When experts have examined distinctions between those adults who develop PTSD versus those who develop more complex adaptations—including difficulty managing emotions, impairments in interpersonal relationships, impaired systems of meaning about self and others, health symptoms and somatic complaints, and fragmentation of memory and consciousness—the evidence points starkly to the role of childhood onset, chronically stressful experiences (van der Kolk, Roth, Pelcovitz, & Mandel, 1994).

Children like Ryan experience many layers of stress, both subtle and overt. Physical abuse and domestic violence—the two exposures in his story that meet the criteria defined as "trauma" by DSM-IV-TR—are only a piece of Ryan's experience. Ryan's life is marked by chaos and unpredictability. There is little reflection or validation of his experience, other than from his grandparents. His actions are dismissed, ignored, or criticized. When frightening things happen, they are most often at the hands of his caregivers, and there is no buffer to protect him. His life has been this way from the moment of his birth. The impact of these layers of experience goes far beyond his ability to metabolize a single, or even multiple, events. His life experiences, like all of ours, have shaped him: in his understanding of himself, of others, and of the world he lives in; in his capacity to regulate his internal experience, his body, his emotions, and his behavior; and in his ability to accomplish the range of developmental tasks that moves beyond survival.

The experience of trauma is complex. Trauma varies in type, source, chronicity, and impact; it is experienced at different developmental stages, within different contexts—family, community, and culture—and in the presence or absence of different internal and external resources and challenges. It is not surprising, then, that disparity exists in our understanding of trauma, in its manifestations, and in its proper treatment.

The focus of this text is on children like Ryan: children who have experienced chronic, often multiple stressors within a caregiving system that is, itself, stressed. We classify these children as having experienced complex developmental trauma. It is our belief that there is no single treatment modality or focus that will work for every child, in every system: No two children are the same, no two families or systems are the same, and no two providers are the same. However, there is research and expert consensus on the core impacts of trauma (Cook et al., 2005), as well as considerable data on those factors promoting resilience and developmental competency (Cicchetti & Curtis, 2007; Masten, 2001). This framework is built around those concepts: core issues known to be both impacted by the experience of chronic and complex traumatic exposures, and those relevant to developmental resilience.

This text is written for the range of providers who work with children who have experienced complex developmental trauma. This range includes individual clinicians but may also include residential systems, schools, shelter providers, foster parents, primary caregivers, and others. We have worked to identify core targets of intervention that translate across the systems in which children and families receive care. An expanded description of the origins of this framework and ways to apply it appears in Chapter 3.

PART I

OVERVIEW

CHAPTER 1

The Developmental Impact of Trauma

Imagine a child, a young girl, 12 years old, who is living with two loving parents in a comfortable home. Her neighborhood is safe, her school is good, her peer group is generally positive, and resources are readily available. She is white, and most of the children in her neighborhood look like her and speak her language. Like all children, she has innate strengths and vulnerabilities. This child is outgoing and personable but struggles with a learning disability. Her parents, strong advocates, have worked with her school to develop an educational plan that meets her needs. Although she sometimes becomes frustrated with classwork and with her school performance, she has received supports and encouragement since her learning disability was first identified.

Take this same child but change one factor. Imagine this same child living, not in a comfortable suburb, but in a family struggling with poverty. Her father recently lost his job, her mother is working two jobs, and the family lives from paycheck to paycheck. How might these circumstances change the course of her development? We can imagine ways in which it builds strengths as well as the many ways in which it layers on challenge. Perhaps her school is less resourced. Perhaps there is less time for schoolwork or for play, as her parents rely on her to care for her younger siblings while they work. She may learn increasing autonomy, but she may also have decreased efficacy in school settings or increased exposure to a higher-risk peer group. Her loving parents continue to play an important role as buffers and containers of stressful experience, but they may be less available or more stressed themselves. Despite all these challenges, with this single—though intense—risk factor, in the context of a safe attachment system, it is likely that this child's development proceeds on task.

Now change more variables. Rather than a member of the majority culture, what if this child belongs to an ethnocultural minority? How might that factor impact her access to resources, her sense of herself, and the perspective taken of her achievements and vulnerabilities by others? Imagine this same child, with the same innate qualities, but with one parent who is impaired or absent. Add the role of an unsafe neighborhood and community violence. Add the role of physical violence by a caregiver and frequent changes in residence or caregiver. How might each of these factors influence this child's development?

Development is dynamic. Developmental tasks build on themselves, with success and mastery at a given stage laying the foundation for potential success and efficacy at a later one. The child, for instance, who successfully negotiates relationships with caregivers in early childhood has learned crucial skills for successful negotiation of relationships with peers in later child-hood. This child has learned how to read nonverbal and verbal cues, communicate effectively, negotiate turn taking, delay gratification, and tolerate and negotiate conflict. Although these skills do not guarantee success in new relationships, they provide a foundation for the develop-ment of newer and more complex skills.

All developmental skills grow, initially, within the context of our earliest relationships and environment. The ways in which we develop are purposeful. Our skills grow in response to the input our environment gives us, so that we can negotiate that environment successfully. In this sense, all of development can be considered adaptive.

USE-DEPENDENT DEVELOPMENT

The extent to which we develop particular skills varies depending on many factors, including our need for a particular skill, our available resources, and the feedback and input we receive from the environment. For instance, a child with a sensory impairment, such as hearing loss, may show advanced development in other sensory areas, such as visual attentiveness. A child in a bilingual home may easily develop facility with two languages, even though that same child might have struggled with learning a second language had exposure not occurred until later, in the school setting. The frequently attended-to youngest child of loving parents may prioritize external soothing over internal regulation capacity, whereas the oldest child of more distant parents may learn to minimize emotional experience.

A key concept in understanding human development is the role of *neural plasticity*: the ability of the brain to adapt and change in response to experience. We are not born with fully developed brain structures and connections; rather, our brains develop and change in response to experience and maturation. Development of our brains is *use-dependent*: Specific changes happen in the brain in response to repeated input, or patterns. There are millions of potential synaptic connections available in our brains at birth; those that are used are strengthened and become increasingly efficient, whereas those that do not receive input are pruned away (Abitz et al., 2007).

As an example, consider the challenge of learning a foreign language. Many of us have had the experience, in adolescence or adulthood, of attempting to learn a second language. As we pronounce a word in this new language, a native speaker corrects our attempts. "It's la silla, not la see-ya." You respond, "But that's what I said!" The native speaker shakes her head and hides a smile. "No, it's not." Human spoken languages contain thousands of speech sounds that vary across cultures. At birth, children have the capacity to discriminate among *every sound in human speech*; by 10–12 months of age this capacity disappears, and we remain able to discrim-inate only those sounds heard in the spoken language or languages surrounding us (Werker & Tees, 1984). Through auditory input alone, our brain improves some connections (those involved in our native language) and prunes away those auditory pathways that have not been used. In this manner, development is purposeful and specific.

Like all other variables, trauma and adversity shape development (Cicchetti & Toth, 1995, 2005; Pynoos, Steinberg, & Wraith, 1995; Streeck-Fischer & van der Kolk, 2000). The experi-ence of complex trauma in childhood has been associated with a host of negative outcomes and risks, some of which are detailed in the Introduction. Rather than framing these as "pathol-ogy," many of these outcomes can be understood as arising from core developmental deficits in *intrapersonal competencies* (e.g., sense of self and self-development); *interpersonal competencies* (e.g., capacity to form and engage in relationships with others); *regulatory competencies* (e.g., capacity to recognize and modulate emotional and physiological experience); and *neurocognitive competencies* (e.g., capacity to engage executive functions and other cognitive abilities to act meaningfully on the world). There are two primary mechanisms through which complex developmental trauma can be thought of as having its impact:

1. The prioritization of certain developmental tasks and skills—typically, those skills relevant to the child's survival.
2. The interference with other developmental tasks—frequently, those most dependent on the availability of a safe attachment system and context.

The Attachment, Self-Regulation, and Competency (ARC) treatment framework focuses on both of these mechanisms by working with children and caregivers to recognize danger signals, differentiate current and past dangers, build skills in managing these responses, and lay the foundation for development of competencies across domains—while supporting caregivers in providing a safe context in which their children may do so.

Our understanding of the developmental impact of trauma, around which the intervention targets of ARC are built, are discussed in this chapter and the next. First, we discuss the tasks of normative development and ways in which developmental trauma may interfere in task completion. Second, we present a three-part model for understanding current behaviors and responses, framing these as adaptive skills and responses that have grown in service of ensuring the child's survival.

TASKS OF CHILDHOOD AND THE IMPACT OF DEVELOPMENTAL TRAUMA

Early Childhood (Infancy through Preschool)— Normative Development

In the first year of a child's life, he or she is busier, by far, than at any other time in the lifespan. The young child is learning the essential building blocks for the remainder of his development. The child is learning that he *exists* as a separate entity from those individuals surrounding him; he is learning the foundations of *connection* in building his earliest relationships within the dyad and familial system; he is building early *affect tolerance and regulation* strategies through the coregulation provided by his caregivers; he is *exploring* his world and establishing the foundational understanding that will serve in problem solving and awareness of objects and space; and he is developing a basic sense of *agency*, or the awareness that he has the capacity to have an impact upon the world.

The earliest understanding of self, other, and self in relation to other grows in the context of the attachment relationship. At birth, a child has little awareness of self as separate and no capacity to discriminate among internal needs and states. As the caregiver responds sensitively and discriminately to the infant's cues and needs, the infant gradually develops a sense of self and an awareness of bodily cues. The infant and young child learn the rudiments of interpersonal interactions, including how to interpret others' expressions and how to communicate needs effectively, within the context of the attachment system (Kelly, Morisset, Barnard, Hammond, & Booth, 1996). Effective communication bids are reinforced when the child's needs are attended to, and the child gradually develops skill with communication. Similarly, understanding of others' communication strategies grows as the child learns to interpret caregivers' facial expressions, vocalizations, actions, and other cues. When these predictably match, the child develops a frame for understanding his or her caregivers' communication. As the child is gradually exposed to a greater number of interactions, his or her repertoire for understanding communication grows. Simultaneously, systems of meaning about self, other, and the world are growing, albeit in a purely nonverbal, emotion-based manner. The child who receives relatively consistent, sensitive responses from caregivers develops a basic sense of safety in the world, an understanding of others as responsive and trustworthy, and an understanding of the self as worthy of care.

Early regulation occurs in the context of coregulation: The infant depends on the caregiver to provide soothing, comfort, and stimulation (Schore, 2001b). Arousal often increases rapidly when immediate needs are not met, and emotional experience appears "splintered"—infants are calm *or* upset, but generally not somewhere in between. It is over time, in response to consistent soothing, that infants and toddlers learn how to flow through emotional states and develop primitive self-soothing techniques. Importantly, it is through this process that infants learn a tolerance for emotional states: When arousal escalates, infants begin to understand that it will not last forever, and that strategies exist for making it settle or disappear.

In a safe-enough system, the young child will begin to explore his or her world. Exploration moves from sensory to physical, as the child sees, touches, tastes, smells, and begins to act on the environment. It is through this exploration that the child begins to develop a sense of *agency*, or a belief in his or her capacity to have some impact on the world. When the toddler knocks over a tower of blocks—and it falls!—she learns that her actions create a *reaction* in the world. When she does it again—and it falls again—she learns that her power is sustainable, and that there is consistency and predictability in external response.

Along with connecting action to response, infants and toddlers are also making connections among sensory stimuli and meaning. The smell of the mother may be connected to comfort, the voice of the father connected to playtime, and the bark of the dog connected to fear. These early connections, laid down prior to the acquisition of language, are solidified and held internally on a nonverbal level, and they may elicit memory and response even much later in life. Many of us have had the experience of walking down a street, smelling something, and being hit by a wave of emotion—often, in the absence of a capacity to identify a specific memory tied to the smell. Sensory connections built early in life are often strong and long-lasting.

There is an increasing focus on agency and independence as young children approach the preschool years and explore the limits of what they are capable of, as well as the limits of the boundaries placed around them. Preschoolers are particularly tuned in to structure, repetition, and security: This is the age when children watch the same movie over and over, prefer the same bedtime story each night, and focus strongly on "rules" as inviolable. The repetition is soothing, but it also provides important information as children are building their understanding of the ways in which the world works.

Preschoolers have little sense of time and space, and their interpretation of the world is concrete and immediate. If something goes wrong, it's because either *you* did something or *I* did something—abstractions do not come into play. Past experiences that are salient may be described as if they happened yesterday, whereas experiences that did happen yesterday, but are not salient, are rapidly gone from the young child's consciousness. Tomorrow, a week from now, and a year from now have equivalent meaning to the preschool-age child, unless anchored in concrete terms.

Early Childhood—Trauma Impact

Bruce Perry, a researcher examining the impact of abuse and neglect on very young children, once stated, "It is an ultimate irony that at the time when the human is most vulnerable to the effects of trauma—during infancy and childhood—adults generally presume the most resilience" (Perry, Pollard, Blakley, Baker, & Vigilante, 1995, p. 272).

Consider the developmental tasks described above and begin to superimpose, for instance, a home that is marked by chaos, in which the child receives inadequate and unpredictable care. There is sporadic response to needs, and the child's communication bids are ineffective. Caregivers' response may be unpredictable, and facial expressions, verbal cues, and actions are inconsistent. The child, then, is left with no frame in which to interpret communicative experience. The child's adaptation may be to communicate more strongly (e.g., frequent fussiness, constant bids for attention) or to minimize communication bids altogether, particularly if these bids rarely lead to response or lead to punishment. These deficits in interpersonal communication continue as the child progresses through toddlerhood and preschool (Coster, Gersten, Beeghly, & Cicchetti, 1989). The child may be overly vigilant to peer and teacher expressions of danger or anger, may misinterpret cues, and may have difficulty negotiating early relationships. Preschoolers may continue to build defenses against emotional experience and/or connection to others, or may become overly clingy and needy with those around them in an attempt to get their needs met (Egeland, Sroufe, & Erickson, 1983; McElwain, Cox, Burchinal, & Macfie, 2003; Vondra, Barnett, & Cicchetti, 1990).

When the child in this stressed environment experiences affective and physiological arousal, soothing and regulation may occur inconsistently or not at all, and in fact the child's affective states may be met with anger or threat. In the absence of adequate self-soothing strategies, and without available external regulation, the child is exposed to overwhelming arousal (Schore, 2001a). As connections and understanding about experience begin to be laid down, the inadequately soothed child learns that emotions, themselves, are frightening, and that arousal in the body is a potential danger. The young child may begin to disconnect from or guard against physical experience, or may express arousal and affect through behavior and action (Erickson, Sroufe, & Egeland, 1985). As the child progresses through preschool age, self-soothing strategies may continue to be primitive, and the building of increasingly sophisticated strategies that are part of normative development does not occur: In the face of ongoing levels of challenging arousal, children must continue to rely on earlier skills.

In the absence of a safe system, the young child's exploration will be impacted. A child of an unpredictably responsive caregiver may sacrifice exploration in service of remaining close to the caregiver, whereas a child of a consistently rejecting caregiver may explore regardless of environmental cues signaling danger. As exploration is impacted, so, too, is agency. The child in the stressed environment has less control, less impact, and a less predictable understanding of the world, and often begins to internalize a sense of helplessness (Crittenden & DiLalla, 1988). This pattern may continue through the preschool age, as the child either continues to sacrifice exploration or begins to develop age-inappropriate independence. Loss of structure and safety—a staple at this developmental stage—will lead the young child to develop rigid control strategies to manage anxiety (Main & Cassidy, 1988). Behaviorally, this may appear as bossiness, lying, or "manipulating."

For the infant and young child exposed to chaos, violence, or neglect, interpretation of sensory stimuli will become infused with danger. At this stage, given nonverbal processing, cues of potential danger will generalize and be solidified without language; later in life, these same cues may trigger a danger response without the child knowing or understanding its origins.

Elementary School/Middle Childhood—Normative Development

During the elementary school years, children expand their worlds beyond their immediate family circle, with gradually increasing ties to and investment in the worlds of school, community, and the peer group. Although caregivers remain the primary target of attachment, there is a gradual increase in the importance of peers.

Children at this age show an increase in independent functioning, paralleled by a strong investment in industry, or personal accomplishments. As children are exposed to the world beyond their family, they discover that they are able to produce, create, and accomplish using internal assets, and the development of pride in these accomplishments plays a strong role in continued identity development. An understanding of individual attributes gradually grows from the concrete and absolute (e.g., "I'm a girl," "I'm smart") to the more abstract and nuanced (e.g., "I'm pretty good at math, but I have a hard time with reading," "People think I'm funny"). During this time period, children are actively building the "filter" through which they will later interpret experience. A child who typically has positive achievements in school is building a belief in the self as academically competent. A child who typically does well in peer relationships is building a belief in the self as interpersonally competent. Continued experiences will expand, be integrated into, or be rejected by these filters through processes of accommodation and assimilation.

Cognitive skills continue to develop, but children throughout the elementary school years continue to rely on concrete information in their meaning making. The power of abstract thinking does not fully emerge until the end of this stage, so interpretation of the world continues to focus on those factors immediately at hand. Similarly, although an early understanding of time and space emerges, children continue to focus largely on present experience.

Elementary School/Middle Childhood—Trauma Impact

As domains of functioning expand through development, so too does the impact of trauma, and children will demonstrate impairments in competent development across domains. Notable at this stage are impairments in peer and school functioning, as these are two primary domains of competence at this stage. Children who have not learned how to successfully interact with their earliest caregivers have greater difficulty developing competent and/or adequate relationships with their peer group or with other adults, such as their teachers (Anthonysamy & Zimmer-Gembeck, 2007; Shields, Ryan, & Cicchetti, 2001). Loss of early exploration and failure to develop a sense of agency may begin to impact children's capacity to perform and sustain performance in the school setting (Shonk & Cicchetti, 2001).

During this stage, competent performance is increasingly reliant on an array of skills. Positive school achievement, for instance, may require cognitive ability but also hinges upon the capacity to concentrate, ability to modulate arousal levels, ability to regulate behavior and control impulses, frustration tolerance skills, and interpersonal relationship capacities. Children who have experienced trauma may have impairments in any or all of these domains. Challenges in these areas may lead increasingly to the experience of felt failure; these experiences then generalize to other arenas, as children overestimate their lack of competence (Vondra, Barnett, & Cicchetti, 1989).

Continued failures of development take an increasing toll on children's sense of self, and the beginnings of a negative self-concept and self-blame are internalized. As with all children, those from stressed environments are actively constructing their filter of self, other, and the world. Repeated experiences of failure or lack of competency in relationships, in academic achievement, and in other developmental domains will grow a belief in the self as inadequate or incompetent (Runyon & Kenny, 2002; Toth & Cicchetti, 1996). Unlike securely attached children, the belief system of children from stressed environments is often more rigid—an adaptive capacity when life involves frequent and absolute discriminations between safety and danger—which means there is less room within belief systems for accommodation and assimilation. Experiences conflicting with a negative sense of self may be rejected as aberrations or exceptions, rather than incorporated. During the latter half of this stage, early signs of helplessness and hopelessness may emerge (Kim & Cicchetti, 2006).

Relationships with others may be similarly rigid: Whereas securely attached children approach relationships flexibly, with differing styles for differing relationships, children from stressed attachment systems may replicate their early attachment styles in new relationships, approaching others with a basic sense of mistrust (Lynch & Cicchetti, 1991). This approach is adaptive: If a child has developed a belief that others are dangerous, through multiple experiences of danger within relationships, it is in that child's best interest to believe that *all* others are dangerous, unless proven otherwise. The result, however, is a significant challenge in building relationships with potentially safe others, including the child's peer group, teachers, and other adults. In the face of the self-protective signals the child puts out, others may respond in kind: For instance, few people want to approach a child who clearly communicates with her behavior, her language, and her facial expressions, "Back off!" In this way, the cycle is perpetuated: The child retains and solidifies a belief that others are rejecting, while the system develops a belief that the child is disinterested in relationships.

Because of the limitations of the growing child's skill set, as well as the restricted circles of functioning, coping with and expressing emotional and physiological experience at this age is largely managed through behavior and interaction. The range of potential behavioral expressions is wide. Children may act out and become aggressive or bullying; may appear hyperactive, silly, or have difficulty managing behavioral arousal; or may withdraw, constrict, and shut down (Alink, Cicchetti, Kim, & Rogosch, 2009; Ford et al., 1999; Hebert, Parent, Daignault, & Tourigny, 2006).

Adolescence—Normative Development

Adolescence is a time period marked by rapid changes: Cognitive abilities develop, social skills and perspective-taking abilities mature, and physiological development changes rapidly. The adolescent must negotiate all of these changes and integrate them meaningfully. Among other primary tasks, the adolescent is actively constructing a coherent sense of identity, a complex understanding of *self.*

The formation of identity happens both in comparison and in contrast: "I am like my peers in this way"; "I am different from my parents in that way." As the adolescent engages in self-reflection and evaluation, others may notice that, like very young children, teens appear self-absorbed. During this developmental period, however, this is less because of a lack of *awareness* of the outside world, as it is in infancy and early childhood, than due to an excruciating awareness of how the outside world may be viewing and focusing on the self.

Along with the growth of a sense of self comes healthy separation and individuation from the early caregiving system. As a means toward accomplishing this, adolescents increasingly turn to their peer group as a source of reference, information, and support. However, while the peer group grows in importance, in a healthy caregiving system, parents and primary caregivers remain an important "safety net" for the adolescent in times of uncertainty and distress.

Because of the desire to define the self, adolescence is often a time of extremes. Adolescents experiment, try on, and discard different roles in a search to discover their own "identity." They play with body image, sexual image, and self-concept. They develop often strong views and judgments, which begin to temper as they move into adulthood.

Adolescence is the first developmental stage in which the future becomes real and meaningful: Unlike younger children, adolescents can draw connections between past, present, and future and can view themselves at a future point in time. Adolescents are not, however, efficient yet at connecting current actions to consequences and the role these play in achievement of goals; this is a skill that develops over time, as cognitive structures become increasingly mature.

Adolescence—Trauma Impact

Adolescence is a particularly high-risk time for youth who have been exposed to trauma (Appleyard, Egeland, van Dulmen, & Sroufe, 2005). In this time of rapid change, self-assessment and self-critique, and extremes of experience, adolescents who have not yet developed the skills to regulate their own experience and interactions may become increasingly disconnected and disenfranchised. For youth who already feel different—and often damaged—as a result of their early experiences, the belief that others are examining them as intently as they are examining themselves can lead to a painful self-consciousness and crystallization of a negative self-identity.

The strong emotions of adolescence place traumatized youth at high risk. In the absence of the more sophisticated strategies normatively developed, traumatized adolescents may continue to rely on more primitive coping strategies. Some adolescents may rely on overcontrol and perfectionism, constricting their emotional experience and their interactions with others. Other adolescents rely on external means of modulation, including substance use, cutting, sensation-seeking behaviors, and sexual interactions (Kilpatrick et al., 2003; Lansford, Dodge, Pettit, Crozier, & Kaplow, 2002). The increased independence that comes with adolescence means that the nature of available coping strategies will carry increased danger: Whereas a 5-year-old may have a temper tantrum in the face of significant dysregulation, a 17-year-old is able to drink to excess and then drive erratically.

Individuation and separation are challenging for adolescents whose internal sense of self is fragmented. Those adolescents whose trauma was chronic or began early in life may continue to rely on dissociative coping, and depersonalization and derealization become prominent at this age (Haugaard, 2004; Putnam, 1997). This disconnect across aspects of experience—and a feeling of separation from the self and the world—may cause adolescents to sublimate their own goals, opinions, and values. Adolescents may be at particular risk for negative peer influence and affiliation, or they may isolate themselves and withdraw from peer interactions. At the extreme, adolescents are at risk for revictimization by both peers and adults (Barnes, Noll, Putnam, & Trickett, 2009). Ultimately, the adolescent's identity may involve splintered aspects of self, which are not integrated into a coherent whole.

Early Adulthood—Normative Development

Although this text focuses primarily on youth, the children of today are the adults of tomorrow, and many clinicians and systems will work with youth into their young adult years. Therefore, brief attention is given to these early transition years into adulthood.

In normative development the transition into adulthood is marked by increasing solidification of a sense of identity: From the 20s to the 30s, adults have a growing consciousness of and comfort with aspects of self. Often, this sense of self evolves into an awareness of self across context and self in multiple roles: as a daughter or son, a spouse, a parent, a worker, a friend. Although the adult may be conscious of ways in which different aspects of self manifest more or less strongly in different environments or in different roles, there is a general coherence in the understanding of self and identity.

In early adulthood there is a growing emphasis on engagement in some meaningful occupation or industrious output, and as time progresses, there is evaluation and reevaluation of life choices. Although the normative time frame for "commitment" to a career path, interpersonal relationship choices, and other life decisions has increasingly shifted, by the late 20s to early 30s, many adults are generally able to visualize and define significant life choices.

During these years, the healthy adult is generally able to function independently, though others will often be utilized as a source of instrumental or emotional support. Attachment targets shift toward partners and children (Dinero, Conger, Shaver, Widaman, & Larsen-Rife, 2008; Simpson, Collins, Tran, & Haydon, 2007), and healthy attachment patterns are typically repeated with the next generation (Benoit & Parker, 1994; van IJzendoorn, 1995). Cognitive and interpersonal capacities increase in complexity, and the healthy adult is able to take perspective, use abstract thought, and link past, present, and future actions and experiences. In fact, having developed fully and prior to the start of any real aging process, executive function and other cognitive capacities are thought to reach their peak in the late 20s (Ostby et al., 2009; Tamnes et al., 2009). As a result, the adult can "think on his or her feet," solve problems, juggle multiple tasks, and engage and concentrate attention.

Young Adulthood—Trauma Impact

As childhood developmental tasks coalesce into the complex functioning of adulthood, the young adult who has experienced chronic early trauma may show significantly impacted functioning across domains. Sense of self and identity may be increasingly splintered and fragmented, with lack of integration across time, experience, and context (Ogawa, Sroufe, Weinfield, Carlson, & Egeland, 1997; Reviere & Bakeman, 2001; Wolff & Ratner, 1999). Self-concept may rigidly incorporate the negative frames developed in earlier childhood, including self-blame, guilt, shame, damage, and powerlessness (Brock, Pearlman, & Varra, 2006; Liem & Boudewyn, 1999).

Interpersonal capacities may continue to be impacted in adulthood. Just as secure attachment patterns repeat across generations, so, too, do anxious ones (Lyons-Ruth, Yellin, Melnick, & Atwood, 2005; Main & Goldwyn, 1984; van IJzendoorn, 1995), and the adult who has experienced early interpersonal challenges may have difficulty forming healthy mature relationships. Relationships may be marked by overdependence and intense need; conversely, the young adult may isolate him- or herself or have relationships that are maintained by keeping others "at arm's length," marked by superficiality or constriction.

Difficulties with the regulation of emotional and physiological states may continue into young adulthood, and in fact may become more extreme or entrenched. With continuing exposure to overwhelming affect and arousal, the young adult may increasingly rely on rigid, primitive strategies for coping (Fortier et al., 2009; Lyons-Ruth, Dutra, Schuder, & Bianchi, 2006; Min, Farkas, Minnes, & Singer, 2007). Vigilance to the environment and intense arousal responses may be followed by numbing and disengagement, such that the adult lives in intense states of hyper- or hypoarousal, or in wildly swinging mood states that vacillate between the two (Ford, 2005; Ford, Stockton, Kaltman, & Green, 2006). Although cognitive capacities are generally complex and nuanced at this stage, the young adult who has experienced trauma may continue to show significant deficits in key capacities such as executive functions and memory (Bremner, 1999; Bremner et al., 1995; Navalta, Polcari, Webster, Boghossian, & Teicher, 2006). Furthermore, these cognitive processes may break down in the face of danger or overwhelming stress, as the survival response prioritizes other capacities. As a result, functioning across domains may be state-dependent, with capacity for accomplishment and positive functioning largely a result of the adult's level of internal regulation. Conversely, the increased cognitive capacities of adulthood may allow the adult to "hold it together," functioning in an apparently coherent way and competent in one or more contexts, while inwardly or in other contexts experiencing significant dysregulation or collapse.

DEVELOPMENTAL RESILIENCE

It would be remiss to discuss the impact of traumatic experience on child development without also highlighting the remarkable nature of human resilience. The concepts of stress and resilience are intertwined; the latter does not exist without the presence of the former. The study of resilience grew from the study of risk, as attempts to understand the impact of overwhelming experience on outcomes highlighted the fact that in *every* population of highly stressed individuals studied by researchers, there were individuals who not only survived but thrived. The field of resilience research grew, as attempts were made to better understand what factors predicted more positive outcomes.

Although many definitions of *resilience* exist, the one that speaks to us is the following: "The process of, the capacity for, or outcome of successful adaptation despite challenging or threatening circumstances" (Masten, Best, & Garmezy, 1990, p. 426). By this definition, every child we have seen is resilient, in some way and on some level. If a child is sitting in our office, then that child has successfully adapted to his or her world—at least long enough to physically survive the circumstances. Successful adaptation may manifest in many ways, and often in ways that seem counterintuitive. For instance, a child who is labeled "manipulative" and a "liar" (common descriptions for a neglected child) is often a child who has successfully adapted to a world in which needs are not met by finding ways to meet those needs. A child who appears emotionally shut down may be a child who has successfully adapted to a failure of caretaking by minimizing access to emotional experience. In the next chapter we discuss why children's behaviors nearly always make sense, given an understanding of the context in which they develop.

Ultimately, though, our goal is for children to do more than physically survive; we want them to adapt successfully to a world that goes beyond the context of danger and deprivation. By understanding factors that promote resilience, we are able to target and support those factors. At core, it is our belief—as individuals who work with children exposed to traumatic stress and given an understanding that trauma derails healthy development—that our primary treatment goal is to build those factors that lead to competent and healthy development.

The Building Blocks of Resilience

Factors that lead to healthy development in children exposed to significant stress can be broken into two broad categories: those that are *internal* to the child (e.g., temperament, specific developmental skills), and those that are *external or contextual*, including both familial and environmental/systemic contributions (Masten & Coatsworth, 1998). Ideally, our work targets both of these levels. Not surprisingly, the relative importance of factors shifts across the course of development: What is vital for an infant will vary from that which is most important for an adolescent. A number of researchers have made significant contributions to our understanding of risk and resilience by studying differential outcomes among high-risk populations, and/or by examining the protective role of developmental assets in population-based samples of youth (Cicchetti & Curtis, 2007; Cicchetti & Rogosch, 2009; Cicchetti, Rogosch, & Toth, 2006; Haggerty, Sherrod, Garmezy, & Rutter, 1996; Masten, Best, & Garmezy, 1990; Masten & Coatsworth, 1998; Urban, Carlson, Egeland, & Sroufe, 1991; Werner & Smith, 1980, 2001; Wyman et al., 1999). We draw from these sources to highlight some of the building blocks of resilience.

Individual/Child Factors

When addressing the developmental assets of childhood, it is important to emphasize that even those factors described as "individual" or internal grow best within the foundation of a safe, surrounding caregiving system. Across developmental periods we see the crucial impact of *working models*, as each developmental period highlights factors relevant to *models of self* (e.g., self-efficacy and independence) and *models of other* (e.g., social orientation and ability to build positive relationships). Also highlighted across developmental stages is the role of the child's ability to regulate experience (e.g., frustration tolerance, cognitive regulation, behavioral control), a set of skills that grow largely from external supports in normative development.

INFANCY

In infancy the strongest predictors of outcome are a positive temperament (e.g., affectionate, good natured, routine sleeping/eating habits) (Smith & Prior, 1995; Wyman et al., 1999) and a secure attachment style, with the latter viewed as both predictor and outcome (Cicchetti et al., 2006; Kim & Cicchetti, 2004; Rothbart, Ahadi, & Evans, 2000). At this stage the caregiving system serves as our primary target for intervention (Lieberman & van Horn, 2008; Scheeringa & Zeanah, 2001).

PRESCHOOL AGE

Two primary factors emerge among resilient preschool-age children: a growing sense of autonomy and some capacity for social orientation. Resilient preschoolers are described as having some sense of self and the ability, to an age-appropriate degree, to provide themselves with structure (Mendez, Fantuzzo, & Cicchetti, 2002). Ability to manage emotions is important, with frustration tolerance particularly predictive (Mischel, Shoda, & Rodriguez, 1989; Shoda, Mischel, & Peake, 1990). In relationships with others, resilient preschoolers are able to seek and elicit support.

MIDDLE CHILDHOOD

The building of a self-perceived sense of efficacy and personal competency is most predictive of outcome at this stage. Across studies, elementary school–age children who have positive outcomes have been able to develop areas of esteem and efficacy (Bolger, Patterson, & Kupersmidt, 1998; Kim & Cicchetti, 2003). Resilient children are able to make use of a reflective cognitive style, taking the time to think rather than reacting impulsively (Cicchetti, Rogosch, Lynch, & Holt, 1993; Shoda et al., 1990; Zelazo, 2001). They have, to some degree, an internal locus of control and believe in their capacity to influence their world (Wyman, Cowen, Work, & Parker, 1991). In the face of adversity, these children are flexible in their use of coping strategies and have a range of ready skills, including the use of humor. With others, these children are socially oriented and have more positive relations with peers and adults than their less resilient counterparts.

ADOLESCENCE

Primary factors predicting resilient outcome among adolescents include a sense of personal responsibility and social maturity. Adolescents who do well have a belief in their ability to exert some control over their own fate, and they have a desire to do so (Campbell-Sills, Cohan, & Stein, 2006). They are, to some degree, achievement oriented and can function independently. They have internalized a set of values and are able to draw on these in decision making. They are able to interact with others, are socially perceptive, and have built relationships (Resnick et al., 1997).

Systemic/Contextual Factors

External factors may include familial context or relationships, peer group, school factors, and/or community supports and resources. The role of relationships appears to be crucial (Werner & Smith, 2001; Wyman et al., 1999). Across studies, perhaps the most consistent predictor of resilience for high-risk children is a safe, nurturant bond with a single person (e.g., grandparent, teacher, sibling) (Chandy, Blum, & Resnick, 1996; Dexheimer Pharris, Resnick, & Blum, 1997; Flores, Cicchetti, & Rogosch, 2005; Wyman et al., 1991). Peer relationships are also important, with resilience predicted for children who have at least one close friend and who are able to maintain friendships over time.

Familial values and socialization practices may be protective. Research highlights the importance of communicating positive expectations to youth, including familial expectations for age-appropriate roles of responsibility—a practice that may foster the child's sense of efficacy (Lipschitz-Elhawi & Itzhaky, 2005). Other family factors include faith or religious practices, reliable emotional support from caregivers, and encouragement of emotional expressiveness (Werner & Smith, 2001).

A great deal of research supports the important contribution of the child's school experience to the building of resilience. Although academic achievement is viewed as a benchmark of competence, equally important in the study of resilience is the child's engagement with and relationship to the school setting (Resnick et al., 1997). Not surprisingly, children who feel positively about their school and their own connection to it do better than those children who do not. School factors that increase this connection include an emphasis on child strengths, awareness of the importance of feedback and praise, availability of roles and tasks that promote trust and responsibility, academic and behavioral standards and expectations, and positive child–teacher relationships.

Beyond home and school, children and families do better when they receive support from and are connected to the larger community. Availability of kinship supports and neighborhood resources may buffer stressed children and families (Jaffee, Caspi, Moffitt, Polo-Tomás, & Taylor, 2007). The importance of youth expectations extends to their role within their larger world, with resilience predicted for youth who feel able to make a contribution to their community.

CHAPTER 2

Child Development, the Human Danger Response, and Adaptation
A Three-Part Model for Understanding Child Behaviors

In the previous chapter we discussed ways that chronically stressed early environments may interfere with normative tasks of development. It is important to bear in mind that child development is responsive to the environment and context in which it occurs, and at the same time that certain tasks and skills are deemphasized, other tasks and skills become increasingly efficient. In this chapter, we discuss a three-part model for understanding the ways that the child's rapid mobilization in the face of danger and inherent drive toward safety interact with developmental challenges to create the behaviors, adaptations, and "symptoms" we typically classify as the complex trauma response. A summary of the model appears in Figure 2.1.

STEP 1: SYSTEMS OF MEANING—THE ASSUMPTION OF DANGER

All human beings have systems of meaning, frames of reference that guide our interpretation and understanding of the world around us, of our own actions and those of others, and of the input our senses provide to us. We develop these frames of reference throughout our childhood, first in the context of the attachment system and later through our experiences interacting with and acting upon the world. As we grow, we add layers of nuance and complexity. Although many of our frames operate in parallel, it is likely that no two of us see the same thing when we view our worlds. We process and make meaning about information on multiple levels, using all aspects of our organism (Tronick, 2007)—interpreting and understanding our worlds through cognition, sensory information, physiological response, and emotional understanding.

Our understanding of the world grows and changes as we develop, and it is strongly influenced by our experiences. Consider variations in cognitive *schemas*, or the ways in which we organize and understand concepts. Schemas may be influenced by developmental factors (e.g., the young child sees all four-legged creatures as *doggy*, the adult sees *cow* vs. *cat* vs. *dog*); by domains of expertise (e.g., *dog* vs. *Welsh springer spaniel*); by context (e.g., *working animal* vs. *companion*); and by personal experience (e.g., *frightening animal* vs. *beloved pet*). As

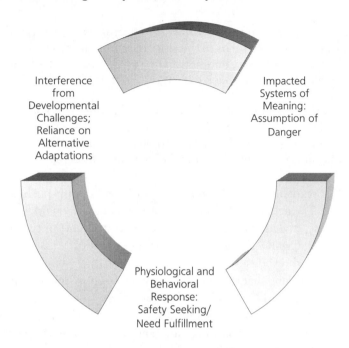

FIGURE 2.1. A three-part model for understanding child behaviors.

described originally in the writings of Piaget, over the course of our development these systems of meaning grow and change through a process of *assimilation* (the interpretation of new information through existing mental structures) and *accommodation* (the expanding and shifting of mental structures to incorporate new information). These mental changes are not random: We build these schemas as an adaptive process, in response to input from our physical and social worlds, and working toward a goal of maintaining cognitive equilibrium. In this way, all children actively construct their understanding of the world (Piaget, 2003, 2008; Piaget, Garcia, Davidson, & Easley, 1991; Piaget & Inhelder, 1991).

The ways in which we make meaning are built upon, and strongly influence, our beliefs about our experiences. This tenet is at the heart of cognitive models of treatment, which operate on the assumption that various mental health disorders (e.g., depression) involve altered or maladaptive cognitions and assumptions (e.g., the tendency to catastrophize: "This is terrible"), and actively work with clients to challenge them. It is also at the foundation of relational and client-centered models of psychotherapy, which emphasize the role of relationship in shifting clients' working models of self and other. It is widely accepted that our beliefs—conscious or not—influence our interpretations, our emotional responses, and our actions. Consider the following situation:

Jimmy is 11 years old, in the sixth grade. During an unannounced fire drill, his teacher stops the lesson and tells the students to line up quickly. The students rush to the door, and, as Jimmy lines up, he feels someone bump into him from behind—hard enough that he falls forward a step before he catches himself.

So . . . what exactly is the situation? Let us consider two possible scenarios:

Scenario A: Jimmy catches himself with his arm against the door, avoiding bumping into the student in front of him. He turns to the student behind him, a new student named Mike whom he's never really spoken to, and says, "Hey, man, be careful—where's the fire?" Both students laugh, and Jimmy turns back to face the front of the line.

Scenario B: Jimmy catches himself with his arm against the door and feels a surge of anger. He's convinced that someone shoved him on purpose—it seems like other students are always trying to start something. He turns and sees that the person behind him is that new kid, Mike, and he shoves him hard, saying, "Hey, man, you better watch out!"

In both scenarios, the available information is the same: A student is pushed from behind. The situation is ambiguous: The action could have been accidental, or it could have been purposeful. In the first scenario, the student assumes benign or neutral intent; in the second, the student assumes malicious intent. Clearly, these assumptions carry very different emotional charges and lead to different behavioral responses.

All of us have assumptions that are formed by the collective pool of our experience in the world, beginning with the working models of self and other we develop within our earliest attachment relationships. As in the above scenarios, these assumptions guide our interpretation of events, particularly when those events are ambiguous or uncertain: When in doubt, our previously developed systems of meaning guide us.

Beliefs that are built upon a foundation of danger may be particularly strong. If you have ever developed food poisoning after eating a particular food, you know that you never quite look at that food the same way again: Even if you logically know that not *all* clams are bad, the distress, discomfort, and fear elicited by that one bad experience is difficult to let go of. Similarly, although someone may have hundreds of experiences of safety as a driver or passenger in an automobile, it may take only one serious accident to build a belief that cars are inherently dangerous. Even when, on a *cognitive* level, you recognize your belief as illogical, your body may continue to react—on a *physiological* level, your belief in danger continues to hold. Thanks to evolution, our brain has a remarkable ability to use life experiences in the service of continued survival.

For children who have experienced repeated stress, chaos, danger, and harm in their relationships and their environment, these assumptions may be rigid and generalized. It is not that *one* individual is dangerous; *all* individuals are potentially dangerous. The belief systems of children who have experienced trauma may include the following:

- "I'm not safe."
- "People want to hurt me."
- "People cannot be trusted."
- "The world is dangerous."
- "If I'm in danger, no one will help."
- "I'm not good enough/smart enough/worthy enough for people to care about me."
- "I'm not powerful."
- "It will never get better."

For children who have a basic and enduring belief that the world is dangerous, it is adaptive and protective to maintain a defensive stance, a constant vigilance for signs of danger. Unlike the clear and concrete cue of a food item in the case of food poisoning, or the car following a motor vehicle accident, when children have experienced multiple and chronic stressors, the cues of danger are widespread and may be overt or subtle. This is particularly true when trauma is experienced early in life because core systems of meaning—and the associated cues of danger—have their foundations in sensory, affective, and visceral experience, rather than in language. For instance, for a child who has been inadequately cared for, cues of danger may include delays in gratification, feelings of deprivation or need, increases in physiological arousal, or perceived rejection or abandonment. For a child who has experienced verbal abuse, cues may include signs of anger, control by others, loud noises, or raised voices. We refer to these cues as *triggers*: those signals that act as a sign of possible danger, based on historical traumatic experiences, and which lead to a set of emotional, physiological, and behavioral responses that arise in the service of survival and safety. Common triggers for children who have experienced developmental trauma include the following:

- Perception of a lack of power or control
- Unexpected change
- Feeling threatened or attacked
- Feeling vulnerable or frightened
- Feeling shame
- Feelings of deprivation or need
- Intimacy and positive attention

It is important to note the subjective nature of many of these triggers: Cues of danger are often not absolutes. Keep in mind the example of Jimmy, standing in line: Was he pushed by accident or on purpose? The "reality" of the situation is not what dictates his interpretation or response, but rather, his guiding assumptions. When these guiding assumptions are predicated on danger, it is the rare person who is not most likely to err on the side of staying safe: in other words, to assume danger until proven otherwise.

Note also that beliefs and associations about these cues are frequently not held at a conscious or verbal level. As discussed above, our brains become increasingly efficient at the tasks they do most often; for a child exposed to frequent stress and violence, this includes the assessment and labeling of danger. Many of these associations were laid down long before language formed and/or were laid down on a visceral, physiological level. It is because of this nonconscious, nonverbal foundation that traumatic assumptions and associations are so entrenched and often so automatic.

Understanding and working with children's triggers and danger responses are discussed in depth in Chapter 5 (caregiver–child attunement) and Chapters 8 and 9 (affect identification and modulation).

STEP 2: PHYSIOLOGICAL AND BEHAVIORAL RESPONSES— SAFETY-SEEKING BEHAVIORS AND NEED-FULFILLMENT STRATEGIES

It is a central tenet of this framework that human behavior is not random: Our behavior and actions are largely functional or else arise to serve some function and continue because no more effective or sophisticated adaptation yet exists. Even the most seemingly "pathological" of children's behaviors may make sense, when understood in light of the purpose they serve for the child.

For children who have experienced chronic and early trauma, two salient factors have helped to shape behavioral responses: (1) the presence or threat of danger, often on an ongoing basis; and/or (2) the absence of sufficient fulfillment of physical, emotional, relational, and environmental needs. As a result, in a highly simplistic manner, many of the behaviors seen in children in the face of cues of potential danger may be thought of as either (1) safety-seeking or danger-avoidance behaviors and/or (2) need-fulfillment strategies.

Safety-Seeking Behaviors

While there are an infinite number of stressors that can cause a subjective sense
of overwhelming stress and distress in a child, there are finite ways that the
brain and the body . . . can respond to those stressors.
                    —MICHAEL DE BELLIS (2001, p. 540)

Over the course of millions of years of evolution, the higher cortical structures of the human brain have developed, advanced, and become increasingly sophisticated. We are able to plan, delay responses, focus attention, integrate information from multiple senses, solve problems, generate novel solutions, form and retain complex memories over long periods of time, and integrate experience across time and place. The subcortical structures of the brain, however, are more primitive. These are the structures which, among other tasks, prioritize our survival. We differ little from other mammals in these structures, and their activation sets off a chain of responses that is hardwired.

Much of the time our behavior and actions are in the control of our higher cortical structures. We engage purposefully in our lives as we act upon the world. As we are doing so, our brain undergoes a constant process of absorbing, filtering, interpreting, and either acting upon or discarding information and input from the world around us. Information that is irrelevant is discarded; information relevant to our task may be acted upon or "filed."

When information is labeled as "dangerous," a rapid mobilization occurs in the body. The brain signals the release of neurotransmitters responsible for rapidly increasing arousal; as these are pumped throughout our body, our heart rate increases, our sensory systems become hyperalert to further cues of danger, and all nonessential tasks—that is, those not relevant to immediate survival—are disengaged. Among tasks considered nonessential in the face of immediate threat is complex thought. Why would this be? Consider the following example:

> It is late evening, and you are walking down a curving side street toward your parked car. Tired after a busy day at work, you are paying little attention to your surroundings. The sidewalks are blocked by snow, but the road is clear, so you walk along the center of the road, knowing that the street is generally quiet. Suddenly, you hear a screech of tires, and you turn to see a car barreling down the road, directly toward you.

In this moment, which part of your brain do you want to have in charge? You can *think*, or you can *jump out of the way*. Most of us, of course, would rather jump first and think later.

In the face of danger, our *limbic system*—the structures of the brain concerned with arousal and emotion—increases in activation, and our higher cortical structures, particularly the *prefrontal cortex*, the part of our brain that engages in executive functions, decrease in activation. In a split second, our body mobilizes for action.

But what if the danger is not really danger? Let's say that, rather than continuing down the road toward you, the car in the example above speeds midway down the road and then suddenly turns right into a side alley. Objectively, you were never in danger: The driver had no intention of continuing down the road. Is your heart pounding any less?

The human danger response does not require actual, physical danger in order to be activated; it merely requires the *perception* of danger. Once your brain has labeled something as dangerous, regardless of "objective reality," your body will respond. In the previous section we discussed the often entrenched and generalized nature of children's "danger systems": For the child who has experienced ongoing chaos, violence, and stress, the array of signals that may be labeled as potentially dangerous is wide. As a result, the danger response may be activated often and indiscriminately, leaving the child at the mercy of frequent surges of arousal, rapid changes in physiology, and loss of access to higher cognitive structures. Although these changes are adaptive and perhaps lifesaving in the middle of the street with a car rushing at you, they are significantly less useful in the middle of math class or while interacting with peers.

Behaviorally, what does this danger response look like? There are three primary categories in which we classify the human danger response: we may *fight*, we may *flee*, and/or we may *freeze*. The response in which we engage depends in large part on the nature of the threat. Fleeing, or escape, often offers our greatest chance of survival: In the presence of a large, unbeatable threat (such as a car), whenever possible, we attempt to escape. When flight is not possible, we may fight: An adult who is being assaulted, for instance, may attempt to fight off an attacker, hoping to eventually either subdue or flee from the threat. Freezing, the least discussed of the danger responses, yet often the one most used by children, is the defense used when neither fight nor flight is possible. It is the danger response most readily available to small animals under attack in the jungle, and to small children under attack by their much larger caregivers. The freeze response is a state of extreme vigilance and arousal, despite a physical stilling and lack of observable physical movement.

Although we use the terms *fight*, *flight*, and *freeze*, actual behaviors used by children in the face of perceived threat or escalated arousal may vary. Examples follow of observable behaviors in children:

Fight: Physiological arousal

- Aggression
- Irritability/anger
- Trouble concentrating
- Hyperactivity or "silliness"

Flight: Withdrawal and escape

- Social isolation
- Avoidance of others; sitting alone in class or at recess
- Running away

Freeze: Stilling and constriction

- Constricted emotional expression
- Stilling of behavior
- Overcompliance and denial of needs

Need-Fulfillment Strategies

Immediate physical danger is rarely the only salient stressor shaping the behavior of the children with whom we work. A lack of predictable fulfilling of the range of human needs—physical, emotional, relational, and environmental—is often superimposed upon other stressors or is the formative stressor. Many factors impair caregivers' ability to provide for their children, including environmental stressors such as extreme poverty and homelessness, social stressors such as domestic and community violence, and individual factors such as substance use and mental health issues. In addition, many children have been affected by attachment losses and placement changes and disruptions.

In the Tasks of Childhood section of Chapter 1 we describe in detail the ways in which the child's development of competencies across a continuum of functioning relies on the sensitive and consistent response of the caregiver. When this response is not available or is inconsistent, the young child will develop his or her own strategies to either maximize the possibility of response or to meet the need in other ways.

Consider the following example:

Susan is 4 years old and lives with her mother, a young, single parent who is experiencing significant depression. Susan's mother spends most of her time curled up on the sofa, watching television or sleeping. When Susan tries to get her mother's attention, her mother generally ignores or dismisses her. Sometimes her mother will hold her if Susan climbs up on top of her, but most of the time her mother pushes her off and tells her to go play. Susan doesn't like to be too far from her mother, though, because she worries that something bad will happen. When Susan feels worried or upset, her mother often doesn't notice, but if Susan starts to cry loudly and throw a tantrum, her mother will generally rouse herself enough to try to comfort her.

For Susan, the lack of attention and care from her depressed mother represents a danger and a significant stressor: Four-year-old children need external soothing, comfort, and care, and Susan is just entering the age when she is cognitively aware of this. The only way for Susan to have her emotional needs met is to maximize the connection to her attachment figure by remaining as close as possible, and to communicate her needs loudly by tantrumming.

Imagine Susan 2 years in the future. She is in kindergarten, where many children are vying for attention from a single teacher. Susan is feeling sad one day, and tries to climb onto her teacher's lap. Her teacher gives her a quick hug, then tells her to return to her seat. For Susan, this perceived rejection serves as a trigger, and Susan copes with the perceived danger—the lack of attention—in the way she has learned: by refusing to return to her seat and then escalating and throwing a tantrum. Her teacher's attempts to deescalate the situation by walking away only increase the perceived danger, and Susan becomes increasingly dysregulated.

It is the rare clinician in this field who has not heard a child with a history of distressed attachment characterized as "manipulative," "needy," or "demanding." Although these behaviors, on the surface, are unappealing, there is an alternative frame for them. A child who is "manipulative," who tries to control the situation, the environment, and other people, is generally a child who is attempting to fill some need, and who has learned that adults cannot be relied upon to fill those needs independently.

Children from distressed early environments often show behaviors that may be categorized as attempts toward *need fulfillment*. Needs may substitute for one another; for instance, a child who craves attention and care may seek out physical objects or sensations, and a child who has been physically deprived may try to fulfill needs through emotional contact. Following are examples of common need-fulfilling behaviors among children who have had inadequate or inconsistent early care.

Emotional/relational needs
- Emotionally demanding behavior (whiny, interrupting, dramatic)
- Seeking negative attention (acting out)
- Poor interpersonal boundaries (e.g., too much sharing)
- Attempts to control the environment; may be described as "lying" or "manipulative"

Physical needs
- Physical nurturance-seeking behavior (e.g., too much physical contact, poor physical boundaries, sexualized behaviors)
- Hoarding or stealing food, clothing, objects

STEP 3: INTERFERENCE FROM DEVELOPMENTAL DEFICITS DUE TO EARLY GAPS IN CARE AND RELIANCE ON ALTERNATIVE ADAPTATIONS

Thus far, our three-part model for understanding behavior points to the role of a *system of meaning* that assumes, and is vigilant toward, prevalent danger, and to *adaptive physiological and behavioral responses* in the face of these cues. The third step in our model highlights the role of developmental deficits stemming from inadequate or distressed early caregiving systems.

As described in detail previously, children who have experienced developmental trauma have invested much of their energy into survival, rather than into the development of competencies. As a result, they may be impacted across domains of development.

Regulatory and Emotional Development

Children who have experienced chronic trauma demonstrate core deficits in the capacity to regulate physiological and emotional experience. They may have difficulty understanding what they feel, where it comes from, how to cope with it, and/or how to express it. The ability to maintain a comfortable state of arousal is impacted such that children may fluctuate from hypo- to hyperaroused states, escalate or constrict rapidly, and/or disconnect from affect and experience. Whichever the case, splintered state shifts and a lack of coherence and connection across emotional states are the result.

Intrapersonal (Self) Development

Children's understanding and perception of self may be strongly impacted. From an early age, children may develop a negative self-concept and a reduced felt sense of competency. Agency is affected; children may feel a lack of power and control over their lives and actions, and they may be more likely to perceive actions as "failures" and to blame themselves, rather than external factors, for those failures. Over time, children will have greater difficulty forming a coherent identity and sense of self, with a lack of integration across experience, a fragmented understanding and manifestation of self and identity, and reduced or absent future orientation.

Interpersonal (Social) Development

Following on the challenges within their earliest connections, children often continue to struggle in interpersonal relationships. Challenges may exist with forming relationships or with maintaining them over time. Children may have (1) difficulty reading social cues, (2) overly rigid or diffuse physical and emotional boundaries, and (3) a basic lack of trust in, or overdependency on, others. In the absence of healthy models of relationship, children may be vulnerable to further victimization or negative influence in their search for connection and attachment.

Cognitive Development

Trauma is toxic to the brain, and the neurocognitive development of children who have experienced chronic trauma may be impacted on a structural level, a biological level, and a functional level. Children may show early lags in receptive and expressive language, as well as difficulty with sustained attention and concentration. Over time, children show delays and impairments in executive functioning, including planning, problem solving, organization, and delaying response. Altered states of consciousness and structural impacts may affect children's memory, resulting in impairment in the consolidation of experience (i.e., transfer from short-term to long-term storage) and difficulty retrieving relevant information in current problem solving. Behaviorally, children may experience increased frustration in the face of challenging task performance, noncompliance with directions, and negative emotional response. Over time, children who have experienced trauma are at significantly higher risk for school disciplinary problems, grade retention, and dropping out.

Alterations in competencies in these domains will interact with, and layer on top of, the child's behaviors and emotions when confronted by signals of danger. In the face of the intense arousal and dysregulation brought on by these triggers, and in the absence of developmentally appropriate skills or external supports, the child is left with no choice but to rely on alternative adaptations—or a range of behaviors and strategies designed to help the child cope with internal and external experience. Common alternative adaptations include the following:

- Emotional numbing/constriction
- Withdrawal/avoidance of others
- Indiscriminate attachments
- Hypercontrol of the environment/rigidity
- Substance use/abuse
- Alterations in eating patterns
- Constricted or excessive sexual behaviors
- Self-injury
- Sensation-seeking behaviors
- Aggressive or other externalizing behaviors

Ironically, it is these alternative adaptations that frequently become the reason for a child's referral and the target of treatment. As a result, well-meaning clinicians invest efforts in treatment of the child's coping skills, rather than core areas of impact: the domains of developmental competency, the systems of meaning, and the lack of safety in the surrounding context.

PULLING THE MODEL TOGETHER

Let us put the various components of the model together, as we consider Janae.

> Janae's mother, a heroin addict, was unpredictable and often frightening. Her behavior changed rapidly: In one moment she might be barely responsive, in another she might be intrusive and emotional, and at certain times she would fly into sudden and volatile rages. Janae learned to be constantly watchful and vigilant. At a young age, Janae learned that her best survival strategy was to remain "invisible," particularly when her mother was in a rage; if she froze and did not move, she was less likely to become the target of her mother's anger.
>
> At the age of 8 Janae was removed from her mother's home and placed in foster care. Her current foster parents describe her as "cold" and disinterested in forming a relationship with them. The home is a somewhat chaotic one, with five children in it, and Janae often appears reactive and irritable, frequently escaping to her room. She is protective of her belongings, and flew into a rage one day when she discovered one of her foster sisters looking through her clothing drawer. When reprimanded by her foster mother, she froze and then tried to run out of the house.

Janae is a child whose early experiences involved chaos, inadequate care, and sudden violence. The unpredictable nature of her mother's behaviors taught her to be constantly alert to cues of danger, and the mother's responses to her emotions and behaviors have led Janae to constrict and shut down her expressions and actions. Despite this apparent constriction, Janae's body operates at a baseline level of high arousal, due to the frequent activation of the danger response and the subsequent chronic dysregulation of her physiology.

Although there is a very wide range of cues that have become associated with danger for Janae, particularly salient ones are unpredictability and anger, especially from women. Janae is also fiercely protective of her space and her property, having been exposed to significant physical and emotional deprivation. In the face of these triggers, Janae's arousal escalates rapidly, and she fluctuates among the triad of danger responses, alternatively raging, escaping, and stilling. Her capacity to cope with her intense arousal is limited; failures within her early attachment system have impacted her ability to regulate her physiological and emotional experience, and the sudden surges in arousal leave her feeling overwhelmed. She has few reliable coping strategies and is unable to view others as potential resources. Her experience has taught her that other people are both untrustworthy and potentially dangerous, and she has little practice expressing her feelings or asking for help. In the absence of either reliable internal strategies or trustworthy external supports, she frequently acts out her distressed emotions with impulsive behaviors.

In Janae's story we see the impact of exposure to significant early stressors, including an unpredictable and often dangerous attachment system. Janae's systems of meaning are infused with danger and chaos, and she is left with little agency or control. Her physiological and emotional experience is, in many ways, as dangerous as external events, as without adequate coping strategies, she is often at the mercy of internal experience. In a new, ostensibly safer caregiving system, her behaviors and actions are misinterpreted, and the misattunement of her caregivers confirms her beliefs about self and others, while forcing her to continue to rely on previously developed safety strategies.

IS DEVELOPMENT FIXED?

It is without question that chronic early trauma exposures may seriously and significantly derail and alter children's developmental pathways. The harm that is done may last not just throughout the child's life, but on into the next generation, as stress, chaos, and adversity are passed down from parent to child (Noll, Trickett, Harris, & Putnam, 2009). Given the wealth of evidence suggesting the harmful nature of these exposures, then, the question arises as to whether developmental pathways can be altered. Can a child whose life has been steeped in danger and survival, who has known chaos, adversity, invalidation, and/or indifference throughout his or her life—and perhaps, from before birth—find peace, health, and joy?

It is our unshakeable conviction, and that of many others in this field, that they can. The literature on resilience is a testament to this, as are the lives of the many children and adults we have encountered in our practice. The potential for resilience is remarkable. We have met many individuals who have managed to harness some factor or factors—an internal quality, an external resource, pockets of strength and competency—and convert them into growth and health, when their histories and experiences should have predicted continued despair and challenge.

As our understanding about the impact of complex trauma grows, so too does our capacity to change outcomes. The factor that itself contributes to the toxic nature of trauma—the plasticity and adaptability of children's brains—is also the factor that highlights the possibility for positive change. We believe strongly that all children have both the capacity for—and the right to lead—joyful, healthy lives, to the best of their abilities, and that the ultimate goal of the child clinician is *not* a reduction in pathology, but rather a targeting and building of the core developmental competencies, the systems of meaning, and the safe, surrounding caregiving system, that will allow the child to continue to build a positive future.

CHAPTER 3

The Attachment, Self-Regulation, and Competency Treatment Framework

Dashaun is 10 years old. His difficulty concentrating and poor academic performance have landed him in an alternative education placement. In his regular fourth-grade class of 25 students, he was one of six children who had experienced violence or abuse within his home. In his current classroom of 10, he is one of nine with some exposure to early violence, neglect, or a significant stressor such as poverty. Dashaun's teacher is not aware of the detailed history of any of her students. She is well intentioned, but often struggles to build a successful learning environment for these challenging children.

Lindsey, 6 years old, is living in a shelter with her mother and her 2-year-old brother. They came to the shelter 4 months ago, after fleeing from Lindsey's stepfather, a violent man who frequently beat Lindsey's mother. There are nine families, with 21 children, living in the shelter. Lindsey's mother must stay with her children at all times or risk losing her placement; she is often overwhelmed and tired by the end of the day, but fears that asking for support will make her look "weak." There are no clinicians on staff.

Jamie is 14 and has just started therapy at a local community health center. Her school pressed her mother to bring her to treatment because Jamie was showing signs of depression and admitted to a school guidance counselor that she cuts herself when she feels upset. In early sessions Jamie's therapist learns that Jamie's mother struggles with alcohol abuse, and that Jamie has a history of sexual abuse by an uncle. Jamie's family has no other supports in place.

Frankie is one of 16 boys in a residential program for youth committed to the state juvenile justice system. Like 14 of the boys in the program, he has experienced early chaos and violence. His father left when he was too young to remember, and his mother entered four successive relationships with violent men. Frankie was physically abused by two of them. He joined a gang when he was 12, and was committed to the state when he was 14. He entered the current program this year, at 15. In the 2 months since he has been here, he has been restrained six times for sudden aggressive behaviors.

Children and families who have experienced stress and trauma show up in every mental health and social service delivery system. They are served by hospitals, primary care physicians, domestic violence and homeless shelters, community health centers, and in specialized school placements. Many children and families receive no special supports, but make up a substantial portion of the population in public schools, after-school programs, and community centers. It is the rare few who make it to specialty, trauma-focused treatment centers.

The reality is that programs that serve children and families are programs that serve children and families who have been exposed to complex trauma. Although trauma exposure is widespread and strongly influences the risk for children and their caregiving systems, many service systems have limited training in, and experience with, provision of trauma-sensitive and trauma-informed care. Similarly, although clinicians in every type of setting work with these children and families, many feel hesitant to approach the role of early trauma exposure in their clients' functioning. Despite these limitations, it is our experience that there is a wealth of knowledge and expertise across service settings and an inherent drive among providers to do good work and to support the clients who are served within their system.

The Attachment, Self-Regulation, and Competency (ARC) treatment framework (Blaustein & Kinniburgh, 2007; Kinniburgh & Blaustein, 2005; Kinniburgh, Blaustein, Spinazzola, & van der Kolk, 2005) grew from an awareness of the above factors. We are both clinicians who have worked in regular and specialized school settings, hospitals, residential programs, and shelter systems, and who came together in a trauma specialty clinic. The ARC framework represents our attempt to capture the work that we do and to translate it so that it remains relevant across the myriad number of systems in which our children and families receive services.

Three primary factors influenced our conceptualization and construction of ARC: the desire to build upon the scientific literature and evidence base, while accounting for the realities of clinical practice; the importance of identifying principles of intervention that translate across service systems; and the wish to remain true to the inherent art and creativity of clinical work, while identifying a larger structure within which to be flexible.

WHAT IS DIFFERENT ABOUT ARC?: THE ROLE OF A FLEXIBLE FRAMEWORK

Evidence-Based Practice (or, How to Fit Real Kids into Scientific Boxes)

Manualized protocols often provide a gold standard for clinical intervention: Careful examination of structured protocols in controlled settings allows the clinician–researcher to study the role of intervention targets for particular clinical symptoms or populations. Challenges exist, however, with the translation of these protocols to "real-world" clinical settings. Clients may present with complex symptom pictures not adequately captured in existing protocols, and the generalizability of many researched treatments to clinical populations has been held in question (Spinazzola, Blaustein, & van der Kolk, 2005). Clinicians may resist or struggle with overly structured intervention formats. Furthermore, a significant percentage of youth who experience complex trauma may not receive intervention in "classic" outpatient settings involving one-to-one treatment; rather, these youth and their families present in a range of settings, including schools, residential programs, shelters, and primary care services.

Increasingly, there is recognition of the value of identifying core components of treatment, rather than emphasizing "one-size-fits-all" treatment models. The ARC framework was designed to incorporate a core components model. ARC identifies key targets of intervention for youth who have been exposed to trauma and their caregiving systems. These targets were drawn from extensive review of the extant literature on the impact of complex trauma as well as factors leading to resilient outcome within this population. We have significant clinical experience with this population in a range of settings, and principles selected for inclusion were reviewed with and modified by input from clinicians and other professionals working in the field.

Translation of Clinical Principles across Settings (or, Bringing the Mountain to Muhammad)

Because youth may present for services in a range of settings, and in recognition of the importance of "whole-systems" intervention, we selected principles that translate across service settings. For instance, when applied in an outpatient setting, ARC principles can be integrated into individual treatment with a child, dyadic caregiver–child treatment, psychoeducation and skills-building interventions with caregivers, and/or child and caregiver groups. In a milieu setting, attachment principles can be integrated into whole-systems intervention, including staff training and milieu structure. Intervention targets can be built into therapeutic groups or applied in more "organic" ways (e.g., incorporation of self-regulation tools into classroom settings). To date, ARC principles have been successfully integrated in diverse types of programs, including outpatient treatment settings, residential schools, locked juvenile justice facilities, therapeutic foster care, youth drop-in centers, and homeless shelters, as well as by a range of individual clinicians in community and private settings.

Staying True to the Inner Clinician (or, Keeping the Art in Treatment)

Every professional is different. Every client is different. Excellent treatment involves a combination of art and science. There are few providers who do not recognize the value of flexibility and the ability to "think on your feet." Good therapeutic work involves a careful assessment of client needs and strengths, recognition of key treatment goals, and the flexibility to approach those goals in a way that works best for a particular client at a particular point in time.

The ARC framework does not attempt to replace clinical wisdom or to supplant individual techniques with a one-size-fits-all model. Rather, ARC identifies key goals for intervention, skills involved in reaching those goals, and examples of ways to get there, with a recognition that many paths may lead successfully to the same destination. One of the best pieces of feedback we have heard is that the framework supports and organizes current clinical practice, rather than replacing it.

SO WHAT *IS* ARC?

The ARC framework is a components-based model that identifies three core domains of intervention for children and adolescents who have experienced trauma and their caregiving systems: attachment, self-regulation, and competency. Within those three domains, nine building blocks of intervention are identified. A 10th target of intervention, trauma experience integration, involves an integration of all other targets, including both external resources and individual skills, addressed within this intervention framework. A visual representation of the model appears in Figure 3.1.

Attachment

Across cultures, the caregiving system, in whatever way it is defined, serves as the foundational context for healthy development. A safe, healthy attachment system can buffer the impact of highly traumatic stressors (cf. Cohen & Mannarino, 2000); conversely, a stressed attachment system can, in itself, create significant risk (cf. Crittenden, 1995; Wakschlag & Hans, 1999).

Given our understanding of the role of attachment in child development, it seems crucial to target the surrounding caregiving system when working with children and families who have experienced trauma. We define the caregiving system broadly: Numerous youth who have experienced complex trauma have exposure to a range of caregiving systems, which may include biological parents or relatives, foster or adoptive parents, school systems, residential programs, caseworkers, and the myriad professionals who interact with these children. As noted, we encourage the targeting of a whole-systems approach, with the guiding assumption that youth can be only as safe as their surrounding system, and that until youth are safe, other aspects of development will continue to be sacrificed.

Our attachment building blocks target two primary factors: (1) the building of a "safe-enough," "healthy-enough" relationship between the child and his or her caregiving system, which requires felt safety within the system itself; and (2) the building of skills and a context that the caregiving system will use to support the child's healthy development.

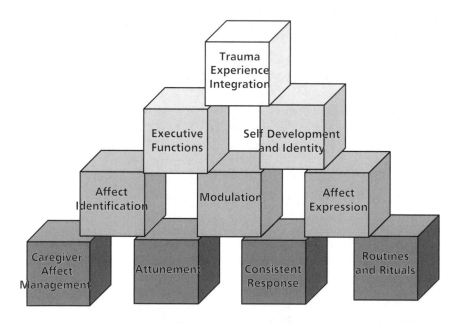

FIGURE 3.1. Core building blocks of the Attachment, Self-Regulation, and Competency framework.

The Attachment Building Blocks

CAREGIVER MANAGEMENT OF AFFECT

As is highlighted throughout the ARC framework, caregivers play a crucial role in child development. Furthermore, the ability of caregivers to support their children in the face of stressors is a key predictor of child outcome. Caregivers' ability to provide support to their children is limited by caregivers' ability to effectively manage their own experience. This section details the role of caregiver affect management in child outcomes, factors that impact caregivers' capacity to manage emotional experience, the crucial role of support for caregivers, and key skills to target in the caregiving system.

Key skills and areas of foci included within this intervention target include (1) psychoeducation about the nature of trauma and normalization of caregiver response, (2) building of caregiver self-monitoring skills, (3) building of caregiver affect management skills, and (4) enhancing caregiver supports. Applications for family systems, milieu, and other substitute caregiving systems, as well as clinician self-applications, are discussed.

ATTUNEMENT

Attunement is the capacity of caregivers to accurately read children's cues and respond appropriately. There are two primary errors that adults make in reading children's cues: We either miss the cues altogether or we react to overt behaviors, rather than "reading" the emotional message underlying the behavior. Children who have experienced significant early trauma may have a particularly difficult time communicating feelings, wants, and needs effectively. This second intervention target emphasizes the particular importance of accurate attunement in the caregiving system of complexly traumatized children.

Key skills and areas of foci within this intervention target include (1) psychoeducation about the role of child vigilance, (2) psychoeducation about traumatic triggers and their expression, (3) building a repertoire for understanding children's communication ("becoming a feelings detective"), and (4) building reflective listening skills.

CONSISTENT RESPONSE

Although research on parenting practices emphasizes that there is no one "right way" to parent a child, studies highlight the importance of consistent response: Children do better when they have a clear understanding of rules and when there is a degree of predictability in adult and environmental response. Successfully parenting a child who has experienced significant trauma, however, has many complications. Children who have experienced considerable chaos may exert rigid control in an attempt to gain some sense of safety, and they may resist or resent imposed rules. Typical parenting practices may trigger strong responses in children with dysregulated emotions. Caregivers may be reluctant to impose consequences on children who have been badly hurt, or they may be overly restrictive in an attempt to keep their children safe. Many caregivers have themselves experienced significant trauma in their own families of origin, and may have no ready model of safe parenting available.

This section highlights key intervention targets for building consistent response. Classic behavioral parenting techniques (e.g., limit setting, the use of positive reinforcement and praise) are combined with education about the role of the trauma response in the use of these strategies. Implementation strategies are framed for caregivers as "experiments," as no one parenting technique will be successful for all children, and process is emphasized over technique. Caregiver felt success in implementing techniques is viewed as essential, and strategies are provided to increase caregiver mastery.

ROUTINES AND RITUALS

Routines and rituals are often the invisible bookends that bracket our days: Most of us have set ways of waking, eating, sleeping, and organizing our time. We notice our routines in their absence more than their presence. Routines provide a sense of coherence and predictability to our days, and a disruption in routine can leave us feeling unsettled. Children and families exposed to complex trauma have often experienced lives marked by extraordinary chaos and unpredictability. As long as their lives continue to be unpredictable, children must invest a significant percentage of their energy in maintaining a vigilance toward continued danger. Increasing predictability builds a sense of safety and allows children to relax and shift their energy from survival toward healthy development.

This intervention target highlights the role of routines and rituals in the lives of traumatized youth and families. Considerations for the building of routines are discussed. Examples of routines at home, in the therapy session, during transitions, and within other key settings are provided. An expanded example is provided for creating routines at bedtime, one of the primary areas of challenge identified by many child clients and their caregiving systems.

Self-Regulation

As detailed throughout the introductory chapters, developmental trauma has a significant impact on the child's ability to regulate physiological, emotional, behavioral, and cognitive experience. Children are affected by failures of the attachment system (our earliest context for the lessons of regulation of the self), by the impact of significant stress on regulatory systems, and by the combination of the two. As a result, we work with children who have significantly dysregulated internal experience, and limited ability to understand, identify, and express that experience.

The self-regulation building blocks target children's awareness and understanding of internal experience, ability to modulate that experience, and ability to safely share that experience with others.

The Self-Regulation Building Blocks

AFFECT IDENTIFICATION

Children who experience early trauma often learn to disconnect from their emotional and physical experience. In the context of a caregiving system that does not provide adequate reflection of and language for emotional states, many children have challenges with differentiating emotions ("I just feel bad"), a lack of awareness of physical and emotional states ("I don't know how I feel"), and a lack of understanding of the connection between emotions and the experiences that elicit them ("I don't know why I feel that way"). In order to regulate emotional and physiological experience in a healthy way, children must first have some awareness and understanding of internal states.

This intervention target highlights a number of skills and points of intervention. Treatment goals include building a feelings vocabulary, providing psychoeducation about the human alarm response and trauma triggers, and normalizing the experience of mixed emotions. Children are taught to be "feelings detectives." Provided exercises and information highlight skill building in children's ability to identify emotions in self and other; to connect emotions to body sensations, thoughts, and behavior; and to understand the links between feelings and internal and external factors.

MODULATION

Complex trauma takes a significant toll on children's capacity to effectively regulate physiological and emotional experience. Overwhelming and chronic stress exposes children to chronically high and dysregulated arousal levels. Caregiving systems, which normatively serve as a buffer and external regulator, may be themselves impaired, leaving the young child alone to struggle with extreme emotional and physiological experience. Most children develop adaptations to help them manage their experience, but these adaptations may themselves leave children vulnerable to ongoing challenges.

This intervention target highlights those skills necessary to help children learn to maintain optimal levels of arousal and to expand their "comfort zone" to be able to tolerate a range of emotional experience. Specific targeted skills include (1) building an understanding of degrees of feelings and (2) building facility with tolerating and moving through arousal states by using strategies that comfortably and effectively increase and decrease arousal. Clinicians are encouraged to develop "feelings toolboxes" with youth, with specific skills and strategies directed toward the energy of the emotion.

AFFECT EXPRESSION

The sharing of emotional experience is a key aspect of human relationships. When there is no comfort in sharing aspects of the self, people are unable to create intimate human relationships, or, often, to get basic needs met. Many children who experience trauma struggle with the ability to safely and effectively express internal experience. Early attempts to communicate may have been met by anger, rejection, or indifference. Children learn quickly that sharing of emotions may make them vulnerable, and they learn to hide or close off this experience in an attempt to gain control. As a result, children either fail to communicate their experience entirely or communicate emotions and needs in ineffective ways. Over time, without effective modeling and experience in relationship building, youth exposed to trauma may be increasingly impaired in their understanding of how to build safe relationships.

The primary goal of this intervention target is to provide children with skills that help them effectively and safely share emotional experience with others, in order to meet emotional or practical needs. Specific targeted skills include (1) identification of safe communication resources; (2) effective use of resources, including how to "pick your moment" and initiate conversation; (3) effective nonverbal communication strategies, including physical space and boundaries, tone of voice, and eye contact; (4) verbal communication skills, including the use of "I" statements; and (5) building a repertoire of self-expression strategies.

Competency

Ultimately, our goal for the children and families with which we work is the building of resources, both internal and external, that allow for ongoing healthy development and positive functioning across domains of competency, including social connections, community involvement, and academic engagement. These intervention targets highlight the importance of children achieving felt mastery and success; receiving the tools to continue functioning as active constructors of their lives; and developing and consolidating a positive and coherent sense of self. Although the building of developmental competency is often relegated to the category of "supportive therapy" or adjunctive treatment when discussing trauma-focused therapy, we view the building of competency as a core component of treatment for children exposed to early developmental trauma.

The Competency Building Blocks

EXECUTIVE FUNCTIONS

Among the most important tasks for a young child is the development of a sense of agency: the knowledge that he or she has the ability to make an impact on the world. Agency develops as we *try*, we *do*, and we *choose*. To some degree, a sense of agency relies on adequately operating executive function skills: those cognitive skills held in the prefrontal cortex that allow us to exert control over our actions by delaying response, anticipating consequences, evaluating outcomes, and actively making decisions. For children exposed to chronic trauma, regular engagement of the "alarm mode" of their brains may lead to inadequate development of prefrontal controls. Research demonstrates impaired executive function abilities in this population, as compared with same-age peers (Beers & De Bellis, 2002; Mezzacappa, Kindlon, & Earls, 2001). Research on resilient youth highlights the role of problem-solving skills in positive outcomes: not surprisingly, youth who are able to make choices effectively, who are active players in their own lives, do better than those who cannot (Cicchetti et al., 1993; Werner & Smith, 2001).

This intervention target emphasizes the development of problem-solving skills, including the ability to actively evaluate situations, inhibit response, and make thoughtful decisions. The classic problem-solving steps are used as the framework for these skills, with added steps to acknowledge the role of the trauma response. A contrast is made between *acting* and *reacting*, and the skills in this section focus on building youth awareness of *choice*. Although problem-solving steps are presented formally, guidance concerning numerous possible entry points in routine conversation are also provided for clinicians and other professionals.

SELF DEVELOPMENT AND IDENTITY

Growth of a coherent and positive sense of self normatively occurs over the course of development: Young children gradually internalize the typical response of others and the environment; latency-age children incorporate experiences across domains and begin to integrate values, opinions, and other attributes; and adolescents actively explore and construct the self, developing an increasingly complex and nuanced sense of identity, including an awareness of future possibilities. Young children exposed to chronic trauma often internalize negative experiences and self-values. Experience may be fragmented and state-dependent. For many traumatized children, there is no sense of future, only a number of disconnected "nows."

In this section, intervention targets four aspects of self and identity. (1) The *unique self* involves an exploration and celebration of personal attributes, including likes and dislikes, values, opinions, family norms, culture, etc. (2) The *positive self* involves the building of internal resources and identification of strengths and successes. (3) The *coherent self* emphasizes examination of self across multiple aspects of experience: self before and after trauma, self with biological parents versus adoptive, self as displayed versus self on the inside, etc. (4) The *future self* involves a building of the child's capacity to imagine the self in the future and to explore possibilities.

Trauma Experience Integration

The final target addressed within the ARC framework is trauma experience integration. Past experiences often interfere with and override children's capacity to engage purposefully in present life. The influence of the past may come in the form of specific intrusive memories, along with associated emotions, cognitions, physiological states, and embedded models of self and other, as well as in fragmented self-states and affiliated patterns of functioning that are elicited by perceived themes associated with the repeated experiences of earlier childhood.

Here we draw upon the range of skills and resources addressed within the nine blocks of the ARC domains and define steps intended to support children in building a coherent and integrated understanding of self and the capacity to engage in present life. The integration of both specific memories and fragmented self-states is framed as a process that occurs over time within treatment, and which is embedded within the caregiving system.

ARC INTERVENTION SECTION GUIDE

Following a great deal of early feedback from the clinicians and other professionals with whom we worked while developing the ARC framework, we have designed the ARC intervention sections to be as user-friendly as possible. Each "building block" chapter is organized around the following sections:

★ Key Concepts

This is the "why" section. These concepts provide the rationale for the intervention principle as well as important teaching points for caregivers.

📦 Therapist Toolbox

This is the "to-do" section; it has three components:

🎬 *Behind the Scenes*

This section describes subtle ways to incorporate the principle into therapy sessions and/or milieu–systemic interactions, important points to remember, and overarching principles.

🛍 *Teach to Caregivers*

Important points of psychoeducation for caregivers as well as specific strategies to build the intervention principle are described here. For the attachment domain, this section focuses on techniques for building safety in the caregiving environment. For the self-regulation and competency domains, this section discusses ways in which caregivers can support their children's skill acquisition. This section also provides a guide for individual and group interventions with caregivers as well as for staff training within a system.

🔧 *Tools*

Often presented in menu format, these tools are specific activities individual and group therapists may incorporate into their sessions. Activities are presented as examples, and clinicians are reminded that creativity is often an essential part of the therapeutic process. Therapists are encouraged to expand on and individualize these examples to fit their clients.

👫 **Developmental Considerations**

In this section particular applications and considerations are discussed for three developmental stages: early childhood, middle childhood, and adolescence. The reader is encouraged to consider, for instance, how attachment principles remain relevant in later adolescence, yet are distinct from these principles as applied in earlier childhood. Given the impact of trauma on development, when planning intervention strategies, readers are encouraged to think in terms of developmental stage rather than chronological age.

🏠 **Applications**

As a flexible framework, ARC is based on principles that translate across intervention settings. This section provides examples of applications of each principle within individual dyadic, group, and milieu–systemic intervention.

🌐 **Real-World Therapy**

Therapy occurs in the "real world." This section discusses the realistic pitfalls and considerations when working on this principle with real kids and families.

🏳 **Cultural Considerations**

Across all sections, cultural considerations are indicated with this mark. *Culture* includes the "thoughts, communications, actions, customs, beliefs, values, and institutions of racial, ethnic, religious, or social groups" (Cross, Bazron, Dennis, & Isaacs, 1989, p. 13). We define culture broadly; it may include self-defined categories such as race, ethnicity, language, country or culture of origin, gender, sexual identity and orientation, community, religion, etc. Culture may also include nuances such as the neighborhood clients grow up in, the particular traditions of the family of origin, or the particulars of the client's generation or current society. As has been pointed out to us, everyone lives in multiple cultures simultaneously (B. Stubblefield-Tave, personal communication, May 18, 2006).

ARC RESOURCES

In the back of this book are numerous resources: educational handouts, clinical worksheets, and expanded examples of individual and group activities. These resources are organized by type and by targeted domain and are often referenced within specific intervention sections. We offer these resources as examples of ways to target specific areas, but we also encourage those who are reading this text to be creative: Often the best interventions are those we come up with in the moment or in context, targeted to the specific child, group, or family with which we are working.

USING THE ARC FRAMEWORK: POTENTIAL STRATEGIES FOR IMPLEMENTATION

As a flexible framework, rather than a structured protocol, practitioners may question (as we often do, when working with complex children and families) where to begin. "I like the framework," we've heard, "but how do I *do* ARC?"

Partly as a response to this question, the intervention sections that follow each contain an "Applications" subsection that describes considerations for implementing the principle in individual treatment, group, and milieu–systems settings. This section highlights, for instance, ways to apply the "Caregiver Affect Management" principle when working with an individual parent versus with the staff in an agency. For the range of practitioners who may be utilizing this resource, we encourage you to consider the following as possible ways of using framework principles, skills, and key concepts.

Integration into Outpatient Therapy

The principles and building blocks of ARC have become, for us and for many of the outpatient clinicians with whom we work, our guide to building individual treatment goals and plans. By examining client and family/system presentation within the context of the 10 building blocks, we can develop concrete treatment goals within each domain.

For instance, if our assessment points to a child with sudden angry outbursts and a caregiver who becomes overwhelmed in the face of these, our treatment goals may include (1) building caregiver tolerance for child affect through development of his or her own coping skills and supports (Caregiver Affect Management); (2) building the caregiver's understanding of the reason for the outbursts through psychoeducation in trauma and developmental expression of emotion (Attunement); (3) building child ability to "read" cues of distress in his or her body and understand where they come from (Affect Identification); (4) building child coping strategies for managing distress (Modulation, supported by Attunement); and (5) building child's ability to use the caregiver or other resources as a support (Affect Expression, again supported by Attunement).

Other ARC building blocks may intertwine in the above goals. For instance, identifying the best strategy to use and ways to plan for potentially stressful situations may involve problem-solving skills (Executive Functions), and targeting the child's feelings of accomplishment in his or her ability to manage internal and behavioral experience may build felt efficacy (Self and Identity Development). Increasing felt predictability around identified "trigger points" may decrease arousal (Routines and Rituals), and helping caregivers learn to "pick their moment" in supporting regulation versus limit setting will target parenting strategies (Consistent Response). The Session Checklist/Tracking Sheet included in Appendix A may be useful in tracking which ARC principles and subskills are addressed within a given session; we have often recommended that clinicians begin with simply tracking, prior to making significant changes. Tracking our "choice points" in session often helps us understand and define what we are targeting with clients—and perhaps, what we are missing.

The intervention sections contain many examples of ways to integrate principles into individual, dyadic, and/or familial treatment sessions. We encourage practitioners to consider both formal exercises as well as informal "tuning in"—in conversation, in play, and in interaction. We also encourage consideration of ways to structure the session so that it integrates these principles in practice. For instance, consider ways to build a consistent session routine; integration of modulation activities into opening and closing portions of session; regularly "checking in" at start and/or end of session to build affect identification and expression skills; integration of competency-building activities; and so on.

Group Treatment

The principles contained within the Self-Regulation and Competency sections translate easily into group activities. Many of the exercises provided as examples in the intervention section menus can be used in group format, and additional activities are described in Appendix C. We encourage practitioners to consider the population with which they are working, including (among other factors) developmental stage, intervention setting, cultural context, treatment focus, and intergroup safety in selecting and developing activities for use in treatment groups. We have worked with a number of programs that have developed groups using ARC principles and have been impressed with the variation we have seen in groups' formats, structures, and foci, while still integrating key ARC principles. In addition to considering specific ARC principles as treatment targets, we encourage consideration of the role of Routine and Ritual when structuring groups for children, adolescents, or caregivers.

Caregiver Support and Education

Four principles specifically target caregiver education and support. In addition, every intervention section contains key concepts, developmental considerations, and "teach-to-caregivers" information. This material may provide a guide for development of caregiver education sessions (either one on one or in groups) and/or caregiver workshops. Included in Appendix B are many caregiver educational handouts and worksheets; some may be of use in your own work with caregivers. Consider these to be a guide; our experience is that written information is helpful for some, but not all, caregivers. Consider other ways to build awareness of the same principles, whether in targeted "education meetings" or—as in work with children and adolescents—as a component of in-the-moment application.

Beyond education, it is important to pay attention to ways to apply the attachment principles, including the caregiver's need for support and felt competency. Consider ways to increase caregivers' supportive resources, whether within or outside of the intervention system; forums to assist caregivers with skills practice, application, and processing of successes and challenges; and ways to increase your own attunement to caregiver responses and behaviors.

Milieu Training, Consultation, and Staff Support

Strategies and considerations for using ARC principles for milieu–systems staff training, consultation, and support are similar to those for primary caregivers. Wherever this framework identifies principles that apply to *caregivers*, substitute the relevant word from your system (e.g., *teachers, counseling staff*). The educational components of the framework may provide a guide for development of staff training. Beyond formal training, however, it is our experience that the greatest systemic shifts occur when learning is made real. So, for instance, rather than just teaching staff about triggers, integrate discussions of triggered responses into conversations about specific child/adolescent behaviors, building of educational plans, and weekly staffing meetings.

As with primary caregivers, it is important to go beyond education and think systemically about ways to build staff support and safety. It is our assertion, repeated throughout this text, that a child will be only as safe as his or her surrounding system—which means that a primary goal is always the building of systemic safety. Consider whether staff within your system, at all levels, are adequately supported; have the capacity to manage emotional experience (both individually and systemically); have forums within which to discuss and process incidents; and have consistency, to some degree, in daily experience and the ability, in turn, to provide that predictability to clients.

Milieu–Systems Applications

ARC principles can be applied in many settings that do not include individual therapy and/or as systemic points of intervention that go beyond individual therapy. The Applications section of each ARC principle includes milieu–systems considerations. However, given the range of settings in which trauma-exposed youth and families receive services, it would be impossible to address all the iterations of ways to implement these principles. Furthermore, we believe strongly that the expertise about a particular system—including best practices for implementing intervention—generally lies within that system. So . . . if you are reading this text and considering ways to implement ARC principles on a systems level, we encourage you to consider the goals, paying attention to two factors: (1) the key concept the principle addresses, and (2) the ways this domain shows up within your setting (e.g., in client presentation, in daily structure). Given those two factors, consider ways to apply the principle in a systemic way.

As an example, the second principle of the Self-Regulation section is Modulation. The primary goal of Modulation is to help the child build skills and strategies for modulating internal experience—physiological, emotional, and behavioral. Although every system may not provide individual skills building with particular children, as might happen within "therapy," there are certainly ways that systems can teach, support, and encourage modulation. A classroom setting, for example, might consider adding a basket of hand-held manipulatives (e.g., stress balls, Play-Doh) available for student use as a way of supporting physiological regulation. A residential program might consider creating a "sensory space" that includes sensory modulation materials (e.g., weighted blankets, soft pillows) in place of, or in addition to, a classic "time-out" room. A family shelter program might consider building daily routine components that encourage child modulation (e.g., evening story hour, with soft music, dim lights, and encouragement of dyadic nurturing). Not every strategy will work in—or be appropriate to—every setting. The best examples we have—including those listed above—come from the individual programs and organizations with which we have worked and the strategies that they have designed to fit their system's needs.

WHO ARE YOU TREATING?: THE IMPORTANCE OF STARTING WITH FORMULATION

As a framework that focuses on the importance of flexibly responding to the individual needs of the child/adolescent within the context of his or her specific family or system, it feels important to include, in regard to the question, "So how do I *do* ARC?," the reciprocal question, "Who are you treating?" In other words, in order to target the individual needs of a client, we must first understand, to the degree possible, who that client is. Any behavior, any symptom, may have many possible contributing factors. Identification of the behavior is not the endpoint; it is merely the first step. *Formulation* is the integration of an array of information (e.g., history, observations, clinical presentation, behaviors, relational style, domains of functioning) into a coherent understanding of the client. It helps us understand, for instance, not just *that* a child is struggling in school, but *why* a child is struggling in school. For one child, the difficulty may be due to poor attention; for another, it may be due to an inability to modulate arousal. For a third, it may be due to challenges navigating the complex relationships in the school setting, and for a fourth, an underlying learning disorder may be its basis. For a final child, it may be a combination of several of the above factors. If we simply target the *outcome* —that is, school performance difficulties—without understanding the root cause, it is likely that our intervention will fail at least some of the time.

Good formulation is often built on a premise that, at essence, people make sense. All individuals function in the way that they function for a reason. These reasons are often complex and multifaceted, and it would be presumptuous to assume that we could break every individual down into the sum of his or her component parts. However, formulation offers us an understanding glimpse into these complexities and supports our empathic comprehension of why a child might be oppositional or clingy, why a child's caregiver might mistrust professionals or parent in a disorganized way, and why a family might struggle to engage in treatment.

Formulation enhances our treatment capacity, as the understanding of *why* leads naturally to an awareness of *what*, along with the flexible capacity to explore *how*. In other words, if the reason *why* a child has frequent tantrums is because of a difficulty regulating arousal, a strong triggered response to lack of control, and ongoing reactivity of the child's caregiver due to her own feelings of being overwhelmed, then *what* treatment is likely to target will include building modulation strategies (coping skills), working with the caregiver to increase the child's felt choice, and supporting the caregiver in building internal and external resources and managing her own emotional experience. *How* we get there may be more challenging and is often likely to involve some experimentation; our hope is that this framework offers some suggestions to support providers with that step.

We have found it useful to approach formulation as a series of related questions that are answered by our evaluation. Evaluation (as well as formulation) should be viewed as an ongoing and dynamic process, rather than as a one-time accomplishment. When working with children and families who have experienced trauma, consider the following questions in organizing your formulation:

1. What has this child/family experienced? Pay attention to both positive and stressful experiences.
2. What other factors have influenced this child and family? Consider the following:
   - Child and family culture (multidimensional)
   - Caregiver functioning (current and historical); intergenerational influences
   - Biological/organic strengths and vulnerabilities, including temperament
   - Economic factors
   - Child role in the family
3. In what ways might those experiences and contextual factors have impacted this child? This family? Consider:
   - Developmental impact: attachment style, self-regulation capacity and organization, relationships, motor skills
   - Beliefs (about self, others, the world)
4. What do the patterns we observe suggest about the child's (or family's) learned adaptations to these experiences? In what way do current behaviors make sense, given historical experiences? Consider not just surface behaviors (e.g., temper tantrums) but core driving issues (e.g., surges of arousal) as well.
5. Do patterns of current behavior give us clues about key triggers or cues of potential danger? If not, based on historical experiences, what might we expect to trigger the danger response in this child?
6. In the face of triggers, what kind of behaviors is the child engaging in? Which current behaviors are we *most* concerned about? (How) Do these relate to past experiences?
7. What other stressors are impacting the current presentation? What other resources are helping to buffer it?
8. What strengths does the child have? Are there ways in which the child has been able to harness these to buffer his or her experiences?

The responses to these questions provide us with a narrative about the child and family. Reread the stories of Ryan, in the Introduction, and of Janae, in Chapter 2, with these questions in mind. Consider the child's functioning in the context of domains of development and trauma impact, as described in Chapter 1, as well as in the context of the three-part model of trauma impact, as described in Chapter 2. Note the ways that the responses to these questions, and our understanding of the child and family, lead into identification of domains to target in intervention as well as areas of strength to support.

CONCLUSION

The previous chapters have provided the background, context, and foundation on which the ARC framework is built. The remainder of this text lays out the three primary domains and 10 building blocks of the ARC framework, including considerations for application across contexts. For each of the building blocks, or targets of intervention, we provide the rationale and key concepts, as well as guidance concerning suggested interventions, components of caregiver education, and developmental considerations. Treatment will necessarily differ from client to client, as each child brings unique attributes, exposure history, context, and presentation. Because of this variation, ongoing clinical assessment is a key component to any intervention.

Keep in mind that, although some skills are prerequisites for others, this framework is not meant to be a step-by-step prescription. Good treatment often involves revisiting key domains at different times in the healing process. As the child grows, enters new developmental phases, or is exposed to additional stressors, previously learned skills may need to be reviewed, and new ones may need to be built.

Many of the exercises included in this book are drawn from clinical wisdom and may be found in other treatment manuals, as well as in classic play therapy workbooks or courses. Some have been modified to address the needs of traumatized children; others appear as they were taught to us in our own training, or as we have used them in our clinical work. Throughout this manual, exercises are given as suggestions; we encourage providers to use their creativity to modify exercises so that they meet the needs of their own clients.

PART II

ATTACHMENT

WHAT IS ATTACHMENT?

- One of the most basic human needs is connection to other human beings. We begin to connect from our earliest moments, and we continue to rely on relationships throughout our lives.

- The earliest relationship(s), built between the child and his or her primary caregiver(s), is referred to as the **"attachment system."** Why is this system so important?

  ♦ The attachment system **provides a model for all other relationships**. Out of this early connection, children form an understanding of *self* and *others*. For instance:

    ○ A child who is loved, cared for, and listened to may believe that he or she is lovable and worthy and that others are generally trustworthy and will be available if needed.

    ○ A child who is consistently rejected and ignored may believe that he or she is unimportant or unlovable and that others are uninterested, unavailable, and likely to reject any attempts to gain support.

    ○ A child who is frequently hurt or excessively punished may believe that he or she is bad and that others are unsafe and potentially dangerous.

    ○ A child whose parents are inconsistently available (e.g., due to substance use or mental health issues) may believe that adults are not able to handle things and are unpredictable in their responses. These children often feel overly responsible for the well-being of others, and may be controlling or clingy in their interactions.

  ♦ The attachment system provides the earliest training ground for **coping with and expressing emotions**.

    ○ When children are born, they do not have the skills to deal with emotions on their own. They rely on parents to comfort them and help them manage distress. When children consistently receive nurturance from their parents, they learn that feelings are not permanent, that distress can be tolerated, and that it will eventually subside. When support is first provided externally, over time, children will internalize these same coping skills. Eventually, children are able to independently manage emotional experience.

○ Children who receive inconsistent, neglectful, or rejecting caregiving have little support in managing the challenging experiences of early childhood. When they feel distress, they must rely on primitive and frequently ineffective or insufficient coping skills. As a result, two primary consequences emerge:

◊ First, the child is unable to develop more advanced coping skills. While other children get better and better at dealing with emotions over time, these children continue to act and look like much younger children in the face of distress.

◊ Second, children may become frightened by or guarded against emotional experience in general, as all feelings may be perceived as potentially threatening and overwhelming.

♦ The attachment system **provides a safe environment for healthy development**.

○ Every developmental stage has key tasks that children work to accomplish. The attachment system provides the safety that gives children confidence in approaching these tasks. Success in relationships, school, identity, and, ultimately, independent functioning all stem in part from the support that the attachment system initially provides.

○ When children do not have the safety net of a secure attachment system, the energy that other children are able to invest in accomplishments instead must be invested in self-protection and survival.

WHAT IS THE CAREGIVING SYSTEM?

• Many children who have experienced chronic/complex trauma spend significant time in alternative systems of care (e.g., residential treatment centers, group homes, foster placements, specialized school placements). They may or may not have a consistent primary caregiver available to them.

• When a primary caregiver is available (e.g., biological, adoptive, or foster parents), treatment may focus on supporting parents in providing a safe environment that fosters children's healing process.

• For children who are in substitute care, professional staff enters into the role of the substitute caregiving system. Because this caregiving system is so crucial to child recovery, it is important to develop a system that is safe for both children and staff. Therefore, intervention will necessarily include a focus on staff-level understanding, behavior, and supports.

• For all children, it is important to also consider the range of adults with which the child will interact and who play a role in the child's surrounding system. This may include, for instance, the clinician, the child's teacher, after-school providers, day care staff, etc. Ideally, intervention will target multiple levels of the caregiving system.

WHY IS IT IMPORTANT TO BUILD SAFETY (FOR BOTH THE CHILD AND THE CAREGIVER)?

• Children who have experienced trauma have a base expectation that the world and others are dangerous. They are chronically in self-defense mode: They anticipate danger and react quickly when they think it is present. In their life, this response mode has helped them to survive. However, this self-protective stance interferes with ongoing healthy development.

- In order for children to move beyond a self-defense mode, they must be in an environment that provides some degree of felt safety. Often, because the danger that these children have experienced is *relational danger*, they are highly tuned in to signs of danger in the people with whom they interact. This makes it particularly important for all caregivers to develop skills to cope with this expectation.

- Maintaining safety with children who constantly anticipate danger is a significant challenge, and can be draining for parents, staff members, teachers, clinicians, peers, and others who interact with them. Because of that, it is important to pay attention to adult safety as well as child safety—and, ultimately, these two things will go hand in hand.

CHAPTER 4

Caregiver Management of Affect

THE MAIN IDEA

Support the child's caregiving system—whether parents or professionals—
in understanding, managing, and coping with their own emotional responses,
so that they are better able to support the children in their care.

★ KEY CONCEPTS

★ *Why Build Caregiver Affect Management Skills?*

- A key role of caregivers within the attachment system is to help children learn skills in self-regulation.

- Before a caregiver can help a child tolerate and modulate affect, however, the caregiver must also be able to tolerate, modulate, and cope with his or her own emotional responses.

- One of the most salient components of a child's emotional climate is the affect of his or her caregivers. All children take cues from caregivers' expressions and learn to interpret the world in part through these emotional reactions.

★ *Trauma Behaviors That Challenge Caregiver Modulation*

- Children who have experienced trauma and attachment disruptions often struggle with intense emotions, difficulty with relationships, impacted systems of meaning, and behavioral dysregulation. The at-times significant needs of these children can be draining for caregivers. Child behaviors and interactional styles that challenge caregiver modulation may include:

  ◆ Triggered responses to caregivers

  ◆ Anger/opposition

- ◆ Demand for attention

- ◆ Patterns of approach and rejection

- ◆ Extreme emotional responses to stressors

- The emotional impact on caregivers is complicated by the role of child vigilance. Children who have experienced trauma are often particularly vigilant to the expressions of others and may interpret caregiver emotion in light of stark dichotomies of safety versus danger, approval versus disapproval, and acceptance versus rejection. This vigilance makes it particularly important for caregivers to monitor and modulate their own feelings. However, this need for ongoing modulation and monitoring can be challenging for caregivers.

- ⏴ It is important to keep in mind that caregivers and families often face additional stressors that impact emotional experience and go beyond their child's specific trauma exposure. Consider the role of experiences such as racism, discrimination, economic challenges, etc., in their impact on the caregiver and family.

★ *Common Caregiver Responses*

It is nearly impossible to capture the full range of potential caregiver responses. Consider the following, however, as examples.

- Challenges that arise in caregiving may lead to the following *emotional* and *cognitive* responses:

  - ◆ **Reduced sense of efficacy** in the caregiving role, for example:

    - ○ For parents: "Why is my child rejecting me?"

    - ○ For teachers: "Why can't I get this child to listen?"

    - ○ For providers: "Why can't I help this child calm down?"

  - ◆ **Guilt and shame** about child experiences: "How could these things happen to my child?"

  - ◆ **Anger and blame** of the child: "She's doing this on purpose! She's trying to manipulate me."

- When faced with intense emotions such as these, it is not uncommon for caregivers, like children, to respond defensively in the service of coping. Common *behavioral reactions* include:

  - ◆ **Shutting down or constricting:** Defending against emotion. This reaction may lead to ignoring or minimizing child and/or child needs.

  - ◆ **Overreacting:** Trying to control or protect the child through overly punitive or authoritative response. This reaction may lead to stifling child expression and/or increasing triggered response.

  - ◆ **Being overly permissive:** Trying to prevent child escalation. This reaction may lead to giving in, in the face of child affect.

▭ THERAPIST TOOLBOX

▰ *Behind the Scenes*

Building the Foundation

- It is an inherently vulnerable situation for caregivers when their own emotions are addressed. Caregivers often approach treatment assuming that the focus will be on the child, rather than on the caregiving system.

- In order to target caregiver affect management, it is important to have a common and respectful understanding of *why* this goal is important.

- It is vital that the provider maintain a nonjudgmental stance. Ideally, the provider is *teaming* with the caregiver (or caregiving system) in the same way that we want the caregiver to team with the child. In order for this to happen, there must be an openness to, acceptance of, and tolerance for the caregivers' thoughts, feelings, ideas, and experience. As an example, if a caregiver states, "Sometimes I hate my child," it is vital that the provider be able to respond in a way that normalizes this experience and facilitates ongoing discussion.

- At essence, the goal is normalization of caregiver experience and support of the caregiving system so that the system is able to support the child.

- Caregiver affect management is a skill that serves as the foundation for all other skills in this framework. For instance, when modulated, a caregiver is better able to attune effectively to his or her child, respond consistently, support regulation skills, and foster competency.

Things to Assess

- What specific situations seem to be the most challenging for caregivers, and when do they feel most comfortable? Work with caregivers to identify patterns of child behaviors and emotions, as well as their own typical responses.

- How much insight do caregivers have about the role of their own response? Be sure to target psychoeducation to caregiver blind spots.

- ▭ How does the caregiver's or family's culture impact caregiver emotional display? It is important to understand what is considered normative within the family. For example, in one family intense speech and raised voices may indicate dysregulated emotion; in another, these same qualities are part of a normative interaction style.

Helping Caregivers Identify Particular Challenges

- For most caregivers the struggle is not with consistent and constant dysregulation, but rather with specific situations that are challenging in some way.

- Consider the following when exploring caregiver's trouble spots:
  - ◆ Areas of insecurity for caregivers in parenting or other role fulfillment
  - ◆ Child behaviors that have, in the past, been associated with crisis or significant events (e.g., hospitalization, assault, self-harm)

- ♦ The caregiver's own trauma history and triggers
- ♦ Areas of discrepancy between child and caregiver (e.g., cultural, generational, values)
- ♦ The role of external stressors (e.g., financial trouble, job stress)
- Work with caregivers to monitor their responses in each of these situations, keeping in mind that "typical" responses may vary widely by stressor.
- Build a plan that identifies specific coping strategies for identified challenge situations.
- Consider the following example to illustrate this point:

> An adoptive mother of two young boys was generally relaxed, attuned, and supportive of her children's needs. When either boy was sad or worried about something, she was able to remain calm and provide comfort. However, she became very anxious when the boys' behavior would become more energetic. In the past, higher arousal had led to sexualized and aggressive behavior by the boys, behaviors that the mother found difficult to cope with, and which led to feelings of helplessness and self-blame. She worried that any energetic behaviors might lead to this same overaroused response. As a result, whenever the boys started to show high energy—even at normative levels for 6- and 8-year-old children—the mother would intervene and separate them.

In this example, although the mother's concerns are valid and real, her actions are communicating to her children that energetic play—an important component of healthy development in young children—is unsafe and unacceptable. In working with this parent, it will be important to (1) validate and help her understand her own emotional response and resulting behavior; (2) build her tolerance for normative, healthy levels of arousal and activity in her children; (3) build tools that will help her support her children in safe play; and (4) build a repertoire of coping strategies for those occasions when high energy might, in fact, lead to dysregulated behaviors.

What about the Therapist?: Managing Your Own Affect

- Because much of this section refers to *caregiver* affect management, it is easy to focus on the parent. However, it is equally important for therapists and other helping professionals to pay attention to their own emotional reactions and to build skills in monitoring and managing them.
- Consider the following parallel process. A child who thinks that she is damaged and unlovable is convinced that she is unable to trust anyone. Placed in a new home, she feels afraid and anxious. Sure the new caregiver will reject her, she self-protects by keeping the caregiver at arm's length. In turn, the caregiver feels ineffective as a parent and rejected by the child. Feeling frustrated and helpless, the caregiver reacts by pulling away. Now what about the professionals working with this family? Faced with the increasing demands of the distressed system, the professionals also begin to feel frustrated and helpless, and to think that they are ineffective and incompetent. Over time, the professionals may feel themselves pulling away, ultimately terminating the therapy. With this, the child's initial prediction of rejection has come true!

- Throughout this section are techniques for teaching caregivers how to monitor their own experience, learn to recognize their vulnerabilities and typical coping patterns, and engage in self-care and other coping skills. It is strongly recommended that professionals practice these same techniques.

A THREE-WAY (OR MORE) PARALLEL PROCESS

	Child	Caregiver	Professional(s)
Cognitions	"I'm bad, unlovable, damaged." "I can't trust anyone."	"I'm an ineffective parent." "My child is rejecting me."	"I'm an ineffective clinician." "This family just needs to work harder."
Emotions	Shame, anger, fear, hopelessness	Frustration, sadness, helplessness, worry	Frustration, helplessness, indifference
Behaviors (coping strategy)	Avoidance, aggression, preemptive rejection	Overreacting, controlling, shutting down, being overly permissive	Disconnection, dismissing, ignoring, therapy termination
The Cycle	"She's going to reject me anyway. I'd better not connect."	"He's just not interested in connecting with me."	"I don't think anyone could make a difference with this family."

Special Concerns

- Many caregivers—parents and providers alike—have their own trauma histories. Be aware that children's traumatic experiences and their resulting responses may act as a trigger and reminder of caregivers' own historical experiences.

- Pay attention to **basic safety**: Are caregivers able to keep themselves and their children safe? Are any red flags present (e.g., significant caregiver depression, substance use, explosive or overly punitive reactions)?

- In the presence of red flags or other concerns, consider whether caregivers may need **additional supports** (e.g., their own individual therapy, increased supervision).

Understanding Vicarious Trauma

- For all individuals who care for someone who has experienced trauma—primary caregivers as well as professionals—there is a risk of **vicarious trauma** and, if unaddressed, **burnout**.

- *Vicarious* or *secondary trauma* has been defined as a process through which the caregiving individual's own internal experience becomes transformed through engagement with the child's (or client's) traumatic material (McCann & Pearlman, 1990).

- Although the vicarious trauma response will differ across individuals, vicarious traumatization leads to a disruption of the same core issues that are impacted by direct exposure to trauma, including disrupted sense of safety, difficulties with trust, impaired self-esteem and self-efficacy, challenges with intimacy, and feelings of loss of control or helplessness (Pearlman & Saakvitne, 1995).

- For providers, understanding, recognizing, preventing, and addressing signs of vicarious trauma represent a primary systems-level intervention in targeting our own affect management. Excellent resources are available that discuss and address the providers' own response (e.g., Pearlman & Saakvitne, 1995; Saakvitne, Gamble, Pearlman, & Lev, 2000; Stamm, 1999).

Considerations in Working with Primary Caregivers

- Caregiver affect modulation should be initially assessed and taught either one on one or in parenting groups.
- After basic skills are mastered, dyadic or family treatment may be useful for practice and coaching in the use of these skills.

Considerations in Working within a Milieu

- In any sort of a milieu system, consider the role of both individual supervision and group/team-level supports.
- It is easy for interventions targeted toward staff affect management to feel inadvertently punitive (i.e., "You shouldn't feel that way"). As with primary caregivers, it is crucial that this process involve normalization of affect, staff supports, and skill building in specific coping strategies.

Primary Components of This Building Block

The primary components of this building block include the following:

- Psychoeducation
  - ◆ Depersonalization of child behaviors
  - ◆ Education about the trauma response
  - ◆ Validation of caregiver experience
- Self-monitoring skills
- Affect management skills
- Building supports and resources

📋 Teach to Caregivers

- *Reminder:* Teach the caregiver the Key Concepts.
- *Reminder:* Teach the caregiver the relevant Developmental Considerations.
- The goal of affect modulation for caregivers is *not* to "fake" their emotions, to pretend that they have no emotional response or to deny internal experience, but rather to monitor affect, to maintain appropriate boundaries, to respond in a constructive, rather than destructive, way, and to communicate to their child that the adults around them can stay safe, calm, and handle difficult experience.

Teaching Point: Normalizing Caregiver Emotional Response

Target	Important points
Depersonalize: Provide education about the impact of trauma.	Teach caregivers basic information about trauma response in children and the impact of trauma on families. See caregiver handout "Introduction: Children and Trauma" (Appendix B).
	Help caregivers understand the normative and adaptive nature of their children's responses.
	Help caregivers differentiate child *triggered response* versus opposition, rejection, etc. Identify: What is the *function* of the child's behavior? Consider: meeting emotional or physical needs *or* coping with perceived danger. Pair with education about triggers (see Chapter 2).
	If appropriate, teach caregivers about the parallel process, and the ways in which it manifests.
Validate caregiver response.	Validate caregiver emotional reactions—as is true for children, all emotions are okay. The goal of affect management is to be aware of and effectively cope with emotional experience.

⚡ Tools: Teaching Caregivers Affect Management

- *Target #1:* Building self-monitoring skills. Help caregivers to identify challenging situations as well as their own typical response. See handout "**Tuning In to Yourself**" (Appendix B).

BUILDING SELF-MONITORING SKILLS

Target	Important points	
Identify difficult situations.	Work with caregivers to identify challenging situations. Consider the following questions:	
	- Are there child behaviors that are particularly hard for you to deal with or that "push your buttons"? - Are there child emotions that you find particularly difficult to cope with or respond to, or which lead to a strong emotional response in you? - What types of expressed feelings or behaviors have been the hardest or highest risk in the past (e.g., led to family crisis, danger to self or other, or need for more intensive treatment)? Do these feelings or behaviors still occur? What are they like? - Are there situations that you know you find particularly hard because they remind you of hard times in your own life? - In what situations do you feel the least effective? - Are any of the child's feelings, behaviors, or experiences particularly hard for you to understand? - What other factors affect your ability to stay centered? (e.g., trouble at work, challenges in your own interpersonal relationships, external pressures)	
Build self-monitoring skills: Teach caregivers to notice their own reactions, across domains.	Physiological	What is the caregiver experiencing in his or her *body*? Teach caregivers to pay attention to heart rate, breathing, muscle tension, numbness, etc. What warning signs does the caregiver's body provide of "losing control" or hitting a danger point?
	Cognitive	What does the caregiver *think* in the face of difficult situations? Consider automatic thoughts about self (e.g., "I can't do anything to help") as well as about the child (e.g., "She's doing this on purpose").

Target		Important points
	Emotional	What does the caregiver *feel* in response to each identified difficult situation? Remember to check for common caregiver responses, as described above.
	Behavioral	What do the caregivers *do* in the face of strong emotion? Do they become punitive? Withdraw? Freeze? Work with caregivers to understand their own behavioral coping strategies.

- *Target #2:* Building affect management strategies. In the Modulation section we discuss "Feelings Toolboxes" for children. It is often helpful for caregivers to have parallel "toolboxes" (e.g., a range of coping strategies) to support their own affect management. Many of the skills included below are described in greater detail in the Modulation section. Also, see caregiver worksheet "**Taking Care of Yourself**" (Appendix B).

- In building caregiver coping strategies, it is important to consider "in-the-pocket" techniques (i.e., those that are used "in the moment" to manage distressing or intense affect) as well as preventive or restorative techniques (i.e., those that are used for ongoing self-care).

USEFUL TECHNIQUES FOR CAREGIVER AFFECT MANAGEMENT

Technique	Important points
Deep breathing	Teach caregivers diaphragmatic breathing techniques.
Muscle relaxation	Teach parents either directed or self-guided progressive muscle relaxation. Also consider practices such as yoga, tai chi, etc.
Distraction	Work with caregivers to self-identify when they are "stuck" (i.e., caught in a cycle of thinking about, worrying about, or doing things that aren't immediately helpful).
	Help them learn to shift their focus through the use of distracting thoughts, activities, etc.
Self-soothing	Help caregivers identify things that are pleasurable or calming.
	Pay attention to both smaller, "in-the-pocket" techniques (e.g., carrying a small grounding stone) and more involved activities (e.g., knitting, going for a walk, taking a hot bath).
	Encourage caregivers to routinely engage in self-care activities.
Time-outs	In order to access affect management skills in the midst of intense emotion or conflict situations, caregivers may need to "take a break."
	Help caregivers differentiate safe versus unsafe situations and ways to separate from these situations.
	Help caregivers develop appropriate ways to communicate this need to their child (e.g., "I'm upset and need a few minutes to calm down. I'm going to go to my room, to take a little space, and when I come out, we'll talk about this.").

- *Target #3:* Working with caregivers to build a support system. For both primary caregivers and professionals, it is important to have supports. Work to actively identify a range of resources.

BUILDING CAREGIVER SUPPORT SYSTEMS

Target	Important points
Identify resources.	*Primary caregivers:* Work with parents to identify their support system. Consider the range of potential resources (e.g., significant others, peers, relatives, clergy, community supports, professional resources). Help parents identify the specific situations in which they are able to utilize particular supports (e.g., to whom can the caregiver go when worried, needing reassurance, needing comfort, needing information). Pay particular attention to caregiver-identified trouble spots.
	Providers: It is important for providers to pay attention to both professional and personal sources of support. Within a system examine the presence or absence of professional supports such as supervision, peer support groups, and training. As for primary caregivers, providers should be able to identify which resources (professional and/or personal) are helpful for specific situations.
Consider the role of caregiver-to-caregiver supports.	Caregiver-to-caregiver support is often particularly helpful. Trauma can be isolating for caregivers as well as children; it is not uncommon for caregivers to feel alone and overwhelmed in the challenge of parenting a traumatized child. Support from other caregivers who have "been there" or are still there is often a valuable addition to the treatment.
Teach good boundaries.	When a support system is inadequate, caregivers may be more vulnerable to placing the child(ren) in the role of support system. However, not all caregiver emotions are appropriate to share with children. Help caregivers identify developmentally or situationally inappropriate experiences to share, as well as more appropriate alternative resources.

🚶 DEVELOPMENTAL CONSIDERATIONS

Developmental stage	Caregiver affect modulation considerations
Early childhood	Young traumatized children are almost completely reliant on adults to provide regulation. Therefore, it is particularly important for caregivers to have support in monitoring and modulating their own affect.
Middle childhood	Modeling of regulation skills begins to become important as children advance in their ability to observe others' experience. Work with caregivers to demonstrate affect regulation skills by naming what they are feeling (and how they are coping); for instance, "I'm feeling a little frustrated, so I'm going to take a deep breath," or "I'm worried about you."
	As children get older, it becomes easier for caregivers to take the time they need to self-regulate before addressing child behaviors and actions. Work with caregivers to find safe ways to delay response.
Adolescence	This developmental stage is often a particularly trying time for caregivers, as their adolescent children progress toward independence.
	Adolescents' repertoire for seeking independence may be limited to rebelling against caregivers, which can lead to heightened caregiver anxiety, frustration, or other strong emotions.
	Help caregivers to understand:
	Adolescents are increasingly able to develop an understanding of the impact of their behavior on others. It is not only appropriate, therefore, but important, for caregivers to be selectively honest about their experience of the adolescents' behavior and actions.
	Phrasing is important, and shame is a large issue for many traumatized teens. Help caregivers balance honesty with empathy.

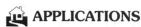 APPLICATIONS

Individual/Dyadic

When working with children and families, normalizing, supporting, and addressing caregiver emotional experience is often a primary and essential starting point. We address caregiver affect management from our first meeting by communicating (1) an understanding of trauma and trauma response, (2) a belief that a child and family can be supported, and (3) a willingness to team with the caregiver in this process. When specifically targeting caregiver affect management, it is often important to meet with the caregiver(s) alone, so that there is adequate safety for the caregiver to explore and verbalize his or her experience. However, the clinician may integrate observations of dyadic or familial processes (e.g., "I noticed when we met together that it was upsetting for you when Jenny started to get really loud in the office. Is that something that happens other places? Is that the kind of situation that tends to be hard for you?").

Building affect management skills is an active process. A primary goal is to help caregivers build active appraisal skills: By stepping outside of the difficult situation, caregivers are able to observe the moment rather than be overwhelmed by it. Work with caregivers to actively monitor difficult situations, their patterns of response, and the use (or lack thereof) of coping strategies. It is important that the clinician notice, name, and celebrate moments of success, even (and particularly) relative successes. As an example of the latter, consider the caregiver who identifies distress at having lost his or her temper. This caregiver has just experienced a moment of success by recognizing and seeking help with an area of vulnerability. When caregivers experience particular difficulties, explore these: What got in the way of using a coping strategy or remaining centered? Troubleshoot ways to cope with these situations in the future.

If there is more than one primary caregiver, it is important to pay attention to differential responses and to normalize these: It is exceedingly rare for two caregivers to have the exact same strengths and/or vulnerabilities. Pay attention to ways that each caregiver's response has the potential to support the other, and ways that these responses may undermine the other. Create a team: For instance, if one caregiver has a particular "push button," use the other caregiver for support; similarly, if one caregiver has a particular strength, tap into this in building parenting strategies.

Group

When appropriate for particular caregivers, support groups and educational workshops offer the significant advantage of being a natural forum for normalizing caregiver response. We provide an example of this from our own work:

> In the early period of developing this framework, we were conducting a training workshop for a group of adoptive parents that was receiving services using an adaptation of this curriculum. While focusing on "surviving the holidays" (the training took place in late November), we spent some time on normalizing the range of caregiver responses, from joy and excitement to anger, frustration, and helplessness. Despite inviting the attending caregivers to share their experiences, the room remained excruciatingly silent (from our perspective!) until finally one caregiver raised her hand. Invited to speak, she stated, "My name is _____, and I've adopted four kids. I love my kids, but I have to admit, sometimes

I really just don't like them." In the aftermath of this statement, the room suddenly came to life: Parent after parent raised his or her hand and spoke of vulnerable moments in parenting and the emotions the parent was reluctant to share. Our normalization of difficult emotion and response was perhaps helpful, but not enough to provide permission; it was only after another parent was able to acknowledge these feelings that the remaining parents felt safe enough to speak.

Caregiver support groups have the potential to decrease some of the most common impacts of trauma: feelings of isolation, disconnection from others, secrecy, and shame. The skills provided in this section, along with those described in the remaining three attachment building blocks (Attunement, Consistent Response, and Routine and Ritual) may serve as a template for building group discussion and activities. A number of handouts provided in Appendix B may be useful.

🏠 Milieu

When working to build affect management within a milieu, the application takes place on a systems or provider level. Providers within systems that serve children and families exposed to trauma face many stressors that challenge our capacity to remain regulated. These include, among others, (1) the exposure to many different clients, all with different presentations, needs, and challenges, and the need to manage internal reaction to all of these and respond appropriately; (2) the frequent unpredictability that comes with working with youth in crisis; and (3) the helplessness that can come from working with systems over which the provider has no control. In systems serving higher-risk clients, such as residential programs or hospitals, affect management may be particularly challenging, given the very real threat to provider and other-client safety that may exist. Given these challenges, it is invariable that providers—like primary caregivers—will experience a range of emotional responses and will have moments of reactivity.

It is important that interventions on a milieu or systemic level feel supportive rather than punitive (i.e., the goal is *not* to send staff the message, "You shouldn't feel the way you feel"). Work to build a programmatic culture that accepts that providers—like our clients—are people with built-in human emotions and danger-response systems. By building appropriate, boundaried forums for staff support, we reduce the likelihood that these emotions and responses will play out in our work with clients. Consider professional supports such as supervision, clinical or staffing meetings, and training. Pay attention to forums that are *process* oriented as well as *task* oriented. This is particularly important in the aftermath of difficult and sometimes potentially traumatizing situations such as restraints or staff or client assaults. Building safe forums in which staff members can explore their own responses and actions—both positive and negative—is crucial to using these experiences as building blocks for future successes.

Beyond professional forums, it is important to pay attention to team building. Working in the field of trauma is too challenging to do alone, and it is important that members of a system feel supportive of, and supported by, their colleagues. In service of this effort, look for ways to explore and build an understanding of common goals and the role of all staff members in working toward these goals. Examine who supports each person on the team at every level. Build and support "fun" activities (e.g., staff retreats and celebrations), recognize and reinforce staff contributions, and normalize and encourage the importance of self-care.

🌏 REAL-WORLD THERAPY

🌑 **Have realistic expectations.** Keep in mind that affect management is hard. Caregivers, particularly those who have an untreated trauma history, may be starting in a very similar place as their children.

🌑 **Build success.** Success will likely be relative. Define realistic goals and take small steps toward reaching them. Offer praise along the way. Don't forget that caregivers need as much praise and encouragement as their children need.

🌑 **Tap into empathy.** When feeling frustrated with caregiver reactions, imagine living in a home with your client 24 hours a day, 7 days a week. Most caregivers have good intentions and are doing the best they can with the skills they possess.

🌑 **Be aware of your own reactions to the caregiver.** Particularly for those caregivers who move slowly, a dual role as advocate for the child and support and educator of the caregiver may lead to frustration and blaming of the parent. Pay attention to your own responses, as well as when it would be useful to bring additional clinicians onto the team.

🏳 **Pay attention to cultural differences.** These may influence your expectations of caregivers, your reactions to their behaviors, their reaction to you, and their feelings of vulnerability in doing this work. Be open to exploring and acknowledging differences as well as common ground.

CHAPTER 5

Attunement

THE MAIN IDEA

Support the child's caregiving system—whether parents or professionals—in learning to accurately and empathically understand and respond to children's actions, communications, needs, and feelings.

★ KEY CONCEPTS

★ What Is Attunement?

- Attunement is the capacity of caregivers and children to accurately read each other's cues and respond appropriately.

- This capacity requires that the caregiver and child be attuned on many levels: cognitive, emotional, behavioral, and physiological.

- Accurate attunement allows caregivers to respond to the emotion underlying children's behavior, rather than simply reacting to the most notable or distressing symptom.

★ Trauma Behaviors That Challenge Attunement

- Children who have experienced trauma often lack the capacity to communicate needs or to identify and cope with difficult emotions.

- Children frequently communicate emotions and internal experience via behavior rather than words. One of the key challenges of attunement work is for caregivers—clinicians, parents, and/or substitute care—to learn how to interpret the function behind the child's behavior.

- Often the behaviors that feel the most distressing to caregivers are simply "fronts" for unmet needs or unregulated affect, particularly those related to trauma.

- **Triggers**, or reminders of past traumatic experiences, may elicit intense emotion and/or numbing responses. Because triggers may not be obvious, it is particularly important to teach caregivers how to identify their children's triggering events and/or typical responses (see Teach to Caregivers, below, for more detail).

THERAPIST TOOLBOX

Behind the Scenes

Things to Assess: Caregiver

- How consistent is the caregiver's response to the child? For instance, does the caregiver routinely have difficulty reading child cues, or is the problem situation-specific? Target intervention to the needs of the dyad.

- Pay attention to caregiver boundaries. Some caregivers are overly involved with their child, whereas others are dismissive or withdrawn. Work to build developmentally appropriate involvement.

- How does the caregiver conceptualize his or her child's symptoms? Consider the following example:

> An adoptive mother of 13 children met with the evaluator of her 9-year-old son. When asked whether her son had difficulties with attention or impulsivity, she stated that he did not. When the evaluator asked more specific questions about the child's daily functioning, the mother described him as "constantly moving"; during a typical family dinner, for instance, she stated that her son might be up and down from the table over 20 times. When asked about this discrepancy, she appeared surprised, noting that she did not consider his behavior problematic.

In this example the family views a behavior as normative and likely would not identify it as a treatment target. However, in other contexts, this same behavior might lead to significant difficulty and, in fact, be a primary reason for referral. This child, for instance, was failing his current grade due to ongoing difficulties with sustained attention. This case highlights one of the common balancing acts in treatment: reinforcing a caregiver's ability to accept his or her child's behaviors and typical responses, while building the caregiver's attunement to the impact of the behavior on the child's functioning in other contexts.

- What level of insight does the caregiver have into the reasons behind the child's difficult behaviors? Does the caregiver understand the contribution of trauma? If not, psychoeducation will be an important part of your intervention.

- What role does culture play in the caregiver's understanding of the meaning and impact of the child's trauma experience? In some cultures, for instance, a child who has been sexually abused may be viewed as permanently damaged and may be ostracized from community members. It is important to work with the child and caregiving system to understand the particular meaning and interpretation of behaviors and experiences.

Things to Assess: Child

- Although the primary goal of attunement work is helping caregivers to accurately read their children's cues, a secondary goal is to help the child accurately read his or her caregiver's responses.

- Traumatized children may be *overly tuned in* to their caregivers, feeling an age-inappropriate responsibility to take care of the adults around them; may be *misattuned*, reading signs of anger, rejection, or abandonment where there are none; or may have learned to withdraw from interaction (i.e., to be *nonattuned*) as a survival skill.

- Although children's ability to accurately identify emotion is covered in greater detail in the Self-Regulation section, it is important to assess the child's attunement style with his or her caregiver, in order to help caregivers adjust their response to that of their child.

Family Norms

- "Attuned" behavior looks different across families, and level of attunement may not always be measurable by surface behavior. Consider two examples:

  Example 1: A single father appears constricted and disconnected in response to his 10-year-old son's affect. Observation and report indicate that he is rarely emotionally nurturing toward his child. However, he frequently spends time teaching his son life skills and other tasks, such as fishing, farming, etc. Over time, the clinician learns that this father's early caregiving environment lacked warmth and affection. Determined to respond to his own child's needs, the father has made a point of spending time with his son. The son describes his father as responsive and caring, citing as evidence a recent day in which his father took the time to teach him how to take an engine apart.

  Example 2: A mother with a 5-year-old daughter appears highly responsive to her daughter's needs. She checks in frequently with her child, often naming affect before the child expresses it. Over time, the clinician notices that the child rarely responds to the mother's statements and often appears to withdraw as the mother becomes more responsive.

- In both cases, the surface behavior is in contrast with the true level of attunement. In the first, the apparently disconnected father is well aware of his son's needs and is providing affection through dyadic tasks—a forum that is comfortable for both him and his son. In the second case, the apparently responsive mother is overly intrusive, often misreading her child's affect and missing the child's cues for distance. The key question in attunement is often the extent to which the caregiver is able to *accurately identify the child's need* and then respond in a manner that adequately meets that need.

- ▱ Cultural background, across dimensions, is one of the factors that influence family norms about caregiver–child interactions. Consider, for instance, the influence of the caregiver's own family of origin on ways of connecting, including beliefs about affection, respect, physical contact, play, etc. It is important for providers to elicit information about clients' cultural norms, rather than making inadvertent assumptions.

Provider Attunement

- Along with helping caregivers attune to their children, providers should practice these same skills. Children and families who have experienced trauma may present with an array of challenging behaviors. As a provider, it is easy to target and respond to the behavior rather than the underlying affect. Children may reenact key relational dynamics with their providers, may play out distress through behavior, and may test the provider in the same way they do their caregivers. Consider the following examples:

  Example 1: A clinician is in session with a 5-year-old boy who has a complex trauma history. After completing a feelings check-in, the boy appears to become increasingly dysregulated, playing with a toy truck and banging it into walls. The therapist, worried about the noise and about safety, tells him to stop banging the truck. In response, the boy begins banging the truck harder, and the therapist warns him that if he does not stop, she will have to terminate the session.

In this example, the clinician was appropriately worried about the child's safety, but got caught in the trap of limit setting and the ensuing power struggle, rather than attempting to respond to the boy's underlying message, "I'm feeling distressed." Although safety is obviously a primary concern, the clinician's anxiety about the child's behavior prevented her from accurately attuning to the dysregulated affect driving his behavior.

  Example 2: A 15-year-old girl in residential treatment is in her room shortly after a phone call with her mother. A passing staff member notices that she is sitting on her bed, kicking her dresser and swearing loudly. The staff member provides a warning that sanctions will occur for swearing and dangerous behavior unless she stops. A minute later, staff hear a loud crash and enter the room to find the girl kicking with enough force that her lamp has fallen off the top of the dresser; she curses at the staff members and tells them to leave her alone. The situation escalates, leading to a physical hold.

In this example, the first staff member appropriately tries to maintain programmatic structure and safety by setting a limit. However, the staff member misses the way that the behavior reflects emotional dysregulation in response to a trigger. Observation of the girl's affect and energy, validation of her experience, and support and cuing in modulation skills may have prevented escalation.

- As is the case with caregivers, affect management is a key first step for professionals in building our own attunement skills. Keep in mind the skills from the previous section, including self-monitoring. Know your own "push buttons" and the behaviors likely to interfere with your ability to respond versus react. Be conscious of self-care strategies and other in-the-pocket coping skills. When regulated and able to respond, the provider may act as an important model of attunement for the caregiver.

- In this section highlighted skills include becoming a "feelings detective" and the use of reflective listening. These skills can be applied to the therapeutic relationship as well as the dyad. Nonverbal attunement exercises, including the examples listed below, may also help to build clinician–child attunement and can often serve as the basis for coregulation.

- A challenge of working with children is often the multiple members of the system with whom the provider is working. As a result of taking on the role of child advocate, we may fall into the trap of demonizing the caregiver. Attunement toward the caregiver(s) is as important as attunement toward the child. More often than not, we are working with parents or other caregivers who are doing their best in often challenging situations. As with children, when a caregiver is unable or unwilling to engage in treatment, learn or practice a new skill, or respond appropriately to his or her child, use your attunement skills to try to understand the caregiver's experience and perspective.

- Therapy with dysregulated children is often a dance; they have varying degrees of ability to tolerate relationship, engagement, play, discussion, etc. Remember to pay attention to behavioral and physical cues that the client is distressed, excited, sad, angry, etc., and modify the session accordingly.

⊨ Attunement is often about more than emotion. Sensitivity to our clients includes an awareness of creating an environment that welcomes and tunes in to diversity. Children and families who have experienced trauma often feel "different." Although it would be impossible to change the therapy room for each new client, clinicians can attempt to create an environment that invites the client to explore, create, and contribute, and that reflects the experience of the child or family on some level. Consider dolls from various cultures, male and female puppets, a tree house in addition to a dollhouse, books that include nontraditional families, etc.

⌂ Teach to Caregivers

- *Reminder:* Teach the caregiver the Key Concepts.
- *Reminder:* Teach the caregiver the relevant Developmental Considerations.
- Keep in mind: Attunement happens on an ongoing basis. It is not just about monitoring and responding to intensive experiences, but also about day-to-day interactions. Teach caregivers to respond to children's cues across situations, whether in play, conversation, or general interaction.

Teaching Point #1: The Role of Child Vigilance

- Child vigilance to caregiver expression may lead to moments of misattunement between child and caregiver. Awareness of the role of child vigilance may help caregivers recognize and respond to these moments.

CHILD VIGILANCE AND ATTUNEMENT

Child vigilance to caregiver expression may result in:
- Misinterpretation of parental cues (e.g., overreading anger).
- Minimizing or denying own needs due to prioritization of caregiver needs (e.g., parenting the parent).
- Feeling overwhelmed by or afraid of signs of caregiver affect.

Help caregivers respond by:
- **Taking the time to understand the child's perspective.** If the child reacts strongly to minor statements, try to understand what brought on the overreaction. What does the child think you're feeling? Saying? Reflect what you see, and elicit the child's thoughts or feelings (e.g., "It looks like you just got really worried when I said that. Can you help me understand why?").
- **Being respectful of what the child is feeling.** Don't argue that the child is wrong—what he or she feels is just that (e.g., "It makes sense that you would feel really worried if you thought I was angry").
- **Correcting misperceptions.** Once the caregiver understands the child's reaction, correct misinterpretations (e.g., "I'm so sorry that you thought I was angry. What I was trying to say was, I'm worried about what would happen if . . . ").

Teaching Point #2: Understanding Triggers

- A primary foundation for building attunement is to help caregivers understand and learn to recognize the child's danger response. Dysregulation brought on by a triggered response is often a primary source of caregiver distress.

- For expanded information and teaching points, see caregiver education handout "**Understanding Triggers**" and caregiver worksheets "**Identifying Your Child's Triggers**" and "**What Does Your Child Look Like When Triggered?**" (Appendix B).

UNDERSTANDING TRIGGERS

What are triggers?	A **trigger**, as commonly defined within the traumatic stress field, is any stimulus that acts as a reminder of past overwhelming experiences and leads to the same set of behaviors or emotions that originally developed as an attempt to cope with that experience.
	Triggers can be *external*—such as a facial expression that reminds a child of a past abuser, or a smell that reminds a child of a lost parent; *internal*—such as feeling hungry, frightened, or highly aroused; or a *combination*—such as an interaction that leads to a child feeling vulnerable.
Common triggers for children who have experienced trauma	Unpredictability or sudden change
	Transition
	Loss of control
	Feeling vulnerable
	Feeling rejected
	Confrontation
	Loneliness
	Sensory overload (too much stimulation from the environment)
	Intimacy (safety, love, security, family)
	Peace/calm/quiet
Intersection between attachment and triggers: What caregivers should know	In the face of strong emotion, children who have previously experienced danger, rejection, or neglect may: • Avoid or withdraw from caregivers. • Become overly clingy and appear unable to take in support. • Freeze. • Appear "manipulative" or attempt to control caregivers. • Engage in conflicting approach and avoidance behaviors.
	When under stress (e.g., after being triggered), one of the biological mandates of human beings is to seek security from the primary attachment figure (i.e., the caregiver). As described above, however, the alternative strategies developed by traumatized children may prevent them from proactively seeking and taking in support.
	Therefore, it is particularly important for caregivers to be attuned to signs that their children are feeling overwhelmed or distressed.

Teaching Point #3: Building a Repertoire for Understanding Children's Communication

- Attunement is a skill requiring parents and caregivers to become "feelings detectives."

- Once parents learn to "read" their child's cues and patterns, they can better respond to the emotion underlying overt behavior, rather than to the behavior itself. Caregivers can then use

reflective listening skills (see Teaching Point #4) to mirror back to the child what they are seeing in an age-appropriate way.

- Caregivers should learn their child's individual communication strategies. What does the child look like when he or she is angry? Sad? Excited? Worried? What are the child's cues? For each emotion, help parents track the following (see caregiver education handout "**Learning Your Child's Language**" and the worksheet "**Learning Your Child's Emotional Language**," Appendix B):

HOW CHILDREN COMMUNICATE

Facial expression	Includes both intense expressions and lack of expressiveness
Tone of voice	Higher-pitched, louder, softer
Extent of speech	Very verbose or very quiet; rate of speech
Quality of speech	Organization, maturity (e.g., regression)
Posturing/muscular expression	What does the child's body look like? Is child curled up, fists clenched, muscles tense or loose, posture closed or open?
Approach versus avoidance	Does child get withdrawn, overly clingy, or both?
Affect modulation capacity	Does child have a harder time being soothed and/or self-soothing? Does child start to need more external comforting? How receptive is the child to soothing—does this change in the face of stress?
Mood	Does child's mood change overtly? For instance, is child normally even-tempered, but becomes more labile in the face of intense emotion? If so, that lability can serve as a warning sign to parents.

Teaching Point #4: Reflective Listening Skills

- Reflective listening helps caregivers actively *hear, validate,* and *communicate support* to their children. Reflective listening skills have their roots in Rogerian client-centered therapy (e.g., Rogers, 1951) and can be used to build caregivers' capacity to actively and empathically respond to their children's communications (whether verbal or nonverbal).

- Teach caregivers reflective listening skills; have caregivers practice in session with you and/or child.

REFLECTIVE LISTENING SKILLS FOR CAREGIVERS

Step	Description
1. Accept and respect all of a child's feelings.	There should never be a hidden agenda to "change" the child's feelings (e.g., *not* "You shouldn't be angry").
2. Show child that you are listening.	Use active listening skills; use eye contact, nod your head, respond verbally, etc.
3. Tell child what you hear him or her saying.	Reflect back what you hear and validate the importance to the child (e.g., "So, you didn't think your teacher was listening to you? Wow, that must have been really hard"). Ask questions if you're not sure which part affected the child.

Step	Description
4. Name the feelings.	Reflect back the child's feelings. If the child doesn't state a feeling, offer a guess (name at least two possibilities), but be prepared to be wrong (e.g., "You seem kind of worried or maybe angry. Is that right?"). Identify the cues—*why* do you think the child seems worried or angry? Always allow the child to correct you.
5. Offer advice/suggestions/ reassurance/alternative perceptions *only* after helping child to express how he or she feels.	Don't jump to problem solving until you've taken the time to hear what the child has to say. Validate the feelings and the situation *first*, then collaborate with the child to come up with a solution, if appropriate. Keep in mind that solutions may simply involve how to express and cope with the feeling.

Teaching Point #5: Putting It Together—What to Do When a Child Is Triggered

- All caregiver skills in this framework provide a foundation and a support for the child/adolescent skills discussed in the Self-Regulation and Competency sections.

- Sensitive caregiver attunement is a primary tool for supporting child self-regulation skills, particularly when a child is triggered.

- As you work with children on self-regulation skills, teach caregivers the following sequence for supporting child modulation. Note how the steps parallel child affect identification, modulation, and expression work.

STEPS TOWARD SUPPORTING CHILD MODULATION

Step	Description
1. Be attuned: keep on your detective hat.	Be aware of shifts in the child's feelings. If you are not sure what the child is feeling, notice the energy: Is it high or low? Withdrawn or active? Look for the cues that were identified during "feelings detective" work (Teaching Point #3), particularly those indicating that the child has been triggered.
2. Keep yourself centered.	Check in with yourself. Use your own affect management skills. Even if nothing else feels in control, you can try to stay in control of your own emotions and actions.
3. Ask yourself:	Where is the child's energy? Where does it need to go (e.g., up or down)?
4. Reflect (simply) what you are seeing.	Name what you see, but keep it simple. Keep in mind which part of the child's brain is in charge. The purpose of reflection when a child is very dysregulated is to cue him or her to use modulation skills (e.g., "I can see that your energy just got really high. Let's see if we can bring it down a little bit so we can talk.").
5. Cue child in use of skills.	Be aware of the range of modulation skills on which the child is working in treatment. Offer simple suggestions of a tool the child might use, either with you or independently (e.g., breathing, sitting quietly, calming down space, stress ball). Early in treatment it is suggested that you engage in these skills with the child in order to both practice regulation strategies and effectively model them for the child.
6. Model use of and engage child in self-monitoring.	One of the primary goals here is to help the child tune in to his or her own physiological experience. In order to support this skill, consider the following example: "When I squeeze this stress ball with you really, really fast, I notice that my heart beats a little faster, my face feels hot, etc. What do you notice?" "Let's see what happens if we slow it down a bit. First, let's take a big, deep breath. Now I notice that something changed. What do you notice?"

Step	Description
7. Reinforce the use of modulation skills.	Be sure to tune in to the child's attempts to modulate (e.g., "I'm really proud of you for trying to calm down your energy"). Remember that success is relative; just noticing that an emotion is dysregulated may be a success for some children.
8. Invite expression.	Once the child is calmed, invite expression/communication. Put the rest of those reflective listening skills to work!

✐ *Tools:* Dyadic Attunement Exercises

- The following exercises can be used in both dyadic and individual therapy. In dyadic therapy the caregiver and child should do the exercises together, with the clinician as observer/facilitator.

- It is particularly important to teach caregivers the material covered in "Teach to Caregivers" prior to engaging in dyadic attunement exercises.

DYADIC ATTUNEMENT EXERCISE EXAMPLES

Activity	Variations	Description
Feelings charades	Basic	Caregiver (or clinician) acts out a feeling state; child must guess. Child then takes turn acting, while caregiver guesses.
	Reverse	Caregiver acts out what child looks like during a particular feeling state; child must guess. Roles are then switched, and child acts out what caregiver looks like.
	Triggering situation (variation 1)	Caregiver and child pick a feeling; caregiver or child acts out a situation that might elicit that feeling, and partner guesses the situation.
	Triggering situation (variation 2)	Caregiver acts out a difficult situation; child must identify potential emotional responses. Roles are then reversed.
	Identify the person	Caregiver and child pick an emotion together. The actor portrays a known individual (e.g., someone in the family) in that emotional state; partner must guess the individual.
	There is an infinite number of variations on this game; target the game to the family's needs.	
Follow-the-leader games	Music	Use drums or other musical instrument. One partner creates a rhythm; the other must follow and/or build on the original rhythm.
	Dance/movement	One partner creates a physical movement; other must follow or build on the original movement.
	Mirroring	Two partners face each other. One partner engages in slow movements; other must follow. Goal is to be attuned to the point that an observer cannot discriminate the leader from the follower.
	Follow the leader	For younger children, pick a fun movement (e.g., walking across the room like a duck); all in the room must copy the movement.
	Classic "follow-the-leader" games	Consider games such as Simon Says, Red Light/Green Light, etc., to build attunement.

Activity	Variations	Description
Parallel "self" books		Work with caregivers and children to create a joint "All about Us" book. The book should contain parallel entries by caregiver and child. For example, pick an event that happened over the past week, and have each describe his or her feelings, favorite part, least favorite part, etc.
Play		Work with caregivers to play *with* their children. Any type of play will work: board games, imaginary play, expressive arts, etc. Teach caregivers to follow their child's lead and not to instruct or direct. Teach caregivers to use reflective listening skills.

ᛟᛟᛟ DEVELOPMENTAL CONSIDERATIONS

Developmental stage	Attunement considerations
General considerations	Teach caregivers what is normative versus atypical at a given age. (As an example: It is normative for 2-year-olds to assert their independence by saying "no"; this is part of appropriate and healthy development and *not* about being "oppositional," as it might be for an older child.)
	⊟ One of the challenges in caregivers' understanding of normative behavior is the impact of ongoing cultural changes in the experience of children at a given age. A 15-year-old in 2010 will have a very different experience than a 15-year-old did in 1975. Acknowledge these differences, and when feasible, invite a dialogue: Allow caregivers and children to teach each other about their lives.
	Regardless of age, language is often difficult for traumatized children. With less practice in safe expression and lower frustration tolerance, traumatized children often have no choice but to communicate their needs through their behavior.
	⊟ Children in substitute caregiving systems may have a different cultural background than that of their caregiver(s). Given the influence of culture on social interaction and emotional expression, attunement may be a particular challenge (both for the caregiver and the child). Again, acknowledge differences and invite a dialogue.
Early childhood	Young children are increasingly able to use language for communication. However, although they become efficient at communicating wants and needs through words (e.g., "I want apple juice," "I want that toy"), feelings continue to be primarily communicated through behaviors and physical states (e.g., temper tantrums as a sign that child is frustrated, upset stomachs as sign child is anxious or worried; shutting down/withdrawing as sign of need for reassurance).
	As children become more sophisticated in language use, adults may overestimate their reasoning ability as well as their capacity to use language to communicate internal state. Therefore, it is particularly important for caregivers to understand where their child is "at" developmentally and to learn to interpret behavioral cues.
	Part of what attunement does for young children is to provide a foundation for the building of affect identification, expression, and regulation skills. By providing verbal labels for children's states, caregivers are supplying the building blocks of emotional knowledge.
	Attuning to children's emotions and helping them to attune to the experience of others also acts as a foundation for the building of empathy and interpersonal interaction skills.
Middle childhood	Children at this age are increasingly tuned in to caregiver expression and feeling states. This can be positive for building empathy and perspective taking, but has multiple pitfalls for overly vigilant traumatized children.
	The elementary school years are the peak age for somatic expression of symptoms (headaches, stomachaches, etc.). Caregivers should pay attention to signs that the child's body may be holding/communicating affect for them.

Developmental stage	Attunement considerations
Adolescence	The key word for attunement in adolescence is *balance*: between connection and independence, privacy and awareness, and so on. Although caregivers often want to know *more* about their children during this higher-risk period, it is normative for adolescents to want to communicate *less*. Some of the negative behaviors, emotions, and interactions that emerge at this point may, in fact, be reconceptualized as the teen's striving for independence and separation.
	Adolescents often have ambivalent feelings about their need for nurturance versus their desire for independence. Because of this ambivalence, it is important for caregivers to provide opportunities for connection while respecting adolescents' negotiation of closeness and distance.
	An important part of attunement at this age is respecting privacy. Negotiate this area actively: Where can the adolescent maintain privacy, and where does the caregiver draw the line in terms of "need-to-know" information?

 ## APPLICATIONS

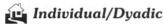 ### Individual/Dyadic

Work with caregivers in individual caregiver education sessions or, if necessary, by phone. Consider using ARC caregiver handouts and worksheets (Appendix B), if appropriate. Intervention in this section involves psychoeducation as well as active exploration, practice, and homework. For instance, rather than simply teaching caregivers about the ways a child may communicate, ask caregivers to track signs of anger or distress in their child over the course of a week, or complete a detailed "detective" worksheet in session about a particular child emotion or experience and the ways in which it manifests. Educating caregivers about triggers and exploring ways in which the child demonstrates triggered responses are crucial aspects of this intervention target.

Once caregivers have a basic understanding of the concepts, it is important to apply this skill "in the moment." For instance, consider the following example. About her adolescent daughter a mother states, "She was driving me crazy this morning—she was all over the place, bouncing off the walls. She wouldn't listen to anything I said, and then got all snarly when I tried to send her to her room." Rather than focusing on the behavior of the child, the therapist might consider working with the mother to go *beneath* the behavior to the likely emotion driving it, the precipitating factors, and/or the function of the current behaviors. It is important, when doing this, to also validate and normalize the caregiver's frustration with the behavior itself, and to explore the caregiver's own use of affect management skills.

Experiential practice of self-monitoring and self-regulation for the caregiver can be a valuable tool. Often the caregivers themselves have had little exposure to the self-care strategies discussed in the previous section. Consider building ongoing practice of dyadic attunement activities and modulation support steps into session routines in order to increase comfort with use of the various skills.

 ### Group

Caregiver groups can be an invaluable way to teach key skills and information, while simultaneously providing caregivers with support from others who have "been there." Use the "Teach to

Caregivers" section as a guide for curriculum content. Active teaching is better than passive: Invite caregivers to share ideas of ways in which their children communicate, evidence they have seen of triggered responses, etc. Hearing from other caregivers often helps normalize behaviors caregivers have observed in their own children. As with individual caregiver education sessions, keep in mind the value of application and practice.

🏠 Milieu

In a milieu system, staff at all levels, and particularly milieu counselors, are in the role of substitute caregivers. Education and training in trauma response and triggers for all milieu staff is crucial. It is important to make this training "real": Rather than speaking in the abstract, apply the concepts to the residents/students/clients served by the system. For instance, pick a particular child and ask staff to consider (1) ways in which that child demonstrates the fight, flight, or freeze response; (2) observations about situations that trigger the child; and (3) strategies that appear to help (i.e., those strategies that increase child felt safety) versus make things worse (typically, strategies that increase felt helplessness or perceived danger). Compare different children: How does Resident A, who has many externalizing behaviors, show a triggered response, and how is that different from Resident B, who is generally quiet and constricted? Help staff to understand the range of ways in which children show their feelings. Integrate these concepts into routine clinical discussions, staff meetings, or other forums in which youth behavior and functioning are discussed. Ultimately, the goal is for staff to develop a repertoire for understanding the "communication strategies" of every resident/client, and to learn to read these messages and respond in a way that supports longer-term goals, rather than reacting to immediate behaviors. Consider building in systematic tools for supporting modulation within the milieu itself in order to increase implementation by both counselors and clients. For example, when possible, create a safe space for use of modulation strategies. Have modulation-related activities readily available to staff and clients. Examples of such activities are discussed in greater detail in the "Modulation" section of this text.

🏠 All: The Value of Misattunement and Mess-Ups

Be sure to pair caregiver affect management skills with efforts to build attunement for all levels of intervention, and to normalize the frequent "misattunements" that occur. It is impossible for a caregiver to remain attuned at all times, and in fact, the missteps can strengthen an attachment bond, if handled well. Support caregivers in backtracking, reviewing difficult interactions, and considering alternative responses. Whether this is done as a supervisor in a residential system with milieu staff, or as a clinician in your own supervision, or with an individual parent, it is crucial to pay attention to safety: Caregivers must feel safe enough to acknowledge the "mess-ups" and the missed moments. Use these constructively: this is all part of a learning process. When necessary, support caregivers in steps toward reparation or resolution. These moments are often as important as the moments that are attuned: It is rare for a child to hear an adult express regret at the way a situation or interaction was handled, so such an experience can be infinitely valuable for both caregiver and child in building real-world relationships.

🌐 REAL-WORLD THERAPY

🌐 **Match the work to the caregiver.** As with other principles in the Attachment section, keep in mind that attunement may be more difficult for caregivers with unresolved trauma. In particular, these caregivers may, like their children, vigilantly attend to others' expressions and/or feel shame, guilt, etc., about their children's emotions. It is important to match up the caregiver affect tolerance work with the attunement work.

🌐 **Have realistic expectations.** Define success in terms of where the dyad has started and build success step by step.

🌐 **Pay attention to vicarious trauma.** Tuning in to strong emotions can kick up difficult emotions in both the clinician and the caregiver. Pay attention to your own self-care needs.

CHAPTER 6

Consistent Caregiver Response

THE MAIN IDEA

Support the caregiving system, whether familial or programmatic, in building predictable, safe, and appropriate responses to children's behaviors in a manner that acknowledges and is sensitive to the role of past experiences in current behaviors.

★ KEY CONCEPTS

★ *Why Is Consistency Important?*

- An important part of building a safe environment is building predictability in caregiver response.

- For children who have experienced trauma at the hands of their primary caregivers, limits may have been associated historically with powerlessness and intense vulnerability. Previous caregivers may have been perceived as out of control, punitive, and frightening.

- Even for children who were not harmed by primary caregivers, trauma itself is often perceived as an unpredictable punishment from the environment.

- A caregiving environment that provides safe, predictable responses to behavior provides children with reassurance that there are meaningful rules and consequences, both positive and negative, for behavior; that there are lines and boundaries defining appropriate behavior; that there are caregivers who are able to keep children safe; and that there are expectations that children are believed to be capable of living up to. As these predictable responses continue over time, children begin to be able to relax some of their vigilance and control, and to invest their energy into tasks of normative development.

★ *Trauma Behaviors That Challenge Consistent Response*

- In the face of unpredictability and chaos, like that associated with trauma, one of the adaptations children often make is to attempt to control their environment and others around them. This controlling behavior is the child's best effort to achieve safety in what is perceived as an unpredictable and dangerous world.

- Although clear, consistent limits and boundaries help children feel safe and are crucial for healthy development, traumatized children may be reactive to and triggered by both limit setting and praise, as these responses are initially perceived as a threat to their own control.

THERAPIST TOOLBOX

Behind the Scenes

- The goals of consistent response are twofold: (1) incorporating the caregiving system's understanding of the role of trauma in child behavior into the caregiver's responses to those behaviors (i.e., incorporating attunement skills into child management strategies) and (2) building a capacity to respond to behaviors in a way that is consistent, appropriate, and sensitive to trauma influences on the child's responses.

- When addressing the area of consistent response in the home environment, the target of intervention is generally the primary caregiver(s), along with appropriate collateral or substitute caregiving systems (e.g., school settings, foster care), and ideally with the collaboration of the child. When addressing consistent response in a system, the target is typically the consistent response within the system as a whole, across and among staff members.

- Norms about what is considered "appropriate" caregiving vary widely across cultures. Behaviors that might be considered abusive in one context are considered acceptable and responsible parenting in another. Research shows, in fact, that effective parenting strategies differ across culture and context. It is important to understand the belief system of your client as well as contextual variables prior to developing treatment targets. Consider the following example:

> Keon was a 12-year-old African American boy being raised by a single father in an urban inner-city area. Keon came to session one day and angrily reported that his father had given him a "whupping" the night before. When the clinician spoke with the father, he acknowledged disciplining his son with a belt after his son brought home a negative report from school that led to a week of detention.

In this example, the clinician is faced with a dilemma. Striking the child with a belt may be considered an incident requiring a mandated report. However, in this family's culture, the father's discipline of his son is considered appropriate, and in fact responsible, parenting. In conversation, the father discusses the discipline he received as a child, his own mistakes during his teen years, and his determination that his son will succeed. In this, as in many situations, clinicians are faced with the challenge of balancing validation of the caregiver's values, belief systems, and cultural norms with accommodation to societal laws and dominant culture.

▷ Our own experience with parenting (as child and as caregiver) may influence our beliefs about what "good parenting" is. Pay attention to your own biases.

▷ When assessing parenting behaviors, it is important to understand not just the action but the intent behind the action. Consider this example:

> A grandfather with significant health issues is caring for his two young grandchildren who have recently immigrated from Cuba; their own parents remain behind. The family lives in a housing project in a dangerous neighborhood, and the grandfather reports significant drug activity and other violence in the building and surrounding area. During an evaluation, the children report that their grandfather frequently sits at the door to the apartment with a belt in his lap and hits them if they try to go out the door. The grandfather reports significant fears for the safety of his grandchildren, and concern that, due to his own physical disability, he would be unable to go after them if they left without permission.

In this example the grandfather's *intent* is to keep his grandchildren safe from the significant violence in their environment. His *action* is one that has raised significant concerns by treaters and child welfare. In working with this family, it is essential to understand and validate the intent behind his actions.

Intergenerational Layers

- Many children who experience chronic, complex trauma have parents or other primary caregivers who themselves have experienced, to some degree, stress within their own families of origin and a lack of appropriate parenting.

- In the absence of a model of appropriate and attuned parenting, stressed caregivers and caregiving systems will make attempts to care for their children, and to manage behavior, in as effective a manner as they are able.

- It is our experience that the majority of parents are doing the best they can, given the resources, supports, and experiences available to them. Given this, it is crucial that the intervener work to develop an empathic attunement to the caregiver. Although as professionals, we must balance this support with our obligation to protect, a crucial foundation of the work described in this chapter is attunement to the caregiver and the understanding that, as with children, *the behaviors of the caregiver make sense*. We are at our most effective in working with caregivers when we first attempt to step into their shoes.

- Along with attunement, it is crucial to maintain an awareness of the importance of caregivers experiencing success as they learn and practice new skills. Behavior management strategies are hard work, when first attempted; build skills slowly and in manageable steps.

- Keep in mind that it will be important to employ these same skills in building safety and predictability in the therapeutic relationship and the therapeutic space. Although limits and rules will necessarily differ from those in the home setting, clear expectations and boundaries in the therapeutic space are essential.

✍ *Teach to Caregivers*

- *Reminder*: Teach the caregiver the Key Concepts.
- *Reminder*: Teach the caregiver the relevant Developmental Considerations.

Teaching Point #1: Guidelines for Use of Praise and Reinforcement

Teaching points	Trauma creates significant distress that impacts individuals and their caregiving systems. Over time, it is not uncommon for a negative pattern to build, in which members focus almost exclusively on difficulties, stressors, and symptoms.
	When overwhelmed by distress, there may be a loss of awareness of the positives. Children (and their caregivers) may begin to identify primarily with the "bad": "I'm a bad kid," "I'm a bad parent."
	This same dynamic may build in milieu treatment settings, as staff begins to focus primarily on stress and pathology.
	This pattern may lead to helplessness and/or hopelessness: *"This will never change!"*
	The use of praise and positive reinforcement can: • Increase positive caregiver–child interactions. • Increase desired behaviors. • Increase attunement. • Increase felt safety. • Build self-esteem and self-efficacy for both child and caregiver. • Increase feelings of child and caregiver mastery.
	Praise and reinforcement must be a conscious choice. Surprisingly, the good things are often *much* more difficult to notice than the hard ones! Noticing the positives often requires effortful focus and selection of behaviors to target.
Selecting targets	**Don't praise everything.** Work with caregivers to be selective. If they praise everything they see, it will feel false to them and false to the child. Pick things that are tangible, that are important, that are goals, etc., and focus on those.
	Start small. Help caregivers pick one behavior to notice. They should consciously tune in to it and praise it whenever it appears. Have caregivers track their use of praise.
	Choose behaviors that are salient and desired. Specifically select targets based on those behaviors that you are trying to build. For instance, if tolerating frustration without tantrumming is an important goal, then any sign that the child is doing this should be noticed and reinforced. Work with caregivers to specifically link the praise to the behavior or effort (e.g., *not* "Good job" but "Wow, I'm so proud of you. I just told you that you had to wait a few minutes before we went outside, and you said 'okay.' I know that can be hard, and I'm really proud of how you handled it.")
	Help caregivers choose targets wisely. If the initial target is the one thing the child never does, neither the parent nor the child will experience success.
	Redefine "success." Help caregivers think in terms of gradual shaping rather than overnight success. If the ultimate goal is for the child not to punch a wall when angry, for instance, then reinforce the first time the child yells and screams but doesn't punch.
	Beyond "being good" Praise should not always be linked to actions. Praise is not just about shaping behavior but about building a positive sense of self. Work with caregivers to reinforce children's qualities and efforts.

Examples of praise statements	Behavior related	"You did a really good job at finishing your homework."
		"I like how well you're sharing with your sister."
		"I feel so proud when you find safe ways to tell me what you're feeling."
	Effort related	"I can see how hard you're working at that."
		"Thank you for trying to compromise, even though it's hard."
		"I can see how frustrated you are, and I'm really proud of you for not yelling."
	Child qualities	"I'm so proud of how kind you are."
		"You're so adventurous—I think it's great!"
		"What a great sense of humor you have."
	Open-ended	"You're such a great kid, I have such fun being with you."
		"I love it when we play games together."
		"It made me so happy to see you smile yesterday."
Reinforcers	Teaching point	One way to increase positive behaviors is to use concrete reinforcers.
	Adult attention is powerful.	Teach caregivers that adult attention is one of the most powerful reinforcers they can use. In building concrete reinforcement systems, don't lose sight of the power of praise.
	Reward charts	Work with caregivers to build concrete reinforcement systems.
		As with praise, choose one or two behaviors on which to focus initially.
		Develop star/sticker charts, point reward systems, etc. Work with caregivers to select developmentally appropriate methods (see Developmental Considerations).
		Help caregivers identify appropriate reinforcers.
	Examples of concrete reinforcers	Special time with caregivers.
		Extra privileges (e.g., computer time, television time, later bedtime).
		Getting to be the leader (e.g., choosing the family movie, choosing favorite food for dinner).
		Activities (e.g., going to the park, playing cards, baking cookies, going out to eat).
		Concrete rewards (e.g., toys, games, books).

Teaching Point #2: Praise and the Trauma Response

- For some children who have experienced trauma, reward and positive attention can trigger a negative response. There are several reasons for this:

    ♦ Praise may be "ego-dystonic." For children who have a strong sense that there is something wrong with them, praise may not match their self-perception and may therefore feel frightening, like a falsehood or a trick.

    ♦ Positive statements can elicit attachment fears. Children who have been impacted by trauma have often experienced multiple losses—of caregivers, of places, and of other important figures in their lives. A positive relationship with an adult may elicit fears that the same things are about to happen. The fear in the child's mind is, "Why attach when someone could take this all away again tomorrow?"

RESPONDING WHEN CHILDREN ARE TRIGGERED BY PRAISE

Don't take it personally.	Help caregivers be aware that praise may be a trigger. If their child responds negatively to being praised, help caregivers separate the attachment fears from relational rejection.
Hang in there.	For many children, part of making meaning about trauma includes self-blame. Praise and reinforcement won't lead to immediate change in this. Help caregivers build tolerance for the emotions (e.g., shame, guilt, frustration) that go along with witnessing negative self-statements by their child.
Don't argue it.	Help caregivers stand by their praise, without arguing. Teach them to keep the response simple. For instance, if the caregiver tells the child that he or she is proud of them, and the child rejects it, a caregiver response might be: "Well, *I'm* feeling proud of you, but it's okay for you to feel however you want."
Stay tuned into child affect.	If a child begins to escalate, help caregivers use their attunement skills to name and respond to the underlying affect. For instance, "I can see that was kind of scary for you to hear. Would a hug help you feel better?"

Teaching Point #3: General Guidelines for Behavioral Management

Teaching points	For many traumatized children, limits in the past have been overly punitive, inconsistent, or nonexistent.
	Children may use rigid control strategies to help them feel safer. Because of this, they may initially resist limits. However, over time, consistent limit setting will increase felt safety in the environment and ultimately allow children to let go of their control.
	Caregivers may be hesitant to set limits with children who have experienced trauma. However, failure to set limits may inadvertently send many negative messages, such as:
	• The child is incapable of controlling his or her own behavior. • The child is too "damaged" to behave. • The child is unworthy of the caregiver's attention. • The caregiver is unable to handle the child's behavior.
	Note that all of these messages increase the child's perception of powerlessness, which can *increase* negative behaviors.
	In contrast, setting consistent expectations and limits sends a different message. It communicates that:
	• Children *are* able to learn behavioral control. • They have the ability to alter their behavior in a way that is appropriate to the situation. • They are worthy of caregiver attention • Their caregiver can keep them safe.
Behavioral management strategies	Ignoring
	Limit setting
	Time-out

Teaching Point #4: Use of Ignoring

Definition	"Ignoring" is actively *not attending* to undesirable behaviors that are not immediately dangerous. The goal of active ignoring is to reduce the occurrence of these behaviors by removing the reinforcing value of attention.

Appropriate targets

Examples of appropriate targets for ignoring include:
- Whining.
- Temper tantrums (unless they include unsafe expression for child or other).
- Pouting/sulking.

When a child engages in behaviors such as those listed above, the caregiver should:
- Acknowledge the feeling.
- Name the negative behavior.
- Name a more appropriate alternative behavior.
- Indicate willingness to engage with the child once the negative behavior stops.

How to

Once the caregiver has engaged in these initial steps, it is important that the following happen:
- Remove attention from the child. Do not continue to give warnings, name the behavior, or engage with the child, once the initial statement has been made.
- Immediately reinforce any positive alternative displayed by the child (e.g., if the child has been whining, immediately praise the child when the whining stops).
- Set limits only if the behavior escalates and becomes dangerous to the child or others. If the behavior continues beyond several minutes, the caregiver may provide additional prompts (e.g., "I'd really like to speak with you, once you're ready to talk in a regular voice").
- If the behavior continues beyond approximately 10 minutes, the caregiver should shift to limit setting (see below).

Example

A 10-year-old boy has been told by his caregiver that he can't have a snack before dinner. He begins to yell and demand a snack.

CAREGIVER: *(Acknowledge the feeling.)* I can see you're mad that you can't have a snack *(name the negative behavior)*, but yelling won't change my decision. *(Name a more appropriate behavior.)* You can tell me how mad you are, or go play with your basketball to help you feel less mad, but while you're yelling I can't talk to you. *(Indicate willingness to engage with child when negative behavior stops.)* When you're ready to talk without yelling, I'll be in the kitchen.

BOBBY: *(Yells for another minute, which caregiver ignores. Then stomps off.)*

CAREGIVER: Good choice; I'm proud of you for listening and stopping your yelling. If you'd like to talk, come let me know.

Teaching Point #5: Setting Limits

Definition

Limit setting involves naming and following through on consequences for behavior. Consequences generally include either removal of privileges or "time-out."

Appropriate targets

Behaviors around which limits should be set will vary according to family or system norms, but generally address those behaviors that are unsafe, aggressive, or violate familial/systemic rules. For instance, hitting, throwing toys at a sibling, yelling or screaming after being given warnings, name calling, and refusal to follow a directive should result in setting of limits.

How to

When initially working with caregivers to set limits, help them select targets and consequences that they can actually carry out. Help caregivers identify specific limits/consequences for specific behaviors in advance. Teach them the following steps:
- Acknowledge the feeling behind the behavior.
- Name the unacceptable behavior.
- Name the limit or consequence.
- Suggest an alternative behavior for current or future use.

Limits

Limits are most effective if they are:
- **Immediate:** Limits should be applied as soon as possible after the negative behavior, particularly for younger children. *Note:* In applying limits, it is important to be conscious of the child's state of arousal; help the child to modulate *before* applying a limit. See "Choose Your Moments," Teaching Point #7.
- **Related:** Understanding the connection between limit and consequence increases when the limit is tied to the behavior (e.g., playing with a ball in the house after being told not to results in losing use of the ball for the afternoon).

- **Age-appropriate:** Limits should be appropriate to the child's developmental stage. See Developmental Considerations.
- **Proportional:** To the extent possible, pair the severity of the limit with the severity of the behavior. Mild behaviors should not be punished with excessive limits.
- **Calm:** Limits should be delivered in a calm tone of voice. Caregivers are less effective if they are frightening to their children. If necessary, caregivers should take the space to calm down before delivering a limit.

Suggested sequence for **applying limits to a behavior that has already occurred** (e.g., unsafe actions)	Teach caregivers the following sequence for addressing behaviors that have already occurred:
	1. "I can see that you are feeling _____, but _____ is not okay" (e.g., "I can see that you are feeling angry, but hitting your brother is not okay").
	2. *Sample options:*
	  ○ "You are showing me you can't be safe right now, so you need to _____ ("go to your room," "sit on the steps," etc.) _____ ("for 5 minutes," "until I come get you," etc.)."
	  ○ "You were told that if you _____, then _____" (e.g., "You were told that if you hit your brother, then you would lose PlayStation for the night. You chose to hit your brother, so now you will not be allowed to use PlayStation until tomorrow.").
	3. "Next time you feel _____, I hope you choose to _____" (e.g., "Next time you feel angry, I hope you choose to come tell me instead of hitting your brother").

Suggested sequence of language for **eliciting behaviors that have not yet occurred**	Teach caregivers the following three-step sequence for eliciting desired behaviors: 1. "Please _____" (e.g., "Please pick up your toys"). 2. "You need to _____" (e.g., "You need to do what I asked and pick up your toys now"). 3. "If you do not _____, then _____" (e.g., "If you do not pick up your toys by the time I come back into the room, then you will not be able to play outside after dinner"). 4. [If the behavior does not occur] "You were told to _____, and you chose not to. Now, _____" (e.g., "You were told to pick up your toys, and you chose not to. Now, that means you will not be able to play outside tonight").
Rationale	This sequence addresses the following: • Provides child with a clear message of desired behavior, as well as consequences for failing to follow through. • Allows the opportunity for the child to connect actions with consequences, and to make a choice about behavior. • Ultimately, removes the power struggle and places the responsibility on the child, as limits are clearly linked to the child's behavior.

Teaching Point #6: Using Time-Out with Traumatized Children

Definition	"Time-out" is a particular type of limit setting that involves the removal of the child from a physical location (and the attention of others within that location) to a space where the child can spend a specified amount of time alone. For younger children, time-out often involves sitting in a specified place (e.g., on a chair, on a step); for older children, similar principles can be used (e.g., sending the child to his or her room for a specific length of time).
Appropriate targets	Time-out is useful for immediately stopping an unacceptable behavior, particularly those that are impulsive and/or unsafe. For traumatized children, time-out may be useful for providing "space" to allow them to calm down from distressing emotion. Appropriate targets, in general, include those listed above for limit setting.
How to	When a child engages in impulsive or unsafe behaviors, the caregiver should: 1. Provide a warning: "If you do not stop _____, you will need to _____" (e.g., "If you do not stop yelling, you will need to take some space"). 2. Following the warning, if the behavior does not stop, restate the negative behavior and name the time-out location and the length of time. 3. If necessary, bring the child to the time-out location. 4. Once the child is in time-out, remove all attention until the specified length of time is over. Often, 1 minute per year of child age is used; caregivers can also specify, "Until you calm down," but the caregiver must clarify what that will look like.

If the child refuses to go to time-out, the caregiver should use an if–then statement to name a consequence if the child does not follow through. It is very important that caregivers follow through on these limits, once they are named.

Once the child has completed the specified time, the caregiver should:
1. Praise the child for following directives and remaining in time-out.
2. Elicit the child's understanding of why he or she was in time-out.
3. Acknowledge the feeling behind the behavior.
4. Give an alternative (or help child think of an alternative) for what he or she can do the next time, instead of the unacceptable behavior.

Example	A 7-year-old girl, angry about having been told that she can't play outside, starts to yell and throw her toys.

CAREGIVER: *(Provide a warning.)* Jemmie, throwing toys is unsafe. If you don't stop, you will need to take some space.

JEMMIE: *(Continues to throw toys.)*

CAREGIVER: *(Restate the negative behavior.)* I told you it was not okay to throw toys. Now you need to sit on the steps until you're ready to talk to me without yelling.

(Takes Jemmie's hand and walks her to the step. Jemmie continues to scream for a few minutes, which the caregiver ignores. After Jemmie has begun to calm down, caregiver returns.) (Praise the child for following instructions.) Jemmie, you're doing a really good job. I can see that you're calming down because you're sitting on the step without yelling. *(Elicit the child's understanding.)* Do you know why I told you to sit on the step?

JEMMIE: No!

CAREGIVER: I told you to sit on the step because you were throwing things, which was unsafe.

JEMMIE: But I wanted to go outside!!!

CAREGIVER: I know you wanted to go outside *(acknowledge the feeling)*, and it made you mad that you couldn't, but throwing toys wasn't a safe way to tell me. But now, you're doing a really good job of using your words to tell me. I'm sorry you're so mad, but it's too late to play outside now. *(Give an alternative.)* Would you like to draw a picture with me instead?

Teaching Point #7: Limit Setting and the Trauma Response

- As with reward and praise, setting limits can elicit strong emotions in traumatized children.

- It is important for caregivers to consider the following in setting limits.

TRAUMA CONSIDERATIONS WITH LIMIT SETTING

Reduce the need for limits.	Traumatized children often feel the need to be in control. Power struggles may be avoided by providing limited choice (e.g., "You can do your homework in your room or at the kitchen table. Which would you like to do?"). This choice provides the child with the illusion of control, while allowing the caregiver to maintain limits around the behavior.
	Have caregivers use their attunement skills to determine the reason behind child noncompliance. Differentiate children who feel overwhelmed by a task from those who are noncompliant with it. Try the following: • Elicit from the child what he or she is feeling and/or name what you are seeing (e.g., "You seem really upset by having to clean your room. What's going on with that?"). • Break large tasks into smaller ones. • Offer to help.
	Compromise. Help caregivers define which rules are essential, and on which they can compromise.
Choose your moments.	When traumatized children are in a high state of arousal, they are unable to access higher cognitive functions, including logic, problem solving, planning, anticipating, delaying response, etc.

When children are highly aroused, caregivers should do the following:
- Name the unsafe behavior, if any.
- Help child to use affect regulation and/or containment skills (including caregiver support), as necessary.
- Apply limits only after child has calmed down.

Be aware of triggers.	All types of limit setting can act as triggers. Time-out and ignoring can trigger fears of abandonment and rejection; setting limits and consequences can trigger fears of punishment, authority, and vulnerability. Although they should not avoid the use of limits for these children, it is important for caregivers to be aware of these possible reactions. The impact can be minimized by:
	• Always naming the rationale for a limit and linking it to the behavior (rather than to the child).
	• Always naming the boundaries around the limit (e.g., length of time in time-out, amount of time privilege is lost).
	• Moving on. Caregivers should not continue to scold, bring up the behavior, or manifest excessive affect after setting the limit and carrying it through. Caregivers should let the child know, explicitly, if necessary, that they still love him or her.
	• Making adaptations to limits for specific triggers (e.g., a child who has been previously punished by being enclosed in a small space might have time-out sitting in a nearby chair, rather than in another room).

🔧 Tools: Consistent Caregiver Response

- A number of techniques can be incorporated when working with caregivers to build consistent response. Consider the following.

Psychoeducation	About why it is often harder to set consistent limits with trauma-reactive children.
	About common caregiver responses and emotions that interfere with consistent limit setting.
Behavioral skills training	Teach appropriate use of reinforcement and consequences.
Practice	Help caregivers to role-play skills in session; target both typical day-to-day scenarios as well as potential trouble spots.
Caregiver coaching	It can be particularly useful to hold dyadic sessions with the child in order to support the caregiver in application of these skills.
Modeling	For caregivers who have difficulty with application, clinicians can model the skills in dyadic sessions.
Homework	Don't just talk about the skills; have caregivers actively practice and track at least one skill (specified in advance) each week.

- The following broad considerations can be useful in increasing the likelihood of treatment success.

Start small and build.	For caregivers to be successful, targeted skills should be realistic. Never target more than one to two behaviors at a time.
	Start by teaching reinforcement rather than limit setting. Target behaviors in which the child already engages, to some degree.
	With limit setting, don't start with the most difficult behaviors.

Collaborate in target selection.	Caregivers need to be engaged in selection of targets. Collaboration is essential for behavioral skills training to be successful.
	Caregivers will often want to target the most distressing, entrenched behaviors first. However, doing so may be frustrating and demoralizing. Work with caregivers to break down difficult targets into smaller steps.
	Balance caregiver identification of the most pressing "wants" with your own assessment of the family's needs.
Use successive approximations.	When targeting difficult behaviors, follow the rule of successive approximation: Success builds in small steps, not large leaps.
	Example: A child consistently punches a sibling when angry. The goal is to reduce *dangerous* expressions of anger, and *then* to build healthier coping, including use of modulation tools and healthier expression.
	Step 1: Reinforce any expression of anger that does not involve physical harm to self or other (e.g., punching a pillow or slamming a door is considered a success in this first step).
	Step 2: Reinforce use of modulation skills, such as those built during self-regulation work (e.g., the child's "Feelings Toolbox").
	Step 3: Reinforce the use of verbal expression—or the child's ability to communicate safely to others—to convey that he or she is feeling angry. Keep in mind that this is the most difficult step.
Predict pitfalls.	Collaborate with caregivers to predict trouble spots. Potential trouble spots may be a result of:<ul><li>Child triggers (e.g., transitions, anniversaries, locations).</li><li>Caregiver "push buttons" (e.g., whining, nagging, lying); in a system, consider individual push buttons as well as systemically vulnerable areas.</li><li>Atypical routines (e.g., vacation days).</li><li>The presence of multiple caregivers.</li><li>The presence of additional stressors, including positive ones (e.g., birthday parties, playdates).</li></ul>
Experiment.	Encourage caregivers to try new techniques. Predict in advance that some may not be successful. (However, keep in mind that nothing will be successful if not applied consistently, over a realistic time frame.)
Assign homework.	Remind caregivers that learning new skills takes practice. Select specific targets and have caregivers practice and track the new skills each day. Check on the application of skills, successes, and trouble spots each week.
	When possible, it may be helpful to be available to caregivers for "on-the-spot" telephone consultation at the start of applying a new skill.
Provide reinforcement.	Work with caregivers to identify and use both verbal and concrete reinforcement with their children on a consistent basis. Help them praise child effort as well as success.
	Be sure to reinforce caregivers for success.
Track progress.	With difficult behaviors, it is often helpful for clinicians to track weekly change (e.g., using charts or tables). Small change is often easier to identify over time with the help of concrete markers.

🏃 DEVELOPMENTAL CONSIDERATIONS

Developmental stage	Consistent response considerations
Early childhood	Young children rely strongly on external markers of success or failure. Because their internal sense of self is not yet well developed, they look to the cues of others to understand whether what they have done is "right" or "wrong." Unlike adults, young children have very little "filter" through which to interpret experience, and they will directly internalize the feedback the environment gives them. The more that feedback is (realistically!) positive, the better.
	Preschoolers are very concrete and have limited capacity to hold information over time. Therefore, reinforcement and limit setting both need to be immediate (if tied to specific events).
	Particularly for young children, praise and adult attention are the most powerful reinforcers.
	Consequences should be mild and immediate. Young children do not retain awareness of the links between behaviors and consequences for a lengthy period of time. Long time-outs or excessive punishments are counterproductive because the child will lose awareness of the rationale very quickly.
Middle childhood	Because industry is such an important developmental task, it becomes important to reinforce successful signs of a child's initiative. Pay attention to efforts outside of the home; caregivers should not just reinforce what they see but also what they hear about from others. Encourage caregivers to build communication with teachers, Scout leaders, after-school people, etc.
	At this age, it is important to begin to elicit self-praise and self-reinforcement: What does the *child* feel good about? Of what is he or she proud? Reinforce the child's positive sense of self.
	Because older elementary school–age children have some capacity to delay gratification, this is a good age to start using point-reward systems.
	Consequences and limit setting become more salient at this stage as children are becoming more aware of the link between behaviors and outcomes.
	Limits can be slightly longer or more involved than for younger children (i.e., a child can receive a consequence at home for something that happened at school, or a consequence that lasts for a longer period of time). However, consequences should remain proportional to the behavior and age-appropriate.
Adolescence	Balance in limit setting is key. Help caregivers pick their battles.
	Natural consequences are increasingly important—the goal is for an adolescent to learn to make appropriate choices and to take responsibility for the consequences of those choices. Therefore, consequences should always be linked, either verbally or through natural flow, with the choices the teen has made.
	Adolescents are moving toward independence, identity development, peer relations, and accomplishments/individual competency. Help caregivers reinforce adolescents' efforts in these areas.
	Because a goal for adolescence is increasing independent control over behavior, it is particularly important for caregivers to reinforce those moments when adolescents pay attention to their own actions and the outcomes. For instance, a teen describes a conflict with a peer that led him to lose his temper. Rather than placing a limit on the action (i.e., loss of temper), reinforce the *self-awareness*.

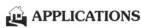 APPLICATIONS

Individual/Dyadic

When working with primary caregivers (biological, foster, adoptive, or kinship), behavior management strategies are often a priority request. Enough with the *concepts*, we hear routinely, "Tell me what to *DO!*" The wish from many caregivers, understandably, is for there to be some formula—an action, a consequence, a statement—that will shift the most distressing child behaviors and make the family's life easier. Although the precise formula does not exist, the one formula to which we can attest is this: REPETITION. Behavioral strategies are most effective when applied over and over, in a responsive and attuned way.

In all homes it is important for rules to be explicit and clear. Work with caregivers to discuss rules with children in age-appropriate terms, and, when appropriate, to post "Family Rules" somewhere visible. The visibility of family rules is particularly important for children who enter into foster or adoptive homes, and who may have experience of rules and consequences being different in different settings; gaining a clear understanding of the rules and consequences is often one of the pressing concerns children have when entering new environments. Keep the rules simple; it is better, in most cases, to have a single rule such as "Be safe," than to have 10 rules outlining "Don't hit," "Don't kick," "Don't throw things," etc.; language can be used to link the behavior to the rule (e.g., "Throwing that toy was an example of not being safe"). (Note: There are always exceptions; for some children, it is important to be clear and concrete when naming rules. Caregivers and clinicians should use their judgment.)

When working with caregivers to build consistent response, it is important to pay attention to their current behavior management strategies, to the context of the child and family, to the caregivers' own parenting histories and beliefs, and to the pattern of child behavior and caregiver response. Pay attention to the "building success" strategies noted above (pp. 87–88). Start small and build; work with caregivers to build success using one tool before moving to another. Practice in session; role-play anticipated child responses and troubleshoot predicted problems. Whenever appropriate, integrate children into this work. For instance, if a parent will be attempting time-out for the first time, explain to the child in advance (i.e., *not* in the moment it is to be used for the first time), in age-appropriate language, what a time-out is and when and how it will be happening. Also when appropriate, coaching in the moment (i.e., in dyadic sessions) can be useful in helping caregivers apply these skills with their children. Reinforce caregivers for their attempts to use these skills, just as we ask caregivers to reinforce their children. Providing active homework is crucial to the success of behavioral management strategies: Integrating new skills depends on practice and consistency, and inconsistent application will increase negative behaviors.

Support caregivers in collaborating with other significant adults in the child's life around responding to the child's behavior. Help caregivers to communicate their goals with teachers and other adults. Similarly, help teachers and other adults communicate any particularly important goals to the primary caregivers. Team meetings are often useful.

Group

Parenting groups are often effective ways to teach behavioral management strategies because caregivers are able to receive both support and concrete suggestions from other caregivers. It is our experience that caregivers of trauma-impacted children have had to learn to be creative in applying parenting strategies, and that a wealth of knowledge often comes from other caregivers who have "been there." Consider the following examples of parenting strategies shared by caregivers in a group education setting:

> An adoptive mother of an 11-year-old girl with a history of significant neglect, whose behaviors escalated whenever the mother attempted to enforce a time-out, described using a technique called "time-in": "She gets too upset to sit by herself in time-out, so I put her wherever I am—if I'm cleaning the room, she has to sit on the bed quietly for 5 minutes, or if I'm cooking, she has to sit at the table. It's still not what she wants to be doing, but she can see me and she knows I'm right there, so she's not yelling for my attention the way she does if she has time-out in another room."

A similar strategy is described by a parent of a 6-year-old boy with a history of significant neglect:

> "We tried ignoring his behaviors, but whenever we did he would get more and more upset. We think being ignored and being put in time-out was really triggering for him, but we didn't want to *not* respond when he got out of control, either. What we finally started doing was having him sit on the sofa, and then one of us would sit next to him. We weren't giving him our attention, but we'd sit with him, with one hand on his knee or shoulder so that he knew we were there, and we'd sit there together until either the time-out period was over or until he was able to be calm enough for the next steps."

A third example involved increasing the child's felt control even in the face of consequence:

> "We built a 'chill-out' space under the table—it was really just a bunch of blankets and pillows, and one of her 'stuffies,' but no other toys. She can use it in two ways: one is, if she just wants to take a break, she can go in there whenever she needs to and take some space. The other is, if she's starting to get in trouble, and we need to set a limit but we can see that she's getting out of control, we give her a choice: You can either go to time-out for 5 minutes, or you can go into your chill-out space. It's really cut down on a lot of the battles, because she gets some control, and she knows it's about helping her calm down."

What all of these examples have in common is a caregiver understanding of the role of dysregulation in child behaviors: In each of these examples, limits are balanced with a goal of helping the child achieve a modulated state. Furthermore, caregivers use their attunement skills to select behavior management strategies that decrease, rather than increase, their child's feelings of distress.

Milieu

Residential and other milieu programs often have expansive and sophisticated behavior management strategies; however, programs may struggle with ways to make these systems trauma-sensitive and trauma-informed. A number of strategies may be useful for milieu programs to consider. Perhaps the most important consideration when applying limits with children who may be in highly aroused or shut-down states is the "two-stage strategy": Stage one involves immediate containment and modulation; stage two, the applying of limits or consequences, along with problem solving and discussion, should occur only after a child has regained some degree of emotional control.

When applying limits in programs, it is important to work with staff to incorporate behavioral strategies that minimize power struggles. For instance, teach staff to use limited choice (e.g., "You can work on your points sheet now or after therapy—when would you like to do it?") and problem-solving language ("Here are your two choices: You can sit in your room, or you can go to school. If you choose to sit in your room, then you will not get your 5 points for classtime. Which choice would you like to make?") to increase youth felt agency and decrease feelings of helplessness. Whenever possible, use positive reinforcement rather than limits to shape youth behavior.

In targeting limits to youth behavior, it is important to pay attention to long-term goals rather than simply to short-term outcomes. In other words, what is the system trying to teach? Although an immediate consequence may decrease a specific behavior in the moment, it is more important, in the long term, to teach and support a youth to make good choices. Work with staff to catch signs of escalation or distress early, prior to significant escalation, and then to coach children and adolescents in making choices that will help them achieve positive outcomes. Pair this skill with youth modulation strategies and executive function skills.

When applying behavioral management strategies in a program, it is important that staff members are in communication with each other, so that response is consistent across staff and across shifts. Consider the following example:

> Jamie, a 15-year-old girl in a residential program, had been increasingly dysregulated in recent weeks, and when upset, had destroyed property and made self-harm gestures. Her clinician and one of the staff members had been working with her to tune in to her feelings of distress and to ask for support when upset. Together, they developed a plan that when feeling upset, Jamie would ask for one-on-one support from a staff member, rather than hurting herself or destroying property. Jamie was able to follow through on the plan when she became upset during the day and had successfully sought time with her favorite staff member, Tricia, on two occasions; she was able to use the time appropriately, make use of coping strategies, and return to her routine. A week into the plan, Jamie became upset late at night, after both her clinician and Tricia had gone home for the evening. Jamie requested support, but the staff on the third shift did not know of the plan and told Jamie that she would have to stay in her room and wait until morning. Jamie escalated and, within 20 minutes, had destroyed a significant amount of property in her room before staff intervened. Because she destroyed property, she was given the consequence of being removed from her current privilege level.

In this example a lack of communication regarding a behavioral intervention plan led to escalating behaviors as well as to unnecessary—and unfortunate—consequences for Jamie. Although the number of "moving parts" in most milieu programs makes it difficult to communicate about everything, it is important for programs to find methods to realistically communicate *key facets* of every individual's behavioral intervention plans.

🌐 REAL-WORLD THERAPY

🌑 **Be realistic.** Behavioral strategies are often very effective, but they require consistent effort and follow-through by caregivers. For a lot of caregivers, shifting their behavioral management strategies is hard, and targeting even a single behavior or skill can feel like the straw that broke the camel's back. Caregivers often need a lot of support, encouragement, and understanding (as well as concrete guidance: Help them make the chart, keep a supply of stickers, etc.) to be able to add new tasks. Keep in mind that ignoring is probably the hardest of the skills and should not be the strategy caregivers try first.

🌑 **Pay attention to your own feelings and be solution-focused.** All clinicians have toolboxes, and we depend on certain interventions as "standards." In child work, caregiver behavioral skills training is often one such standard, and we rely on it as a tool that can invariably help with identified behavioral problems. When a family is unable to use these techniques— particularly when we believe they can make a difference—it can be very frustrating. It is easy to fall into the trap of becoming angry at or blaming the caregiver. It is important to try to take the family's perspective; failure of these techniques is often less about caregivers rejecting the techniques than it is about their feeling overwhelmed. Work to identify (with family members) the barriers to implementation and help problem-solve and adapt the techniques.

🌑 **Predict the problems.** When new limits or rules are applied, children may rebel: Their behavior may get worse before it gets better. Predict this "worst case" for caregivers, and help them find strategies to deal with both the behavior and their own response. Be a cheerleader for the caregiver.

CHAPTER 7

Building Routines and Rituals

THE MAIN IDEA

Work to build routine and rhythm into the daily lives of children and families.

★ KEY CONCEPTS

★ *Why Build Routines?*

- The experience of trauma is often associated with unpredictability, chaos, and loss of control. In the aftermath of trauma, felt experience of these elements (i.e., unpredictability) may become powerful triggers, or cues, of possible danger.

- Parents, clinicians, educators, and others involved in the lives of children who have experienced trauma often describe children's strong reactions to change, difficulty with transitions, and rigid attempts to control themselves, others, and the world around them.

- Consistent routines and predictability are often helpful in decreasing the insecurity and feelings of vulnerability carried by traumatized youth.

- Predictability can increase a sense of safety in relationships and in the environment. When children feel safe, they are able to shift their energy from survival to healthy development. Ironically, it is often the presence of predictability that allows children to eventually relax their own rigid controls and to achieve comfort first with day-to-day experience and ultimately with flexibility and spontaneity.

★ *What Are Routines?*

- In normative development, routines are typically generated and organized first by the attachment system: Caregivers structure their young children's lives in a way that builds rhythm and predictability, through responsive schedules of feeding, interaction, and sleep. By young childhood, children begin to internalize a reliance on structure and predictability: Most people have known a 4-year-old who wants to hear the same story repeatedly, or a 6-year-old who corrects your actions because, "That's not the way Mommy does it." This predictability helps young children learn about and organize their worlds.

- As development continues, the young child's focal reliance on structure often relaxes into a subtler appreciation of rhythm in daily life. Most people's lives are guided, to some degree, by routinized experience. We wake at certain times, sleep at certain times, and have familiar routines that are so built into our day as to be invisible.

- We often notice our routines only in their absence: when our typical morning schedule, for instance, is disrupted by unexpected demands. Most people can relate to the unsettled feeling that comes with the loss of an expected daily routine. Even though most of us do not have days that are structured and planned out minute to minute, the subtle routines in which we engage are grounding.

- For the children with whom we work, this "unsettledness" has often been part and parcel of their daily experience—lack of predictability has been the rule, rather than the exception.

- Building routines and rituals in the life of a child who has historically experienced chaos requires merely a shifting of focus to increase the presence of these invisible, yet predictable, routines.

- Routines should target areas of vulnerability or difficulty, such as bedtime or mealtime; often, these are triggers because in the past, they were associated with danger, fear, and/or deprivation.

★ *What about Rituals, Traditions, and Celebrations?*

- Daily routines offer one type of predictability and coherence over time. Another important source of coherence is *ritual*: the repeated practice of traditions, celebrations, patterns of behavior, or experiences. Rituals are often passed among members of a family, culture, or community, and may repeat across generations.

- ▱ Rituals offer a connecting thread, not just of the individual to him- or herself over time, but to other members of the family, community, or culture who share the same ritual. Rituals may be specific to a family (e.g., the singing of a particular song or eating of a particular food on special occasions) or to a larger community (e.g., attendance at midnight Mass on Christmas).

- ▱ Shared rituals may provide a sense of belonging, of being part of a larger whole. Many groups and organizations, including schools, service organizations, clubs, religious/spiritual centers, etc., have developed varied rituals and traditions, from songs and chants to handshakes to traditional celebrations and activities.

- The exploration, celebration, and creation of rituals with children and families, as well as the larger communities in which children are often embedded, may provide a way to celebrate the threads of connection among and across the child and members of his or her surrounding system.

⬛ **THERAPIST TOOLBOX**

🎬 *Behind the Scenes*

Home and Milieu Routines

- A primary goal is to work with caregivers to build routines into the home or milieu setting. In Teach to Caregivers, below, we discuss examples of areas to target when building routines.

- When working to build routines, it is important to consider the goal: Establishment of routines is *not* about structure for the sake of structure; rather, it is about supporting children, families, and systems in establishing predictability *in the service of modulation and felt safety.* Given this larger goal, it is important to strike a balance between structure and flexibility; as with all targets and skills within this framework, we encourage caregivers to consider the question: What is it that you are trying to help the child achieve? If enforcing a routine consistently increases, rather than decreases, distress and arousal, perhaps it is time to consider shifting the routine. Similarly, if flexibility on the caregiver's part seems to increase controlling strategies by the child, it may be important to consider increasing structure. Use attunement skills to observe the intersection between routine, structure, and child functioning over time.

- Routines will necessarily change over time as children shift across developmental stages, as felt safety in an environment grows or decreases, and as natural changes affect daily experience. For instance, a younger child may rely on a caregiver's external soothing at bedtime, whereas an older child or adolescent may have the capacity or preference to use more internal self-soothing strategies. This change is often organic, but it is useful to tune in to changes in routine and/or to the need for them.

- Although routines often form an umbrella under which many individuals function (e.g., within a milieu system or a family), it is important, to the degree possible, to account for individual needs. For instance, although all residents within a milieu may typically be expected to transition from school to a community activity, a particular resident may need 20 minutes of "downtime" following the highly stimulating school day before she can be successful in group activities. Similarly, whereas older siblings may be expected to complete homework immediately after school, a child who struggles with arousal and attention may require active engagement in high-energy activities before he can focus on this work. Consider ways to utilize routines—and the exceptions to them—to help children be most successful.

- In any setting, involve children, as developmentally appropriate, in the creation of routines. Consider the child's particular needs, wants, opinions, and preferences, as well as the realities of the home or system. For instance: What elements will be most important to incorporate into bedtime routines? What level of independence and/or support will the child want or need in carrying out scheduled activities? How important is the particular routine to caregivers? Engage children and other members of the system in developing daily/weekly routines that are realistic and helpful.

THE IMPORTANT ROLE OF MODULATION

A primary goal in working with children who have experienced trauma is to support regulation of experience. As noted above, routines themselves are often modulating because they add predictability to daily life. However, there are ways to more directly address modulation in the daily routine through a focus on *daily rhythm* as well as on *explicit inclusion of modulation strategies* in the daily schedule:

DAILY RHYTHM. Many children struggle to manage arousal effectively over the course of the day. In structuring the daily schedule, it is important to consider the child's "energy needs." For instance, limit highly arousing activities near bedtime; consider adding focusing activities (e.g., rehearsal/discussion of daily schedule, mindfulness exercises) prior to the start of the school day or other structured time periods; and build in activities that let the child expend energy when transitioning out of those times.

EXPLICIT MODULATION STRATEGIES. We have seen many families and systems experience positive outcomes by building specific modulation strategies (e.g., relaxation or yoga groups, deep breathing, jumping jacks) into key moments—transitions, mealtimes, and bedtime—of daily routine. By preemptively including strategies that target the child's arousal level, rather than solely using strategies in reaction to dysregulation, the child may increasingly be able to maintain effective arousal levels. Consider the following example:

> Elena, a 9-year-old girl adopted from an orphanage in Romania at the age of 3, presented as highly aroused. Her parents described her as "perpetually in motion," and she became both easily excited and easily distressed by daily experiences. She had particular difficulty settling into focused activities such as classroom time and homework. Her parents had reported that a number of strategies seemed helpful when Elena was upset, such as giving her a blanket to wrap around herself and playing soft music. They also reported that "speed dancing" (dancing to fast music in a cleared-out room in the house, an activity enjoyed by Elena) seemed to help her expend energy when she became overly excited and started to get out of control. The parents began to build these activities into Elena's daily routine in an effort to help her modulate her arousal: In the morning, before leaving for school, they had "cuddle time" with the blanket and soft music; they worked with her school to allow Elena to engage in similar strategies in the nurse's office, both midday and "as needed" when upset; and they added "speed dancing" time into her after-school schedule. After a month, they reported that these strategies seemed to help Elena's daily modulation; in particular, they reported that she seemed less easily upset by minor stressors during the school day and better able to transition home in the afternoon.

Therapy Routines

- In addition to in-home ones, routines can also be incorporated into the therapy setting. Consider the following:

- Therapy routines can be as simple as what happens on the walk between the waiting room and the therapy room, using an age-appropriate "check-in" to start every session, and creating a predictable transition at the end. See the table below for examples. Some children will need the entire session to be structured; others need greater flexibility.

- Young children who have a high need for control may initially appear resistant to therapy routines. It is our experience, however, that routines are ultimately comforting: By providing predictability in the therapy setting, children are able to achieve a sense of safety and a sense of control because they know what to expect. Don't assume that a child who complains about your routine truly hates it. Consider the following example:

> Tamika, 5 years old, regularly complained about the "feelings check-in" built into the start of her weekly therapy session. Each week, she would arrive for session, sit at the small table in the room, and ask, "Do we need to do those stupid faces today?" The clinician would respond in the affirmative, Tamika would complete the check-in about her feelings and experiences that day, and then the two would transition to the symbolic play that Tamika loved, or to other activities.
>
> One day, the clinician entered the room with Tamika and immediately began to address an issue to which Tamika's mother had alerted her in an earlier phone conversation. After about a minute, the clinician noticed that Tamika was shifting in her chair and appeared tearful. When asked by the clinician whether something was wrong, Tamika burst out, "We didn't do those stupid faces!"

In this example, the clinician received a reminder of why we engage in routines: Even the ones that are "hated" on the surface offer predictability. Although we invariably have times when routines change or are disrupted, explicit naming of these disruptions, whether in advance (e.g., "Next week we're going to do something a little bit different") or in the moment (e.g., "I know we usually have free play right now, but there's something we need to talk about. Let's talk first, and then we can have free play right after, okay?") may be important in reducing distress.

- Consistency of the therapy room space itself may be an important "invisible" ritual; when possible, use the same location. If this is not possible, it often helps to have consistent portable materials (e.g., the child's therapy folder, toy bag).

- Rules are an important part of therapy routines and of establishing felt safety. Consider, particularly with young children, identifying some basic therapy rules. We often suggest rules that target (1) safety: for example, "When you have big feelings in here, it is important to be safe" (elaborate on safety); (2) child control over therapy topics and the child's own personal boundaries: for example, "It's okay for you to say that you don't want to talk about something that I bring up. If you don't want to talk about something, it's all right to tell me that you don't want to talk about it"; and (3) the child's right to give feedback to the therapist: "If I say something that you don't like, it's okay to tell me that I said something wrong."

- Consider developmental and individual needs. We have found that younger children often prefer greater structure (and explicit naming of this structure), whereas older children and adolescents prefer subtler or "invisible" routines. However, every child is different. Allow children to contribute to the creation of therapy routines.

- Pay attention to pacing in the structuring of therapy sessions. Allow time to transition *into* the session, time to cover specific therapeutic material and tasks, and time to wind down and contain arousing material at the end.

- *Transitions are important.* Keep in mind:

    - Be aware of time—try not to start or end late. Punctuality builds boundaries and predictability around the treatment session.

    - Location may be an important concrete facet of the transition into the therapy room (e.g., the child who always wants to start at the art table).

- ♦ When needed, use time cues. Some examples:
  - ○ Make an in-session schedule.
  - ○ Use a timer to concretely break up session activities.
  - ○ Provide cues when limited time remains.
- ♦ Support children in developing or engaging in rituals that help them achieve felt safety when transitioning into or out of a session. For instance, consider the use of transitional objects (from home, brought into session; and/or from session, brought to home), dyadic portions at start and end, modulation activities, etc.

Celebrations and Rituals

- Although much of this section focuses on daily routine, rather than larger rituals, traditions, and celebrations, we encourage providers to support families and systems in identifying and celebrating familial, cultural, and systemic traditions. This work often varies in relation to the context:

- With biological/kinship families, the work may involve expression of curiosity about, and exploration of, the various traditions, norms, and celebrations in which the family currently (or historically) engages. In families in which celebrations are limited and/or have become associated with negative, rather than positive, experiences, providers can work with family members to create new traditions or celebrations.

- In foster and/or adoptive families, children and caregivers often bring multiple, and sometimes disparate, traditions and celebrations to the system. Younger children may not have the capacity to hold the continuity of previous traditions; older children may be reluctant to engage in them, due to a fear of disruption, a wish to engage fully in a new family, or a concern about caregivers' response. Consider the following example:

> Leon, a 14-year-old African American boy, was placed at age 12 and adopted at age 13 by a Jewish couple. Early in their treatment, close to the winter holiday, Leon's new clinician asked him if he would be doing anything for Christmas, a holiday Leon had described celebrating as a young child. Leon shook his head quickly and said, "I don't celebrate any of that stuff now. My family does Hannukah." On further exploration, Leon was able to state that he made a decision "to give all of that up" when he joined his current family, because he wanted to be "one of them."

This example illustrates both strengths and challenges: Leon's wish to integrate into his family and his willingness to do so speak to his desire and capacity for building relationship. A primary concern, however, is his felt understanding that, in order to do so, he needed to give up some aspect of self that may (or may not) have been important to him.

Work with family members to share and explore each other's traditions. New parents of a younger child may need to independently explore and incorporate aspects of his or her culture and tradition, whereas parents of an older child can work collaboratively with him or her to understand and share common and different experiences. Families may wish to create new "melded" or original traditions that combine aspects of all members' experiences and that are unique to the new family system, as well as to incorporate intact the traditions most important to each family member.

- Milieu systems (e.g., schools, residential programs) often have their own unique culture and traditions. Making these explicit can contribute to community engagement and involvement. For instance, the monthly barbecue, the school song, the weekly election of a resident who exemplifies the program's strongest value, and the annual Halloween celebration are all ways to foster continuity and connection for both children and staff. As with families, milieu systems are often comprised of individuals with a diverse range of cultural experiences, including language, food, religion, race, gender, etc. It is important for milieus to integrate opportunities to celebrate diverse cultures in addition to establishing a unique milieu culture.

- **A word of caution about rituals:** For many children and families who have experienced trauma, some rituals and traditions have become associated with negative experiences—for example, the Christmas when Dad became drunk and violent, the birthday when Mom did not show for her visit, etc. For children from nonmainstream cultures, dominant cultural rituals may enhance feelings of difference or loss. For many people currently struggling, times of celebration are experienced as particularly difficult. It is important to understand the meaning of specific holidays and other larger rituals for each individual and family.

✐ Teach to Caregivers

- *Reminder:* Teach caregivers the Key Concepts.

- *Reminder:* Teach caregivers the relevant Developmental Considerations.

- Work with caregivers to create appropriate daily routines. Remember to choose targets selectively and to work with the caregiver(s) and child to identify trouble spots. See the following table for examples of common routine targets.

Morning	The morning transition is often difficult for everyone, but particularly for highly stressed, chaotic households or for busy systems. Support caregiving systems in creating consistent and realistic morning routines.
Mealtimes	Meals are often a forum for communication and a place for family "together time." In systems, meals provide an opportunity for less structured peer interaction and conversation. Mealtimes can support the development of social skills, turn taking, manners, and interest in others' activities. Work with families or systems to come together for meals that are part of a daily routine as often as possible. • Food choice is a common area in which children exert their need for control. Work with caregivers to avoid power struggles. Find a middle ground between too much flexibility and too much control. For instance, provide a predictable alternative (e.g., child can eat family meal or eat a peanut butter and jelly sandwich).
Play	Play is a child's natural means of expression. Caregivers should be encouraged to play with their children, and time should be allocated during the week for "family play" as well as solitary and peer-to-peer play. Although often mistakenly considered less important than chores, homework, or other task-oriented components of experience, play is a vital part of healthy development. In addition, play also provides a forum for socialization and skill building. • "Together time" should *not* be tied to rewards or consequences (e.g., "If you don't clean your room, you don't get to spend time with Mom"). For children with histories of neglect and abandonment, in particular, such a statement can be triggering. • Work with caregivers to build one-on-one time with each child in the family as well as to schedule full family times.

Chores	Performing chores helps to foster a sense of responsibility and self-efficacy. Of course, chores should be age-appropriate, but it is okay for even very young children to have expectations regarding their areas of responsibility. Such an approach conveys the idea that all family or community members are integral to the successful functioning of the system, and that the child makes an important contribution. Work with caregivers to develop child-appropriate and realistic daily expectations.
Homework	School achievement/success is an important area of competency for children. Caregivers can contribute by emphasizing the importance of homework, providing an appropriate environment to support homework completion, being available to provide help or encouragement, and emphasizing effort over success. Work with caregivers and children to identify child and family needs.
Family together time	It is important to build into daily family routines a time for caregivers and children to come together, formally or informally, to share experience. For instance, some families may consider holding a weekly "family meeting" to share significant events; it may be incorporated into mealtime, bedtime, etc. Regardless of the forum, it is important that there be opportunities for family members to share their experiences on a routine basis.

- Bedtime may be particularly important to target. See expanded example in the following table.

BEDTIME ROUTINES

Teaching points	Bedtime is often a difficult time for traumatized children and adolescents, particularly those whose abuse occurred at a similar time or in the place they are now expected to sleep.	
	It may be hard for children whose arousal is high during the day to calm their bodies in preparation for sleep.	
	Bedtime routines help children decrease their arousal and learn to transition into sleep.	
Support caregivers in:	Developing a consistent bedtime routine. Have child put on pajamas, brush teeth, have quiet time, etc.	
	Problem-solving ways to keep bedtimes and their routines as consistent as possible. Pay attention to location where child is sleeping; work with caregivers to help child sleep in the same place each night. Pay attention to familial and individual obstacles.	
	Identifying nighttime boundaries and coping with nighttime fears. For example, what will caregiver do if child awakes during the night? Work with caregivers to be consistent in follow-through.	
	Minimizing child's engagement in highly arousing activities near bedtime. Decrease child's involvement in activities such as video games, overstimulating television shows, loud music, active play, etc.	
General activities	Nurturing	Read a story, cuddle, or listen to soft music together.
	Bathing	Have child take a bath or shower about an hour before bed; this may help bring down arousal. Pay attention to issues of privacy, boundaries, and the possibility of these being a trigger.
	Safety check	Help children feel safe. Leave on a nightlight, hang a dream catcher, check under beds or in closets, rub on "no-monster" lotion, etc.
	Relaxation/quiet time	Allow child to read, listen to quiet music, etc.

Bedtime routines: developmental considerations	Early childhood	Routines at this age should include the caregivers. Nurturing activities (e.g., reading a bedtime story) are a good way to build attunement and relax the child.
		Night is a time when generalized fears often emerge. Predictable nighttime routines are particularly important during this developmental stage.
	Middle childhood	Although children at this age will desire greater independence, bedtime is a natural place for nurturance, and traumatized children may show some developmental regression around bedtime.
		Developmental changes may shift the mechanics of bedtime: for example, may involve caregivers reading *with* their child instead of *to* them; may include independent activities (e.g., child brushes teeth, showers, gets in pajamas) as well as together time (e.g., caregiver enters room to say "good night").
	Adolescence	Balance is very important at this developmental stage. Some important areas to balance: • *Independence versus nurturance:* Adolescents need privacy. However, like younger children, they may also experience developmental regression around bedtime. Check in with your teen before bed—for instance, does he or she want a good-night hug? Allow some control, but don't assume that your older child no longer needs nurturance. • *Flexibility versus limits:* Although adolescents are independent, don't lose sight of the need for limits. Maintain expectations around bedtime (e.g., must be in room by 10:00 P.M.), but allow flexibility (e.g., can have quiet time—read, listen to music—and turn off lights when ready).

⫻ Tools: Building Routines into the Therapy Session

- The following table provides examples of ways to structure therapy sessions. Keep in mind that routines can be overt or subtle (e.g., a check-in can be very concrete and structured, or it can be as simple as, "So, how'd the week go?").

- The relative balance and ordering of each of these "therapy sessions" will necessarily vary for every child. Some children may engage in structured activities for much of the session; others will have limited tolerance (or less need) for structured activities, and will need more extensive "open" time. Be flexible; every routine is child-specific.

- Pay attention to the child's need for control when creating routines. For instance, while there may be an expectation that each session has a "therapist choice" and a "kid choice" time, the clinician may consider allowing the child to choose which comes first. To minimize power struggles, be sure to specify how long each will last and provide cues before transitioning.

- Consider ways to incorporate caregivers into therapy routine. For instance, consider involving caregivers into a dyadic check-in, or inviting them in for a closing "therapy summary."

THERAPY ROUTINE EXAMPLES

Opening check-in	Feeling faces ☺ ☺ ☹	Point to face(s) on poster or handout that are closest to current feeling.
		Draw a picture of "feeling(s) for today."
	Ball toss	Roll or toss a ball back and forth and take turns telling one new thing that happened since previous session.

	Today's news	Have child name one good and one not-so-good thing that happened today; draw a picture or talk about it.
	Thumbs up/ sideways/down	Pick one event from the past week: Was it thumbs up (positive), thumbs sideways (neutral), or thumbs down (negative)? Why?
	Energy check	Use thermometers, numbers, or other scales to check in on energy. Where is the child's energy at right now?
Modulation activity		Use age-appropriate modulation activities at the start and end of each session. Consider the child's needs. For instance, a high-energy child may need activities that help her expend her energy and then focus (e.g., balancing peacock feathers, jumping up and down at higher, then lower, energy levels); a lower-energy or withdrawn child may need a mutual engagement activity such as throwing a ball back and forth. Most children prefer to have some choice—allow the child to pick from among two or more activities. Check energy level before and after the modulating activity: Has it gone up or down? How can the child tell? (See Modulation section for further discussion of this concept.)
Structured activity ("therapist choice")		Include a structured or focal task in each session. Draw from attachment, self-regulation, and competency domains, and consider individual child needs and goals. Activities can be brief or comprehensive and often extend across sessions.
Free time ("kid choice")		"Kid choice," or open time, is an important part of therapy sessions. During open, unstructured time adolescents often engage in conversation, young children engage in rich symbolic play, and/or children of any age engage in activities that help them naturally modulate and balance the more challenging work of therapy (don't discount the importance of board games for helping children engage in the rest of "therapy work"!).
Closing check-out (note that closing routine often parallels opening)	Feeling faces	What face (on the poster or handout) is closest now to child's feelings? What has changed?
	Ball toss	Roll/toss ball back and forth; have child and therapist each pick one thing that you and he liked or disliked about therapy today.
	News wrap-up	Keep a running list: Of what did child feel proud in therapy today?
	Thumbs up/ down	What was the child's favorite or least favorite thing from today's session?
	Energy check	Where is child's energy now? Is it the same or different as at the start of session?
Modulation activity		Based on where the child's energy is now, build a closing modulation activity into session. Consider incorporating caregivers, as appropriate, into closing routines.
Clean-up	Contain it!	Clean-up is an important part of the session as well as a closing ritual for purposes of containment. **Always** actively involve the child in putting away therapy materials.

🏃 DEVELOPMENTAL CONSIDERATIONS

Developmental stage	Routine and ritual considerations
Early childhood	This is perhaps the most crucial stage for building rituals and routines: 1. Younger children rely almost completely on caregivers for provision of structure. 2. Structure is a particularly salient need during this developmental stage. Young children love predictability: This is the age when children watch a video over and over until it breaks, notice when caregivers skip a word or a page in a favorite book—despite the fact that they can't yet read—and ask to hear the same stories over and over again.

Developmental stage	Routine and ritual considerations
	Most rituals and routines will be dependent on caregivers, and individual/self-structuring will likely be minimal. The goal here is not to foster premature/age-inappropriate independence, but to encourage growth of agency and exploration within a safe structure provided by caregivers.
	Having said that, there are certain independent routines that are age-appropriate. For instance, even very young children can develop self-care routines, such as brushing teeth or washing hands, with parental guidance. Age-appropriate chores may include picking up toys or helping parents place clothes in the laundry basket. These routines can build feelings of independence and industry, crucial over time to the development of agency. It is key, however, that there is family support for individual achievement, and most routines at this age are best accomplished with parental involvement and monitoring.
	Most young children have limited attention spans. When developing routines, keep this in mind. For instance, at-home activities, unless highly engaging, are likely going to need to shift regularly to keep the child's focus and attention; minimize expectations for lengthy independent play. Therapy sessions can be broken into 5-minute chunks (rather than 20-minute).
Middle childhood	As children get older, there are increasing demands on their time: They enter school, join after-school activities, spend time with friends, etc. With the intensified daily schedule it is important for families to make an extra effort to schedule times to come together.
	Older children can begin to take a more active role in the creation of individual and familial routines and rituals. In addition, older children can be more autonomous in carrying out daily routines. However, caregivers should remain involved in the creation of expectations for routines, as well as in providing support for follow-through.
Adolescence	Family routines are increasingly challenging to adolescents. Teenagers normatively desire time outside of the home, greater flexibility, and more independence. They will take a larger role in creating autonomous routines outside of the home setting. Adolescents and their caregivers tend to travel in "nearby orbits," each with their own busy lives. It is still important, however, for these orbits to overlap on occasion, and in routine, expected ways.
	Regular communication is both important and challenging in adolescence. Teach caregivers that adolescents will have things about which they do and don't want to talk. There can be expectations around communication even when family members don't see each other (e.g., leave notes). Work with caregivers to appropriately monitor adolescent activities.

APPLICATIONS

Individual/Dyadic

As an outpatient provider, the goals of this target are twofold: (1) supporting caregiving systems and children in building or maintaining appropriate routines that foster healthy child development; and (2) building routines into our own work with children and families. Throughout this section are many examples of targets and considerations when working with families to create routines. When exploring the role of routines in daily life, it is important to be realistic and to consider the individual needs of the family. Extensive structure in a home that has comfortably operated in chaos will likely fail; pick targets carefully and selectively and work with families to develop routines that fit into the organic structure of each family's day and that target current areas of difficulty (i.e., don't build a routine solely for the sake of building routine). Predict difficulties: As with any change, new routines may sometimes be met with resistance. Consistent application is important before determining that a routine is successful or that it doesn't work.

In our own work we have found that bedtime and nighttime sleep patterns are the most commonly identified times of distress and/or difficulty for children, across the developmental span, from early childhood through later adolescence. Given this common area of difficulty, it is worthwhile to assess early in treatment a child's sleeping–waking patterns, as well as the family's typical schedule and process around bedtime. Although there are many important targets of treatment, basic physiological regulation (sleeping, eating) is crucial for competent daily functioning. It may be important to assess for potential triggers associated with bedtime, including specific and more generalized triggers. For example, clients have identified feelings of extreme vulnerability associated with decreased arousal levels and sleep states.

When working with families, it is important to acknowledge individual differences and the role of "comfortable chaos": Many of us have spent time (and continue to spend time) in environments in which a degree of chaos and spontaneity added to the richness of daily experience. The goal is not to replace spontaneity with rigid structure, but rather to buffer and surround experience with threads of continuity. It is important to provide psychoeducation for clients about the particular role of routine in the lives of children who have experienced danger in their young lives, the varying developmental need for predictability, and the ways that predictability can, over time, foster comfort with flexibility.

A similar issue has arisen when we discuss routines with other clinicians. Many clinicians, from a variety of theoretical and training backgrounds, have made rich use of child-centered methods (play, talk, sandtray, etc.) that emphasize following the lead of the child client. These clinicians have raised questions about whether integrating routines will diminish the fertile work found in spontaneous engagement with client material. Our perspective is that the two are not mutually exclusive, and that in fact, while not naming them as such, most clinicians will find their work guided, to some degree, by invisible routines and rituals. Indeed, routines often provide the subtle "surrounding structure" of sessions, but can be flexibly determined to account for the differing styles of our practice. Particularly with children who struggle with safety in relationships, we encourage clinicians to observe the subtle patterns that define their therapy process, and, as indicated, to "try out" simple additions to their therapy routines. Finally, it may be useful to bring those subtle patterns and invisible routines to the attention of our clients so that they can be active participants in the process of determining routines and rituals.

🏠 Group

As with individual therapy, group processes are often most successful when an element of routine and predictability is incorporated into session structure. Many groups offer predictability in the organic coherence over time that is associated with group themes. Beyond the coherence provided by content, we encourage group leaders and curriculum developers to consider the important role of routine in structuring group sessions. As with individual sessions, consider the role of opening check-ins or icebreakers, modulation activities, and internal structure. In creating routines, consider the content focus of the group: For example, in a group focusing on coping skills, opening exercises might include a modulation activity or affect identification check-in; in a group focusing on identity, opening activities might include an icebreaker question related to the self; and in a group focused on interpersonal relationships, dyadic or group cooperative activities might begin the session.

Groups vary widely depending on their nature (structured, content-focused, process-oriented, psychoeducational, etc.). All groups, however, share the common element of having a beginning, a middle, and an end. We encourage group leaders to consider either subtle or overt strategies to mark these transitions as a way to facilitate children's (or caregivers') capacity to successfully enter into, and transition out of, groups. Consider also, within the group time, the balance between activities that rely on active versus passive engagement with material, between higher- and lower-energy activities, and between independent and cooperative engagement. Strategize about ways to create and incorporate routine in a way that helps group members be most successful (in modulating, engaging, building safety, etc.). It may be easier, for instance, for a child to follow a natural "bell-curve" progression of lower to higher to lower energy over the course of a group, then to move rapidly among low-, then high-, then low-, then high-energy activities. Early in a group, it is important to be flexible and to tune in to specific group needs: A structure that worked well for one group, for instance, may be more challenging with a different group. Be willing to adjust or enhance structure, as needed, to respond to the particular needs of individual group members or group dynamics.

Milieu

As in home settings, milieus offer a rich environment in which to provide predictability in experience. Many programs rely on rules, routines, and structure to organize daily experience, and this structure often supports children who have faltered in more relaxed or unstructured settings to succeed and build competency. It is not uncommon to hear of the child, for instance, who evidences extreme behaviors in the home setting but who thrives in the structured environment of school. Much of what has been discussed in regard to the building of routines in home settings similarly applies to milieu programs. This includes identifying specific targets of focus (e.g., bedtimes, transitions), the role of modulation both in daily rhythm and in the incorporation of specific activities, and the incorporation of routine and predictability into key facets of daily experience.

With respect to building structure, we have observed two primary areas of vulnerability in milieu systems: (1) an overemphasis on structure and rules in the absence of understanding individual child needs; and (2) inadequate understanding of the impact of disruptions in routine on child functioning. Both areas are challenging: It is inevitable that there will be moments of disruption in a larger system, and it can be difficult to be flexible around individual child needs when trying to address the needs and safety of many children at once. Despite these challenges (and with full empathy), we encourage those who work in systems nonetheless to focus on both of these areas.

In terms of the first: Systemic routines are important because they provide continuity in daily experience. Most children will adjust and adapt, at least to some degree, to the requirements of the system. Some children, however, will struggle, to greater or lesser degrees, with some aspect of daily routine. When a child has consistent difficulty (e.g., with a transition, with some component of the schedule), consider, to the degree possible, ways to adapt that routine to the individual needs of the child, keeping in mind the ultimate goal of building child success.

In terms of the latter: As structured as many programs are, many things will introduce disruption (and, occasionally, chaos) into daily routine. Although it is not possible to account for all these disruptions, it is possible to anticipate that changes may stir reactions and difficulties. When planned variations occur, work to provide advance notice and troubleshoot possible reactions. When unexpected changes occur, train staff to anticipate increased reactivity by children who may be sensitive to disruptions. Use caregiver affect management skills to manage staff's own responses to these reactions, and use attunement skills to support children in regaining equilibrium.

Children living in milieu settings are particularly vulnerable to common triggers such as felt rejection, abandonment, and loss due to separation from their primary caregivers. It is important to build routines around phone calls, visits, and family work, when applicable, in order to support modulation of associated arousal. For children who do not have caregiver involvement, it may be important to create individualized rituals when celebrations take place with other residents' family members. For example, have specific staff members assigned to a particular child, or offer the child an alternative to participating in the group celebration.

In milieu systems that are focused on teaching self-regulation skills, it may be important to create a routine approach to supporting modulation. Programs that we have worked with have modified their behavior management structure in order to incorporate this idea. For example, consider implementing a break system (to be distinguished from time-out) in which children can take self-directed and/or staff-directed breaks when dysregulated. It is helpful to build a structure around the break process. For instance, a break might include an initial check-in, practice of a modulation strategy (or strategies), and a check-out; the content of the check-in and check-out may vary based on the needs of each program. Modulation strategies might include talking to staff, using a sensory tool, or taking a walk (if possible). See Modulation section for further examples of potential tools.

In terms of larger systemic culture and rituals: Milieus offer a positive forum for the incorporation of rituals from a variety of cultures as well as for the building of community-specific rituals and traditions. Pay attention to integrating celebrations from the many cultures represented by the individuals who are part of that system. Invite children to share their traditions— whether individual, familial, community, or cultural—with other members of the larger community. Build community-specific traditions and capture these concretely—in photos, on bulletin boards, in weekly newsletters, etc.

🌐 REAL-WORLD THERAPY

🌐 **Don't overdo.** The goal is not to rigidly structure every moment of a child's day, but rather to create a subtle sense of predictability. In fact, given the rigidity that many traumatized children bring to their interactions, comfort with flexibility is an important goal. Rituals and routines can be thought of as the "bookends" that contain the daily living that happens in between.

🌐 **Be realistic about expectations.** Know where a family or system is currently "at." Attempting to build overly expansive or inflexible routines will often be a set-up for the child and for the caregivers to fail. Build slowly, and with the input of the child and the caregivers. As with any intervention, early success is essential.

🌐 **Don't get discouraged.** Don't forget that the most common targets of routine are frequently those areas in which the child has developed what appear to be the most idiosyncratic behaviors—frequently in the service of anxiety management. Don't expect predictability to occur overnight; it is often in retrospect, after a lengthy period of "hanging in there," that the child's internalization of the routine becomes apparent.

🌐 **Hang in there.** Predictability isn't always formal. Consistency is often as simple—and complicated—as sticking around, meaning what we say, and saying what we mean. With so many of the kids with whom we work, disruption of attachment becomes a regular occurrence as they are moved from placement to placement to placement. For this reason, it is quite adaptive of them to protect themselves from further loss by rejecting others. Part of attachment work is sticking with these kids who present as oppositional, unlikable, inconsistent, etc., in order to prevent further rejection. When you say you will show up—and you do—it is powerful. When you say you will remember to bring the glittery markers next week—and you do—it is powerful. Working and living with children who have experienced loss, over and over, is often about the long haul, about sticking it out for the journey. Don't underestimate the impact you have by just *hanging in*.

Beyond Attachment

The Role of the Caregiving System in Building and Supporting Regulation and Competency

- Although the first four building blocks of ARC specifically target the caregiving system, caregivers continue to play an essential role in supporting child regulation and competency skills. In fact, a primary goal in building caregivers' capacity to modulate affect, attune to the child, and develop consistent responses and routines is to provide a safe foundation and container for addressing the remaining ARC targets.

- Consider the following in understanding the role caregivers may play:

BEYOND THE A: THE ROLE OF THE CAREGIVER IN ARC TREATMENT GOALS

Goal	Caregiver role
Affect identification	The caregiver uses attunement skills to mirror and reflect the child's experience. Through the process of reflection the caregiver is able to support the child in learning to recognize and verbalize emotional experience. Over time, accurate caregiver attunement and response will support the child in developing a more sophisticated understanding of both internal and external cues, as well as the situations that generate them.
Modulation	The caregiver provides a source of physiological organization by modeling effective self-regulation, supporting the child in his or her use of modulation skills, acting as a modulation resource, and fostering a sense of both internal and external safety by providing consistency and routines.
Affect expression	The caregiver is able to act as both teacher and communication resource. Key skills of affect expression can be taught, modeled, and reinforced by the caregiver. The caregiver is able to foster self-expression by providing routine forums for communication as well as effective communication strategies.
Executive functions	The caregiver models and supports a calm approach to problem solving, or simply remains calm in the face of a problem or stressor. Additionally, by responding to behavior in a consistent manner (either by offering praise/reinforcement or by enforcing limits/ consequences), the caregiver teaches important lessons about choice and agency.

Goal	Caregiver role
Self and identity	The caregiver acts as a source of unconditional positive regard, a resource for formation of a coherent self-narrative, and a foundation from which the child can grow through exploration of interests, values, and self-concept.
Trauma experience integration	The caregiving system offers the reflective and supportive context within which a child is able to process and explore overwhelming experience and to integrate trauma into the broader narrative of self. Caregivers may provide external modulation and support, and often are active participants in the process of trauma experience integration.

• When working with caregivers—whether parents or providers—it is vital to articulate the important role the caregiver's skills play in supporting the healthy development of the child.

PART III

SELF-REGULATION

WHAT DOES IT MEAN TO "REGULATE"?

- *Self-regulation* involves the capacity to effectively manage experience on many levels: cognitive, emotional, physiological, and behavioral.

- Successful regulation of experience may involve many different things, including:
  - ◆ Some degree of awareness of internal state
  - ◆ The ability to tolerate a range of arousal and affect
  - ◆ The ability to engage in action or cognition to modulate arousal and affective state
  - ◆ An understanding of the interconnections among aspects of internal experiences (i.e., sensation, feeling, thought, behavior)
  - ◆ An understanding of the factors that influence internal experience
  - ◆ The capacity to effectively communicate experience with others

DEVELOPMENTAL SHIFTS IN REGULATION

- The earliest self-regulation challenge involves basic physiological organization: patterns of sleeping, alert interaction, eating, and eventually toileting.

- Over time regulation of experience moves from being primarily externally structured (i.e., soothing as provided by caregiver[s]) to primarily internally directed, although we continue to use significant others as modulation resources throughout our lives.

- All skills involved in regulation develop from a very basic level to an increasingly sophisticated one. For instance, awareness of internal state for a young child may be as simple as "I feel bad," whereas an older adolescent may be able to identify such nuanced states as "I'm feeling disappointed and concerned."

THE IMPORTANT ROLE OF THE CAREGIVING SYSTEM

- The caregiving system plays a prominent role in the successful development of all aspects of regulation.

- Many caregiver behaviors contribute to the development of healthy self-regulation over time. Among others, these include:

  ◆ *Reflection:* Reflection of the child's experience can be verbal (e.g., "You look like you're getting sleepy now") or behavioral (e.g., the caregiver who responds to the child's laughter with a smile). The mirroring of the child's experience through the caregiver's facial expressions, words, and actions supplies the earliest **lens through which the child learns to interpret his or her experience**.

  ◆ *Modeling:* Caregivers' own expression and modulation provide both a **visual language** for understanding affect as well as a **model of coping**. The child learns to "read" and understand facial expressions and other verbal and nonverbal cues of emotion, along with their associated experience, by observing the ways in which caregivers' expressions pair with actions (e.g., the appearance of a loving expression paired with soothing) and experience (e.g., an expression of pain after touching a hot pan). Caregivers' actions in the face of distress serve as a demonstration of modulation strategies and affect tolerance (e.g., the caregiver who appears frustrated and then takes a deep breath and smiles).

  ◆ *Stimulation and soothing:* When provided in an attuned manner, the caregiver is able to support a child in achieving **optimal levels of arousal** by alternatively providing stimulation and soothing. By responding appropriately when energy levels become overwhelmingly high (i.e., intense distress) or low (i.e., sleepiness), the caregiver's words, vocal tones, and behaviors become a source of physiological organization. Gradually, the young child internalizes these skills and begins to be able to independently maintain a comfortable state of arousal.

- When caregivers are unresponsive, inconsistent, or abusive, infants and young children must rely on primitive modulation skills (e.g., rocking, thumbsucking, dissociation) to soothe their own affect. Lack of reflection and modeling leave children with no emotional language with which to interpret their own or others' experience. In the absence of reliable supports, and particularly in the face of ongoing stress and distress, children will continue to rely on primitive coping, which leaves them unlikely to develop more sophisticated self-regulation strategies.

WORKING WITH SELF-REGULATION IN HISTORICAL CONTEXT

- Shame, isolation, secrecy, and feelings of damage are often central to the trauma experience.

- Children and adults who have experienced trauma may believe that there is something wrong with them; that they are different from others; and that strong emotions are representative of "craziness," "being bad," or a loss of control.

- The elephant in the room:

  ◆ It is not uncommon for treatment to target specific areas of "deficit" or "pathology" (e.g., oppositional behavior, anxiety) in the absence of an organizing frame or context.

- ♦ Well-intentioned clinicians and other providers who do hold an awareness of the role of trauma in a child's presentation may hesitate to name it. This hesitancy often stems from a belief that a child must be fully "safe" before approaching historical experiences.

- ♦ When treatment occurs in the absence of an understanding of the role of history, the link between past and current experience is not addressed, and the self-perception of shame, damage, isolation, and secrecy may actually increase.

- Naming the elephant: When working with the child who has experienced trauma, consider the following:

  - ♦ **Acknowledge the child in his or her entirety:** past experiences, current reality, strengths, vulnerabilities, possibilities, interests, etc. Although it is important to understand the child in context, every child is more than the sum of his or her experiences. It is important to communicate from the start that we are interested in the whole child.

  - ♦ **Validate the adaptive nature of (often distressing) behaviors.** Identify the role these behaviors may have played in the child's life. For instance, for a child who engages in frequent aggressive behaviors with peers, we might say, "It seems as if it's pretty important to you to show other kids how strong you are."

  - ♦ **Educate the child about the trauma response, triggers, and the links between past experience and current response.** Understanding the human danger response and its current role in dysregulated or self-protective behaviors is a vital step toward providing the child with some measure of control and also decreasing stigma. Links to past experiences can be kept simple, especially early in treatment (e.g., "When kids have really hard things happen like what happened with your dad . . . ").

  - ♦ **Differentiate past and present.** In working with children to understand, be aware of, and manage their current emotions and behaviors, it is important to explain that behaviors that were protective and adaptive in the past may not be as helpful in the present. Explore these with the child and family. For instance, keeping feelings from showing may have helped protect a child from a violent caregiver, but may currently be keeping the child from getting his or her needs met. Examine the role of context: There may still be situations where the child needs to engage in self-protective behaviors.

TARGETING CHILD NEEDS: UNDERSTANDING THE FUNCTIONAL NATURE OF MODULATION ATTEMPTS

- Many of the distressing behaviors and symptoms that lead to a child being referred for treatment can be understood as the child's attempts to cope. For instance, oppositional behavior may be a preemptive strike to cope with anticipated rejection; self-injury may be an attempt at self-soothing; and sexualized behaviors may be attempts at control or connection.

- All symptoms have many possible origins. A crucial first step in working with a child or family is to try to understand the function(s) underlying behavior. Skill building can then be targeted to the child's specific needs.

- Although it would be impossible to capture all possible child presentations, three common presentations are offered here to serve as examples.

Presentation #1: The Overly Constricted Child

Presentation	Overly constricted children are often quiet and have difficulty initiating conversation, activities, and interactions in general. They are not oppositional and, in fact, may be overly compliant. These children have difficulty describing any emotions; a typical response to "How are you doing?" is "Fine" or "I don't know" (which, for these children, is a realistic response). Constricted children appear defended against emotional experience in general, and often lack an understanding of how to connect emotionally with others. A common adaptation to overcome this limitation is to engage in "other-pleasing" behavior: Constricted children may appear to subordinate their own needs, opinions, etc., to others. In younger children this difficulty with self-expression may include failure to engage in imaginary play. At times these children may show explosive outbursts of emotion in response to what appear to be minor stressors, as their intense control becomes overwhelmed or challenged. In the aftermath of this intense emotion, however, these children return quickly to a constricted state and have difficulty acknowledging or processing the emotional experience. This appearance is often consistent with that displayed by the avoidantly attached child and is common among children who have experienced some degree of emotional rejection and/or neglect (including that created by caregiver impairments, such as depression).
Primary skills deficits	• Limited emotional vocabulary • Limited awareness of internal experience • Restricted range of tolerance for arousal • Limited skills to cope with and manage emotional experience, including positive emotions • Deficit in ability to seek social support, particularly in the sharing or management of emotional experience
Function of this adaptation	Constriction represents a child's strategy for coping with overwhelming emotion. In the absence of regulation skills and/or social support, the child relies on denying and withdrawing from emotional experience.
Therapeutic considerations	• Initial work should be displaced; gradually shift from external to internal (e.g., help child identify affect in a television show or book character). • Help child identify cues associated with the affect. Behavior is often a good starting point, and it is less threatening than the feeling itself. Other children may respond to identification of body states or thoughts.

Presentation #2: The Externalizing Child

Presentation	Externalizing children rely on a "front" to prevent others (and, often, themselves) from awareness of vulnerability, perceived damage, and an often deep sense of shame and self-blame. These children generally have access to the "powerful" emotions—anger, injustice, blame—but little ability to acknowledge more vulnerable feeling states such as fear or sadness. They may readily acknowledge being angry at someone or upset about something that has happened that day, but will deny feeling hurt or worried about the incident. These children frequently externalize; emotions are generally connected to outside events rather than to their impact on them. Perceived injustice is often a powerful trigger for these children, and injustice will likely be perceived relatively frequently. Their presentation may be oppositional or argumentative with people in authority, although they are often able to build relationships with people they perceive as less threatening or demanding. These children appear to desire connection but seek it in ineffective ways (e.g., as the "class clown," through negative behaviors). They have a profound sense of mistrust in relationships and have difficulty believing that others truly care about them. Because of this stance, these children may "test" relationships to see if others will abandon or harm them. This relational reenactment may represent their attempt to control anticipated negative interactions as well as to confirm their perceived sense of self and other. This presentation is often associated with children who have experienced explicit harm (e.g., physical, sexual, or psychological abuse).
Primary skills deficits	• Acknowledging and coping with vulnerable emotions • Modulating intense emotion, particularly in the face of key triggers such as injustice, shame, etc.

- Accepting responsibility for actions in social conflict
- Engaging empathy and perspective-taking in difficult relationships

Function of this adaptation	Externalizing emotion and responsibility allows children who feel intensely shamed or damaged to protect themselves from those overwhelming feelings. With limited skills to cope with intense affect, these children are unable to tolerate any feelings that threaten their already fragile sense of self.
Therapeutic considerations	• Forcing these children to acknowledge difficult emotions before they are ready is likely to lead to power struggles and increased shame. • Normalizing denied emotions is a key intervention with these children. Often, this is done via displacement (e.g., "I could understand how someone might be very worried if _____ happened to them"). • Providing psychoeducation about triggers and the trauma response may be very important for normalizing the anger response and may serve as a foundation for helping children learn to differentiate "true danger" from perceived danger.

Presentation #3: The Labile Child

Presentation	The labile child's presentation is changeable. These children are strongly affected by environmental triggers, others' emotions, and internal states. Clinical assessment is often complicated, because their presentation can vary from day to day and hour to hour. Their emotional reactions appear unpredictable and may be disproportionate to the apparent stressor; they may go from 0 to 60 in a matter of moments, or completely shut down just as quickly. Presentation in therapy is therefore inconsistent: On some days these children may appear very well put together, whereas on others they are reactive, withdrawn, or overwhelmed. Distress is experienced as diffuse, with difficulty differentiating both the type of emotion and its source. In addition, they have difficulty judging degree of emotion—irritability feels like rage, and sadness feels like despair. Emotional states are disconnected, and it is difficult for these children to access an emotional experience when no longer in the midst of it. When they are in the midst of it, however, they are unable to think past it. These children's lives are driven by emotion, but they have little cognitive framework for understanding it or ability to cope with it in healthy ways. These children have frequently experienced interpersonal trauma over an extended period of time and have relied heavily on dissociative coping. As a result, their sense of self—and therefore of their emotional experience—is fragmented.
Primary skills deficits	• Inability to modulate emotional experience (rapid escalation or numbing, with difficulty returning to baseline) • Misreading of environmental cues; low threshold for perception of threat • Inability to integrate experiences into a cohesive narrative and/or sense of self
Function of this adaptation	These children have developed a heightened biological alarm system. In the face of *any* emotion-inducing stimulus (internal or external), their bodies provide them with the fuel they would need to survive if they were in true danger. However, this response has become as likely to occur presently with mild input as it did in the past with threatening. Their physically intense reactivity leaves these children at the mercy of their emotions.
Therapeutic considerations	• The goal with these children is not to necessarily alter their emotions, but to reduce the intensity to a realistic level, so that it is tolerable/manageable, and to help them identify where it comes from. Therefore, it is important to normalize their emotions, teach them to recognize shifts in degree of feeling, and provide concrete emotion management strategies. • Experience is state-dependent for these children; they may be able to discuss their emotions and alternative coping skills in the aftermath of an incident, but they will have a much harder time applying those skills in the moment, when their primary concern is survival. Because of this state-dependent aspect, repetition of skills and external cuing in their use are essential.

CHAPTER 8

Affect Identification

THE MAIN IDEA

Work with children to build an awareness of internal experience, the ability to discriminate and name emotional states, and an understanding of why these states originate.

★ **KEY CONCEPTS**

★ *Why Target Affect Identification?*

- Traumatic stress overwhelms the limited emotion management skill set available to developing children, often forcing them either to disconnect from their feelings or to use rudimentary or unhealthy coping skills.

- Children who have experienced inadequate early caretaking and/or insufficient emotional support may have never developed adequate skills in identifying and expression emotion.

- Other children may have developed limited skills that became overwhelmed and splintered in the aftermath of trauma, particularly if the trauma has had a substantial impact on the emotional functioning of the entire family unit.

- Because of these factors, children who have experienced trauma are frequently disconnected from, or unaware of, their own emotional experience.

★ *How Does Trauma Impact Affect Identification?*

- Difficulty with identification of emotions may present in many different ways. Common presentations include those described in the Self-Regulation introduction. In general, children may have:

♦ Trouble accurately discriminating among their own emotional states.

  ○ For example, children who report a single emotional experience ("I'm fine")

  ○ Reliance on "power" emotions ("I'm mad")

  ○ Diffuse distress

  ○ Lack of access to emotional experience ("I don't know" as a valid response to "How do you feel?")

♦ Physiological or behavioral expressions of emotional experience.

  ○ Playing out of disconnected affect through impulsive behaviors, hyperactivity, or silliness

  ○ Disconnected somatic distress such as headaches or stomachaches

♦ A lack of understanding of the connection between physiological states and the experiences that elicited them.

  ○ Inability to process in the aftermath of experience

  ○ Feeling "victimized" and targeted due to lack of awareness of the link between behavior and the responses they elicit from others

  ○ Baseline state of hyperarousal and rapid escalation with distress due to defense against *any* emotional experience

★ *Hypervigilance and Affect Identification*

• Difficulties with affect identification are frequently about more than identification of the child's own emotions; many children who have experienced trauma have as much difficulty reading others' cues as they do understanding their own experience.

• As a result, some children may expend a great deal of energy working to read the emotional cues of others. Children may be:

  ♦ Selectively hypervigilant (i.e., overly tuned in to cues of potential danger)

  ♦ Insufficiently attuned (i.e., miss cues that others are frustrated, annoyed, proud, etc.)

  ♦ Inaccurate in reading cues, with overperception of negative affect (e.g., interpret a caregiver's fatigue as anger or a peer's joke as rejection)

• This skill deficit may have an impact on peer relationships and caregiver–child attunement. Children may be reactive to perceived danger, rejection, and other slights, or may miss cues of positive response.

THERAPIST TOOLBOX

Behind the Scenes

• Affect identification work targets the child's understanding of emotional experience in both **self** and **other**:

- ◆ *Identification of emotion in self:* the child's awareness of what he or she is feeling and where the feeling comes from.

- ◆ *Identification of emotion in other:* the child's ability to accurately perceive others' feelings; relies on ability to accurately read cues such as body language, voice tone, eye contact, etc.

- • Within each of these domains, understanding of emotions (and therapeutic tasks) will involve two primary goals:

  - ◆ *First*, support children in **building a vocabulary** for emotional experience in self and other.

  - ◆ *Second*, help children **build connections among identified emotion and internal and external experiences**, including precipitating events, physiological states, behaviors, and coping styles and eventually to the impact of past experiences on current situations:

    - ○ *Connection of emotions* to:

      - ◊ *Body sensations:* Ability to identify how a feeling shows up in the body

      - ◊ *Thoughts:* Identification of thoughts that are associated with feelings

      - ◊ *Behavior:* Identification of behavioral manifestations of feelings

    - ○ *Contextualization of emotion:*

      - ◊ *External:* Factors in the environment that precipitate the feeling; this may include identification of specific triggers

      - ◊ *Internal:* Internal factors (i.e., being tired, being hungry) that contribute to the development of different feelings

- • Affect identification work often occurs in stages, moving from basic to more nuanced.

  - ◆ In early stages the goal is **development of a language that encompasses emotional experience**. Intervention may include:

    - ○ Inviting the child to share daily emotional experience (e.g., "How are you feeling today?").

    - ○ Naming emotions in the context of specific experiences (e.g., "How did it feel when *x* happened?").

    - ○ Inviting observation of the experience of others (e.g., "How do you think Jimmy was feeling when . . . ?").

    - ○ Reflecting the child's observable affect and behavior (e.g., "It looks like you may be feeling kind of worried").

    - ○ Normalizing affective experience (e.g., "I would imagine a lot of kids might feel kind of upset if something like that happened").

  - ◆ Both embedded in and as a more advanced version of this first stage, providers and other caregivers can work with children to **connect emotions to other aspects of experience**. These connections can serve as clues or cues of emotion (e.g., "I know I'm happy because I have a warm, tingly feeling in my stomach"). Interventions may include:

○ Feelings detective work in self or other (e.g., "What makes you think Jimmy is feeling mad?").

○ An understanding of the range of ways in which people express emotion (e.g., "How does your mom look when she's mad? How is that different from how your dad looks?").

○ An understanding of variations in the child's own expression (e.g., "Sometimes when I'm mad I want to shout, and sometimes I want to be by myself").

♦ In later stages, for children who have a demonstrable vocabulary for internal experience, the work will focus increasingly on **an understanding of the context of emotions**. This includes an exploration of environmental and internal factors and precipitating events. As with other types of affect identification, this work may range from basic to sophisticated. For instance:

○ A child at a basic level of understanding may simply identify the precipitating event: "I was sad and mad because my teacher yelled at me."

○ An older child or one with a more sophisticated understanding may work to identify not just the event but associated historical experiences and behavioral response: "I was upset when my teacher yelled at me, and it kind of kicked up old feelings from when my mom used to yell at me, so I started to feel freaked out and like I had to get out of there."

• Considerations in affect identification work:

♦ In order to address modulation, children must be able to label different internal experiences. Keep in mind that a vocabulary for internal experience does not have to be initially sophisticated: It may be enough for a child to say that he or she feels "bad," "good," "charged up," etc. Pay attention to building a language for energy and arousal as well as emotion.

▱ Language plays a key role in the communication of emotional experience. Children or families may use words to describe feelings that are unfamiliar to the clinician because they are particular to that child or family. Work with caregivers and children to understand the different labels they apply to emotional experience. Consider the following example:

> A 10-year-old girl was completing a feelings check-in with her clinician. The clinician drew standard faces and left several circles blank for the child to fill in with additional emotions, if desired. The child quickly filled in one face, naming it as "attitude." When filling in thermometers to indicate the extent of her feelings that week, the child indicated having had a high level of "attitude," along with "sad" and "worried." Over the next several weeks, the child reported feeling "attitude" at each check-in.

In this example, a child uses a word, *attitude*, to label emotional experience that may have a number of possible interpretations. In working with her, it is vital that the clinician seek to understand the meaning of this term to the child, rather than making assumptions about its interpretation. In this case, the clinician was able to eventually gain an understanding of *attitude* as referring to the angry front used by the child to cope when feeling hurt and upset; the predominant internal experience for the child was one of vulnerability, although the external display was of a "power" emotion.

♦ Because therapeutic techniques that assist children in understanding the connections among feelings and internal/external experiences may elicit strong emotions, it is often important to address affect modulation techniques (as detailed in the next section) simultaneously.

- Keep in mind that many experiences elicit a **range of emotions**.
  - ♦ In helping children identify emotion, it is important to acknowledge that there may be more than one feeling.
  - ♦ Normalizing "**mixed feelings**" is particularly important for children who have had conflicting feelings in the past (e.g., loving a parent while being afraid of him or her), and who have learned to splinter and separate out those states from each other.
- In addition to formal exercises, affect identification work often happens "in the moment."
  - ♦ **Tune in to signs of affect in statements, interaction, and play.** When these appear, name the affect and link it to concrete observations. For example:
    - ○ In play:

      (*The child is manipulating doll characters; one is placed to the side, and the child makes crying noises.*)

      THERAPIST: Oh, that doll looks really sad. He's crying and sitting by himself. I wonder why he's so upset?

    - ○ In interaction:

      THERAPIST: It kind of seems like you're mad or upset today.

      ADOLESCENT: No, I'm fine.

      THERAPIST: Well, you haven't talked much since you got here, your hood is up over your head, and you're all scrunched up in your chair. That's not how you usually are, so I was curious if something was going on.

    - ○ In statements:

      CHILD: So we have these stupid science projects we have to do, and we have to have partners, and no one wants to be mine. Science is stupid anyway.

      THERAPIST: Wow—that sounds hard. I can imagine some kids would feel sad or worried if they didn't have a partner.

  - ♦ When naming affect for a child, be aware that he or she may disagree with you. Allow for this, but consider discussing any potential discrepancy between observed affect and content.

⏏ *Teach to Caregivers*

- *Reminder:* Teach the caregiver the Key Concepts.
- *Reminder:* Teach the caregiver relevant Developmental Considerations.
- Caregiver attunement skills should be used to support the child in affect identification. Consider doing caregiver attunement work and child affect identification work simultaneously.
- Reflective listening skills will be an important support for emerging child affect identification skills. Work with caregiver(s) to practice and apply these skills.

⚡ *Tools:* **Affect Identification Tools**

Teach to Kids: Psychoeducation about Feelings

- Examples of how to speak with children about key teaching points are provided. Keep in mind, however, that psychoeducation should be provided in a developmentally appropriate way, so language will vary from client to client.

- The following represents a guideline for speaking with children about affect identification. Not all teaching points will be relevant to all children.

UNDERSTANDING FEELINGS

Teaching point	Important information as sample language
Everyone has feelings.	"Everyone—kids and adults—has a lot of different feelings. It's normal for things in our life to make us feel different ways."
	"There are no 'wrong' feelings—no one can tell you how you should or shouldn't feel about something."
	"There are lots of ways that feelings can show up, and if we don't know what our feelings are, they can come out in ways that hurt us or other people."
Feelings come from somewhere.	"Most of the time, feelings are not random—something causes them. Feelings can be caused by *thoughts*, *people*, *situations*, and *internal sensations*." (Clinicians should provide concrete examples of ways in which each of the above can be linked to feelings.)
	"Special kinds of situations are the ones that feel dangerous. There are a lot of different kinds of situations that might feel dangerous to kids' brains. Once our brains decide that something is dangerous, our body gives us the fuel we need to deal with it. This fuel helps us react fast, move quickly, protect ourselves, and get to somewhere safe. When we go through danger over and over, our brains learn to recognize clues that danger might be coming (like sounds, smells, or things we see), so that we can react really fast. Sometimes these clues happen when there isn't really any danger. When that happens, we call these clues 'triggers.' When there is a trigger, our brain sets off our danger alarm to try to help us stay safe, even though there really isn't any danger around. It's important to learn to recognize triggers and our danger response, so that we can take the time to *think*, instead of just *reacting*." *Note:* Significantly expanded psychoeducation about triggers and the danger response appears in the next chart.
It is not always easy to know what we feel.	Experiencing really hard things can interfere with kids' ability to know what they are feeling. There are a lot of reasons for this: • "A lot of kids learn about feelings from their moms and dads when they're babies or very little. [Can help to give examples—for example, picking babies up and rocking them.] Sometimes, though, parents have a hard time helping their kids with their feelings. This could happen because . . . [may be useful to give examples or tie to kids' own experiences]. When that happens, kids have to learn all those skills later on." • "One of the ways kids may cope with trauma is to shut off or avoid feelings. This can help in the moment, but when kids do this often enough, they can start to lose touch with what their feelings are." *Note:* It is important to use language appropriate to the client. The word *trauma* may be too abstract or triggering for some children. Use terminology that resonates with the child's and/or family's experience. • "Trauma can also create feelings that are so big, it can be hard to tell one feeling from another. So, for example, feeling mad can feel just like feeling excited." • "Sometimes feelings can come up so suddenly that it can be too confusing to know what they are or where they came from. This is especially true if something is triggering them."

Teaching point	Important information as sample language
There are cues that can tell us what we are feeling.	"Feelings show up in lots of different ways. They may show up in our behavior, our bodies, our facial expressions, our thoughts, our tone of voice, and in other ways."
	Behavior: "Sometimes our feelings come out in what we do, what we say, or how we act with other people. Feeling angry might make some kids hit someone, it might make other kids say mean things, or it might make kids act rude or refuse to do what they're told."
	Behavior: "Other times, feelings show up in what we *don't* do. For example, some kids, when they're upset, don't want to play or be with other people. They may hide out in their rooms or skip school."
	Body: "Feelings may show up in our bodies. We might get a stomachache when we're worried, or a headache when we're really angry or upset. We might notice that our muscles feel really relaxed when we're happy, or that we feel full of energy when we're excited."
	Facial expressions: "It's harder for us to see our own facial expressions, but what we feel will often show up on our face. We may smile, glare, curl our lip, show our teeth, or roll our eyes, depending on what we are feeling."
	Thoughts: "What we are thinking may give us information about how we are feeling. Sometimes our thoughts are about ourselves—for instance, we might think 'I did a terrible job at that' when we are sad or disappointed—and sometimes our thoughts are about other people—for example, we might think 'He's such a jerk' when we're mad."
	Tone of voice: "How we feel may show up in how we speak. Some people get really loud when they're angry, and others get really quiet. When we're really nervous, we might speak kind of softly, and when we're excited we might be louder."
It is important to be a "feelings detective."	"Knowing about our feelings can help us in a lot of different ways. When we know what we feel, it can help us to understand the situation we're in—for example, angry feelings may tell us we don't like something, and worried feelings may tell us we have a problem we need to try to solve. We can try to do something to manage or change the feeling if we don't like it or if it's too big or too small, and we can share the feeling with other people.
	"One of the things we are going to work on is becoming 'feelings detectives': We are going to work on understanding what different feelings are, how they show up, and what we can do with them."

Teach to Kids: Understanding Triggers

- It is important for children to understand the impact of the trauma response on their current emotional reactions. An important component of building affect identification and modulation skills is psychoeducation about the trauma response and triggers.

- The following chart provides key teaching points and sample language for speaking with children about triggers. Keep in mind that language should be geared toward the developmental stage and individual needs of the child client.

UNDERSTANDING TRIGGERS

Target	Description
The body's alarm system	*Teaching point:* The human brain has built-in systems that recognize danger and help to keep us safe.
	Sample language: "Everyone has a built-in alarm system that signals when we might be in danger. One reason why human beings have been able to survive over time is because our brain recognizes signals around us that tell us danger might be coming. This helps our bodies prepare to deal with danger when it comes."

Target	Description
Normative danger response	*Teaching point:* The human danger response is completely normal.
	Sample language: "When our brain recognizes danger, it prepares our body to deal with it. We have three major ways to deal with something dangerous: We can fight it, we can get away from it, or we can freeze.
	"What we pick to do sometimes depends on the kind of danger. So, for example, if a really small squirrel is attacking you, you might fight it, because you're bigger and stronger than it is. If a car comes speeding at you, and you're standing in the street, you'd probably run, because you can't really fight it, and if you stand still, you'll get hit. If you saw a big bear or some other animal nearby, you might freeze, because you can't really fight it, and you're probably not fast enough to run away."
Link between danger response and increased arousal	*Teaching point:* The fight–flight–freeze response is associated with an increase in arousal level.
	Sample language: "When it's time for our body to fight, or run, or freeze, we need a lot of energy to do any one of those things. So, when the brain recognizes danger, the "action" or "doing" part of our brain sends a signal to our body to release a bunch of chemicals, like fuel for a car. Those chemicals give us the energy we need to cope with the danger."
Overactive alarm	*Teaching point:* Overactivation of the alarm system occurs with chronic exposure or extreme exposure to danger.
	Sample language: "When the danger signal goes off, the 'thinking' part of our brain checks out what is going on around us. If it is a false alarm, and there is no real danger, the 'thinking' brain shuts off the alarm, and we can keep doing whatever we were doing. If there is danger, the 'doing brain' takes over and gives the body fuel to deal with whatever is going on.
	"Sometimes, though, the danger alarm goes off too much. That usually happens when kids have had lots of dangerous things happen—like their parents hurting them, or someone touching them when they didn't want it, or someone yelling or fighting a lot. For kids who have had to deal with danger a lot, the 'thinking brain' has gotten tired of checking things out and just assumes that the signals mean more danger. So now, when the alarm goes off, the 'thinking brain' stays out of the way and lets the 'doing brain' take over."
Triggers	*Teaching point:* The false alarm goes off in response to reminders, or "triggers."
	Sample language: "False alarms can happen when we hear, or see, or feel something that reminds us of bad things that used to happen. Those reminders are called 'triggers.' Our brain has learned to recognize those reminders, because in the past when they were around, dangerous things happened, and we had to react pretty quickly.
	"Different people have different reminders. So, if someone got yelled at a lot, hearing people yell might activate the alarm and make the 'doing' part of the brain turn on. If someone didn't get enough attention when they were little, feeling all alone or scared might turn on the alarm."
	Note: It is important to use examples that are relevant to the child.
How triggers manifest	*Teaching point:* The triggered response can be connected to dysregulated behaviors and emotions.
	Sample language: "Once our alarm turns on, our brain prepares our body for action. When that happens, our body fills with 'fuel' to prepare us for dealing with danger. This is really important if it's real danger—like a bear, or a speeding car, or a really mean squirrel—but it's not so helpful if it's a false alarm, and there isn't really any danger around. Imagine if you were in math class and something felt dangerous—suddenly, your body is filled with fuel.

Target	Description
	"Remember that the fuel gives us the energy to fight, or get away, or freeze. When our body has all that energy, we have to do something. So—some kids will suddenly feel really angry or want to argue or fight with someone. Some kids just feel antsy or jumpy. Some kids want to hide in a corner or get as far away as they can—and sometimes they don't even know why. Other kids will suddenly feel really shut down, like someone flipped a switch and turned them off. All of these are ways your body is trying to deal with something it thinks is dangerous.
	"Sometimes, though, what set off the alarm isn't really dangerous—it's just something that feels bad or reminds us of something bad that happens. When kids have a false alarm like that, it can be hard for other people to understand what just happened and to help. Sometimes kids even get into trouble."
	(*Query:* "Are there times you've suddenly had a lot of energy, or felt really mad or upset or scared, and couldn't quite figure out what was going on?")
Recognizing triggers	*Teaching point:* Link to skill: Building recognition of triggers.
	Sample language: "We're going to work on learning about what kinds of reminders might feel dangerous to you and how your body reacts when those reminders are around. Everyone has different triggers and different ways to respond when the alarm goes off. If we know what sets off your alarm and how you respond, we can get your thinking brain on board to help figure out when danger is real and when it's a false alarm."

- See child education handout "**The Body's Alarm System**" and child worksheets "**My Body's Alarm System**," "**My False Alarm Goes Off When . . . ,**" and "**Identifying Triggers**" (Appendix D).

Exercises for Building Affect Identification Skills

- The menu includes activities in multiple modalities; choose activities based on child preference.

- Some activities may be more arousing than others; pay attention to helping children wind down before the end of session.

- When doing Affect Identification exercises, pay attention to identification of triggers and triggered response.

- Consider ways that all activities described below can be adapted to the child's current level. For instance, for a young child or a child with a limited feelings vocabulary, feelings flash cards might focus on "basic" emotions (e.g., happy, sad, mad, worried); with an older child, there might be exploration of nuance (e.g., angry vs. frustrated vs. enraged).

- There are numerous worksheets in Appendix D that may be useful for helping children learn to recognize and understand their feelings.

- The following activities each target one or more of the skills involved in affect identification. The following key is used to identify potential targets:

  - ◆ **I-S**   *Identification of emotion in self*
  - ◆ **I-O**   *Identification of emotion in other*
  - ◆ **C-Bod**   *Connection to body sensations*
  - ◆ **C-Th**   *Connection to thoughts*

◆ **C-Beh**   *Connection to behavior*

◆ **C-Ext**   *Contextualization—external:* factors in the environment that precipitate the feeling

◆ **C-Int**   *Contextualization—internal:* internal factors (e.g., fatigue or hunger) that contribute to the development of different feelings

AFFECT IDENTIFICATION EXERCISE EXAMPLES

Activity	Targets	Description	
Feelings flashcards	I-S, I-O, C-Ext	Suggested materials	Create flashcards using drawings, magazine/book pictures, etc., that depict a range of emotional expressions. Cards can be created solely by clinician or jointly with the child.

		Techniques	• Have the child identify and label what he believes that he is seeing in the picture.
			  ◆ Progress from basic to subtle:
			  ◆ Start with pictures that contain obvious affect.
			  ◆ Start with a limited number of basic emotions (e.g., sad, mad, happy, worried).
			  ◆ Expand to subtler emotions and/or variations on a single emotion (e.g., a series of cards that depict frustration, irritation, anger, rage).
			• Have child identify possible reasons for each emotion (e.g., "What do you think happened to make him feel _____?").
			• Have child identify personal experiences that might elicit the same or similar feelings (e.g., "What kinds of things might make you feel _____?").

		Considerations	• *Pacing:* Build slowly and pay attention to child distress. Moving from external to internal, over time, may help the child develop comfort with this skill.
			• *Relevance:* Use materials appropriate to the child's world. Consider issues of:
			  ◆ Cultural/ethnic background
			  ◆ Child likes/dislikes (e.g., sports figures)
			  ◆ Degree of displacement needed (e.g., photographs vs. cartoons)

Feelings charades	I-S, I-O, C-Beh, C-Ext	Suggested materials	Prompt cards may include: • Feelings • Scenarios (with three or more people) Some children prefer to use puppets, dolls, stuffed animals, etc.
		Techniques	Can be used one on one, with families, or in groups. Consider the following: • Select feeling; one person (child, clinician) acts out feeling, and the other must guess. • Person guessing names cues that led him or her to identify specific feeling. • Select scenario; two people act it out, and the third must guess emotion of each player. With larger groups, can be reenacted using different feelings. • Use puppets, dolls, or stuffed animals to act out feelings and/or scenarios.
		Considerations	*Relevance:* Clinician should use scenarios appropriate to the child. *Reading level:* Assess child's ability to read card.

Activity	Targets	Description	
Word play	**I-S, I-O**	Suggested materials	None, or cards with neutral words. Suggested words include "Oh," "Really?," "Yes," "No," "Hmmm." May be helpful to have a list of feelings for prompting.
		Techniques	• Pick a word (e.g., "Oh"). • Model saying the word in different states (e.g., "How does 'Oh' sound when it's angry? Excited?"). Pay attention to use of cues such as voice tone and volume, body language, eye contact, posture and muscular tension, etc. • Have the child guess the feeling; point out or elicit from child the cues that led to feeling identification. • Take turns identifying which feeling the other is showing.
		Considerations	None.
Feelings detective	**I-S, I-O, C-Beh, C-Th, C-Ext, C-Int**	Suggested materials	Paper or whiteboard writing tool
		Techniques	Help children identify connections among feelings, thoughts, behavior, and experience. • On paper or whiteboard write a list of emotions (start with basic; if appropriate, move to advanced). • Talk or write out ways that feelings may show up in behavior. • Talk or write out different thoughts that might lead to a feeling. Note that thoughts are frequently harder for children to identify; provide general examples (e.g., "If I thought that no one liked me, I might feel sad or worried."). • Talk or write out different situations that might lead to the feeling. Again, it is often useful to provide examples. • As children become proficient with these skills, begin to apply them to real-world situations. For instance, if a parent reports that the child seemed angry last night, ask the child to use his or her feelings detective skills with you to identify what was going on.
		Considerations	*Introduction of technique:* Help children understand the rationale for this technique. Here is a sample introduction with younger children: "Kids are very good at telling grownups how they are feeling with their behavior. Words are sometimes harder for kids. You probably know a lot about kids because you are a kid. Maybe you can teach me some more. What kinds of behavior do you think kids use to show grownups that they are sad, mad, or happy?" Allow the child to be the expert.
Body awareness	**I-S, C-Bod**	Suggested materials	• Large rolls of white paper *or* standard letter-size paper • Markers or other drawing materials in a variety of colors

		Techniques	• Provide basic psychoeducation about how feelings are held in the body. Help children understand that one way to identify and differentiate emotions is to learn how different feeling states are held in their body.
			• Do a body drawing: On standard paper, draw a silhouette figure of a body *or* have the child lie down on large sheet of paper and trace the child's body.
			• Make a key.
			  ♦ Have children identify emotions that they sometimes have; if they deny having a range of emotional experience, consider asking them to simply generate a list of emotions or to generate emotions that kids might have.
			  ♦ For each emotion on the list, have them assign a color that represents that emotion; create a "key" on the same or separate page.

Activity	Targets	Description

- Locate the emotion in the body.
  - Provide an example of how emotions might show up in the body. For example: "Feeling worried might make your stomach feel funny, or feeling angry might make your fists clench." Elicit examples from children of where their emotions show up in their bodies.
  - Have children color specific areas of the body to indicate each emotion's location. Keep in mind (and name) that:
    - Some feelings may be held in more than one part of the body (e.g., *Mad* might make your fists clench and your face hot").
    - More than one feeling can be held in the same place (e.g., "Both *scared* and *excited* might make your heart beat faster").
  - Work with children to expand details about the physical sensations associated with the feeling. For instance, muscles can be tense or loose, body temperature can be hot or cold, fists can clench or hands can be numb. Pay attention to feeling states marked by *lack* of sensation (e.g., for some children, anger may be marked by a sensation of numbing throughout the body).
- Work with children to learn to tune in to and recognize these different physiological states. For many children, this will act as a "clue" in their feelings detective repertoire, as it may be easier for them to recognize physical states than thoughts, triggers, or specific emotions.
- Over time, incorporate this exercise into your feelings check-in (e.g., "What is your body feeling today?").

| | | Considerations | - Keep in mind that working with the body has implications for traumatized children. Consider: |

- Keep in mind that working with the body has implications for traumatized children. Consider:
  - The body may act as a *trigger*. In particular, a full-body tracing may not be appropriate for some children, depending on the degree of discomfort that they have with their body and/or the degree to which their history includes physical violations. Always offer a child a choice between using the silhouette and the full-body trace.
  - The body trace may also be an issue for children with sexualized behaviors and for those who have difficulty maintaining appropriate physical boundaries. For these children, the silhouette should be used.
- Help children tune in to physical manifestations of emotions by commenting on them when they are visible in the therapy room. For instance, if, after a known stressor, a child appears hyperaroused (e.g., jumpy, fidgety, having a hard time sitting still), say, "I notice that your body has a lot of energy today [state your observation]. You've been pretty jumpy since you got here, and you've tried a bunch of different toys without being able to focus [be specific]. What do you think your body might be telling you? [elicit child's participation]." Help children draw on previously learned feelings detective skills.

| What is in your head? | **I-S, C-Ext, C-Int** | Materials | Paper or whiteboard, markers or other drawing materials in variety of colors. |
| | | Techniques | - Draw a silhouette of a large head. Do not include features; simply draw the outline.
- Select a specific emotion to target. Classically, this exercise is done with *worry*, but it can be used with other specific emotions. |

Activity	Targets	Description	
			• Provide psychoeducation. Teach children that all of us have many different things going on in our head at the same time. Some things take up a lot of space (and therefore a lot of energy), and other things take up less space. The goal of this exercise is to help identify what kinds of thoughts or experiences lead to a specific emotion (e.g., worry), and how much of our energy they are currently taking. Note that this exercise both links experience to feeling and provides a foundation for affect modulation techniques. • Make a key. ♦ Have children identify specific thoughts, experiences, or people who are linked to a specific emotion. Note that this may be simplistic and/or concrete: for example, "My mom," "School," etc. ♦ Have children select a different color to represent each identified eliciting event. • Have children color in a portion of the head, with the amount of space colored used to represent the amount of energy or "space" that thought takes up. Using this technique, a big worry should take significantly more space than a small worry; something that makes a child feel very excited should take up more space than something that feels only a little bit exciting.
		Considerations	• This technique may be useful for initial and/or ongoing clinical assessment. • Keep in mind that the representations of different "worries" (or other emotions) will likely change over time. This exercise is a useful tracking tool and can be used to help children tune in to and become aware of changes in their experience over time.
Feelings book	**I-S, I-O, C-Bod, C-Th, C-Beh, C-Ext, C-Int**	Materials	White paper, colored construction paper, pens or pencils, drawing materials, materials to bind book (e.g., file folder, binder clips, ribbon). Note that book should be bound in such a way that it is easily altered/reorganized over time.
		Techniques	• Introduce the exercise. Tell children that they will be creating a book that is all about them. • Create a front and back cover using two sheets of construction paper. Allow children to be as creative as they would like with their cover. Consider suggesting that they include things that represent their interests, personality, etc. • Insert blank pages in between the cover pages. Additional pages can be added over time or included from other therapy exercises. • The feelings book can be used in many ways. The following are some suggestions: ♦ Daily check-in. ♦ Emotion drawings. Have children generate list of emotions and draw a picture about one emotion each week. ♦ Emotional experiences. Have children use feelings detective skills to write about one experience each week that elicited an emotion (positive or negative). Help them identify thoughts, behaviors, body sensations, etc., associated with the feeling.
		Considerations	• Be creative in the use of the feelings book; tailor it to the child. • The book is most effective if it is incorporated into the therapy routine on a weekly basis. • Review the book with children on a semiregular basis. For instance, notice with children if their emotions are changing, if they have experienced the same feelings for weeks in a row, if the same experiences keep eliciting strong feelings, etc. • The book can be useful for ongoing clinical assessment.

Activity	Targets	Description	
Examples of other exercises	All	Books	Use child's favorite stories and/or books (available in the therapy room) to discuss the emotions of identified characters. Pay attention to thoughts, behaviors, somatic expression, context, etc.
		Television shows	Use child's favorite television shows and/or television characters to discuss emotional experience. Again, pay attention to thoughts, behaviors, somatic expression, context, etc.
		Modified board games	Incorporate affect tasks into board games. For instance, while playing Candy Land, assign a feeling a particular color space. Any time someone lands on that color, name an experience that elicits that emotion.
		Deck of cards	Create a deck of cards with four emotion faces, rather than four suits. Use numbers to represent intensity of emotion. Select cards from deck and act out situations, etc.

🚶 DEVELOPMENTAL CONSIDERATIONS

Developmental stage	Affect identification considerations
Early childhood	Tasks at this age should be concrete. The focus is on differentiation of basic feelings rather than subtle variations. Initial exercises should use the four basic feelings (happy, mad, sad, scared, or worried).
	A significant amount of affect identification work can be done via children's spontaneous play. Elicit from child and/or name what characters are feeling, doing, expressing, and why.
	Remember that the emotional cues of younger children are frequently somatic (e.g., stomachaches) and/or behavioral (e.g., irritability, opposition).
Middle childhood	During this stage, children are increasingly able to use words to describe their experience. Balance drawing techniques with those that help children put words to experience.
	Children are increasingly able to connect internal sensations, feelings, and experiences. Keep in mind, however, that this age group is less likely to play than younger children, and less able to hold sustained conversation like adolescents; therefore, structured tasks are often the primary therapeutic tool during this stage.
Adolescence	Adolescents have an increasingly sophisticated grasp over the nuance of language and affect. They can identify subtler types of feelings, as well as multiple feelings at the same time. They may have a particular preference for verbal and/or written techniques.
	It is common for traumatized children to vacillate between, or remain in a single pattern of, emotional constriction/avoidance and/or intense emotional expression. For adolescents, these extremes may be particularly heightened.
	Some adolescents will rely on their newly developed verbal and analytical skills as an avoidance strategy. Rather than connecting to a feeling, they will invest their energy in discussing and analyzing it. For these adolescents, it is important to continue to help them gently connect back to internal experience.
	Other adolescents will become easily aroused and overwhelmed by feelings and unable to access higher cognitive functions to explore emotional experience. It will be important to help these adolescents learn how to tune in to signs of intense emotion and utilize calming techniques.

Developmental stage	Affect identification considerations
	Adolescents may be able to self-identify typical behavioral patterns in response to emotions. Help them describe things they usually do if they're angry, upset, sad, etc. Use these as cues to help them identify emotions and triggering situations.
	Adolescents are more likely than younger children to use coping strategies (e.g., alcohol, substances, sex, cutting) in the face of emotion that adults find unacceptable. It is important that adolescents know that they have permission to talk about these matters in the therapy room. Link these less healthy (but often effective) strategies to underlying emotions, thoughts, and eliciting experiences.

APPLICATIONS

Individual/Dyadic

Identification of emotions and internal experience is generally a cornerstone of our work with children who have experienced trauma. Because dysregulation of experience is such a prominent impact of trauma, learning self-modulation becomes a primary task. In order to modulate, however, a child must first be aware of the presence of a feeling or arousal state.

In our experience almost all individual sessions incorporate, in some way, the naming and exploration of internal experience. Particularly with younger children, consider building structured "feelings check-ins" into the session routine. It is often helpful to include a check of both emotion and energy/arousal, as this will support modulation work. With older children and adolescents, check-ins can be less structured while still exploring significant weekly events (e.g., by using a "thumbs-up" and "thumbs-down" event-of-the-week method). Consider, when appropriate, incorporating caregivers into weekly check-ins; this is particularly helpful for building an understanding of affect identification in others.

For children who have a limited feelings vocabulary due to age or deficits in self-expression, building a language for emotions will be a key component of the work. Incorporate activities such as the ones described above into sessions. Pay attention to the child's comfort level (e.g., initially use displaced figures, such as magazine faces, rather than exploring the child's own affect to increase tolerance for this work). Beyond structured activities, much of affect identification work happens in the moment. If affect identification is a goal for a particular child, pay attention to moments that lend themselves to naming, normalizing, and exploring internal experience. It is particularly important to pay attention to moments of mixed emotion.

Psychoeducation about triggers and triggered responses is often a key component of this work. Worksheets and educational handouts provided in Appendix D may be helpful. Keep in mind, however, that discussion of triggers and their origins is often affect provoking for both the child and the family. Pay attention to the child's response, normalize associated affect, and incorporate modulation strategies, as needed, into the work.

When appropriate, incorporate caregivers into sessions in some way. Support children in sharing emotional experience directly with caregivers. Work with caregivers to use their attunement skills, including reflective listening, outside of the treatment setting as a support for affect identification.

🏠 Group

Many identification tasks lend themselves well to therapeutic groups, either as a focus of the group or as part of session routine. Consider incorporating check-ins at the start of each group (e.g., by asking each group member to identify current emotion(s), level of intensity, or level of energy/arousal). Role plays and improvisation are a great group activity for identifying feelings, feeling "clues," and feeling context. Group leaders can portray a scenario or invite group members to act out a situation; other group participants can identify players' feelings, possible thoughts, facial expressions, triggers, and behavioral responses.

When there is familiarity and safety among group members, they can support each other in identifying cues of emotion in self and other. For instance, group members can provide information about how they know when another participant is angry or happy.

Clips from movies and television shows offer a useful forum for teaching about and exploring triggers and triggered responses (along with other aspects of emotion). Look for moments of fight, flight, and freeze responses and explore the function of these responses. Pay attention to participant vulnerability in these discussions and to the importance of validating the range of responses. Consider the following example:

> A group of adolescent boys in a juvenile justice facility were shown clips from a movie about a young teenage boy with an abusive father. In one scene the father enters the house, having clearly been drinking. The boy freezes on the stairs and remains still and watchful as the father yells and throws things at him, before exiting the room. After the group leader paused the clip, one of the boys stated, "Man, I would have punched that a**hole!" The group leader acknowledged the wish and asked the participants what they think would have happened if the boy had punched the father. The group agreed readily that the boy—small for his age and no match for his father—would have been beaten. After a discussion of why the boy would stay still instead and how that stance might have protected him, the group watched a second clip, shortly after the first scene, in which the boy is yelled at by someone outside the home and has a rageful response, destroying property and punching a wall. The boy who had made the first comment stated, "Bet he wishes that was his dad."

Through exploration of the danger response in film, these boys were able to tolerate a more vulnerable discussion than they might otherwise have been able to do. When possible, it is important to take the next step and to explore participants' own possible triggers and danger responses.

🏠 Milieu

Milieus offer a natural forum to support youth affect identification. Work with staff at all levels to observe and reflect youth behaviors and emotions. Pay attention to positive as well as challenging emotions; it is equally important to observe and celebrate a child's positive affect as to notice and support a child in coping with distress. Set as a goal the identification of early cues of dysregulation (e.g., what a particular child looks like or does *before* the explosion), name these when they appear, and support the youth in using modulation strategies. Consider the role of affect identification in youth reactions to staff. Be aware of the potential for miscues; explore these (e.g., "What did you think my reaction meant?") and clarify them.

Consider incorporating check-ins into daily routines (e.g., at the start of class, during meals, at the end of the day). Create an environment that acknowledges affect, using visual cues, posters, and/or bulletin boards. It may be helpful to create "themed" bulletin boards (e.g., pictures of "happy moments," examples of activities that people might do when sad, etc.).

Affect identification work may play an important role in conflict resolution. Use identification skills to support perspective taking (e.g., asking, "What do you think Sean might have been feeling when he said that?"). It is important to pay attention to timing in this work; it is difficult to have perspective (a skill requiring the "thinking brain") when a child is not modulated. Once calm, use reflective listening skills (Attunement) and problem-solving skills (Executive Functions) to support children in understanding their reactions, associated situational precipitants and triggers, and potential solutions.

🌐 REAL-WORLD THERAPY

🌐 **Kids have their own agendas.** Some children reject structured feelings activities. Keep an eye on the goal, even if you can't do the specific activity on which you planned.

🌐 **Be true to the context and to provider and child preference.** This section has provided an array of sample activities as a way of stimulating ideas about possible useful techniques. Keep in mind two points:

1. There are no limits to the number of potential exercises you can create. Use your imagination and create feelings-relevant activities that will match the interests of the child with whom you are working.
2. A lot of this work happens in the moment, and in conversation, rather than through structured therapeutic activities. Tune in to opportunities to explore affect in the material children are already bringing to you.

CHAPTER 9

Modulation

THE MAIN IDEA

Work with children to develop safe and effective strategies to manage and regulate physiological and emotional experience, in service of maintaining a comfortable state of arousal.

★ KEY CONCEPTS

★ *Why Target Modulation?*

- The ability to safely and effectively modulate emotional and physiological experience is often a key challenge for traumatized children. Two primary historical factors influence this difficulty with affect modulation:

  - *Attachment.* Young children initially rely on their caregivers to act as "external modulators" by providing comfort and soothing during times of distress. Often this is done through positive sensory experiences such as rocking, swaddling, sucking, singing, etc. Over time, they internalize these experiences and develop skills for self-soothing. Children who experience unresponsive, inconsistent, or abusive caretaking may fail to develop healthy age-appropriate skills, and instead must rely on primitive regulation strategies.

  - *Traumatic stress response.* When children are exposed to overwhelming stress, particularly chronic stress, they must cope with high levels of arousal. In the face of overwhelming emotion, children attempt to employ whatever modulation skills are available. Often these are inadequate for reducing arousal. As a result, children either fail to regulate or regulate to the extremes (e.g., constriction).

- In the face of current stressors and triggers, children often move rapidly into "danger mode." Even minor stressors may derail children because their early experiences provided insufficient supports for the development of physiological organization. Their ability to remain regulated is impacted by sudden surges of arousal, shifts in neurological control from cortical (frontal) to subcortical (limbic) areas, and desperate—and unconscious—reliance on rigid and often primitive strategies to manage internal and external experience.

★ *How Does Trauma Impact Modulation?*

- Children who are unable to modulate may attempt to (1) overcontrol or shut down emotional experience, (2) manage their arousal through physiological stimulation or behavior, or (3) rely on external methods to self-regulate. Often, none of these is a conscious process.

   ♦ Some children **overcontrol or shut down** emotional experience via:
      o Constriction/numbing
      o Avoidance
      o Isolation
      o Distraction
      o Fantasy/daydreaming

   ♦ Other children **manage arousal through behavior or physical stimulation**:
      o Physical movement: jumping, running, etc.
      o Primitive self-soothing: rocking, thumbsucking, hair twirling
      o Aggression
      o Sexualized behaviors

   ♦ When emotion management strategies fail, children may **rely on overt methods to alter or control physiological states**:
      o Substance or alcohol use
      o Eating control/dyscontrol
      o Self-harm

- Note that these methods are not mutually exclusive; coping strategies used by a child may vary over time (e.g., depending on developmental stage) and within different contexts.

THERAPIST TOOLBOX

Behind the Scenes

- Many children who have experienced trauma feel at the mercy of their emotions, which they experience as overwhelming, unpredictable, and powerful. Emotional experience is intricately linked with arousal; modulation (and dysregulation) often occurs on a physiological level. A great deal of modulation work can be done without ever referencing "feelings." The ultimate goal of this work is to help children learn to maintain optimal levels of arousal.

- Modulation, or the ability to move toward optimal levels of arousal, involves a number of different strategies and skills:

- ◆ The ability to identify initial emotional or physiological state and the degree to which it is comfortable and/or effective. *Awareness of current arousal level, whether high or low: "I'm feeling really charged up." "I'm feeling really shut down."*

- ◆ The ability to identify and connect to subtle changes in state. *Awareness of shifts in arousal: "I just started to feel a little calmer."*

- ◆ The ability to identify what it feels like in the body to experience subtle changes in state. *Recognition of the cues of state changes: "I can tell I feel calmer because my stomach is churning a little less."*

- ◆ The ability to identify the ways that different emotional experiences impact the body's energy and level of arousal. *Recognition of the link between emotions and energy or arousal changes: "Whenever I get mad, I get really revved up."*

- ◆ The ability to identify and use strategies to manage those state changes. *"When I breathe really deeply, it helps my stomach start to feel better."*

- Modulation is bidirectional: It may involve increasing arousal (i.e., "up-regulation") or decreasing arousal (i.e., "down-regulation"). Every child will have a different "comfort zone," or range of comfortable arousal. It is important to partner with children in learning about and exploring their own preferred arousal state.

- What is *comfortable* for a child may be different from what is *effective*. In teaching and supporting modulation skills, both of these constructs will need to be explored.

  - ◆ *Comfort zone.* One key goal of modulation is to help a child feel comfortable in his or her body. As discussed above, every child will have a different comfort zone. Trauma can have a significant impact on a child's comfort zone. For instance, some children may feel most comfortable at very high states of arousal because long-standing "danger readiness" and hypervigilance have allowed their brain to feel "ready for action" and therefore less helpless or vulnerable. For other children, a highly constricted state may be most comfortable. For these children, who often have few effective coping strategies, arousal in their bodies may feel quickly overwhelming, and they may expend significant energy to keep their emotions and arousal state at very low levels.

    In addition to exploring and *identifying* a child's comfort zone, our work may involve (*slooooooowly* and carefully) *expanding* a child's comfort zone. Be cautious as you go: If you try to bring down the arousal too quickly of a child who lives in the upper ranges, he or she may feel unsettled and engage in some behavior designed to increase arousal back to comfortable levels. Similarly, if you try to increase the arousal of a constricted child before he or she has the tools to manage the arousal, the child may shut down further in an attempt to manage these feelings. Consider the function of a child's comfort zone in your selection of modulation activities. For example, begin with activities that allow a child to stay within that comfort zone and then slowly modify and/or change the activity to expand the zone.

  - ◆ *Effective modulation.* A second key goal is to help children achieve a level of modulation that will help them navigate their world most effectively. Effective modulation is often about context. An appropriate level of arousal in a classroom, for instance, is different from an appropriate level of arousal on a playground. Additionally, for children who live in dangerous communities, arousal levels connected with vigilance to danger may be essential to their safety. It is important that skill building in modulation incorporate an understanding that no level of arousal is "wrong"; however, the ability to manage arousal may help children effectively navigate the current moment (e.g., modulating in service of (1) effectively relating or communicating, (2) effectively getting needs met, (3) effectively and safely completing tasks). If a child's comfortable state of arousal is higher or lower than situations routinely require (e.g., the highly energetic child who must frequently work to bring down his or her energy), it is important that the child have alternative places or moments in which to safely experience the preferred energy state.

♦ In order for children to tune in to variations in arousal, clinicians need to concretely support them in eliciting changes in state. Achieving state changes can be done through fun activities (e.g., tossing a ball, dancing) or through more targeted regulation (e.g., deep breathing). Work with children to notice their own physiological reactions to these activities. A key teaching point is that children have the power to change their own physiology. Over time, the goal is for them to be able to autonomously implement these strategies.

♦ Not all modulation activities will be effective—or enjoyable—for all children. Frame the activities as experiments and allow children space to actively explore their own reactions. What may be down-regulating for one child may be up-regulating for another. Consider concrete measures of children's reactions: Have them practice appraisal skills, including monitoring heart rate, pace of breathing, body temperature, and level of muscle tension, before and after activities. Providers can practice their own self-monitoring skills to model this process. Additional techniques include using charts, scales, etc., to track degree of arousal, positive versus negative experiences, and so on. Be mindful that even referencing "the body" may increase vulnerability in some children.

• It is important for children to practice modulation techniques when they are calm to gain mastery over the skills and internalize an awareness of how their body feels at different states of arousal. Initial practice of these skills should not be paired with significantly distressed or constricted emotional states. Over time, these skills can be actively applied in the moment to manage arousal.

• To apply these skills successfully in the moment (e.g., when upset or shut down), children will often need cuing (from caregiver, clinician, teacher, etc.). Essentially, the caregiver (or whoever) will need to act as the "external modulator" by modeling, cuing, and **actively participating** in the modulation activity with the child.

• A note about *connection*:

♦ It is important to note that modulation involves the ability of the child to *tune in to, tolerate,* and *sustain* connection to emotional states or arousal.

♦ Often, children will appear to have the ability to modulate, because they either are able to talk about emotions in a calm manner or are observed to shift from high arousal to calm.

♦ However, constricting or shutting down affect suggests that the child is unable to tolerate it rather than using healthy modulation skills. Similarly, verbalizing emotion without a connection to affect may indicate a lack of tolerance for the internal experience of that emotion.

• When connecting modulation skills to emotion, build on the vocabulary developed with the child during affect identification exercises. For instance, if a child talks about getting "really hot" when angry, think together about ways to "cool down."

- In addition to formal exercises, affect modulation work can often be done in the moment.

    ◆ In session, tune in to and notice signs of state modulation or state shifts. When appropriate, build on reflection by engaging the child in active attempts at modulation.

        ○ In play:

            ◊ Play behaviors

            (The child comes into session calm, but when asked about her day, starts pulling out multiple toys, and is now slamming figures around the dollhouse.)

            THERAPIST: Wow, all of a sudden your energy got really big—there's lots of toys on the floor, and those dolls are really looking busy. It seems like being asked about your day might have kicked up some feelings.

            If distress continues: THERAPIST: Let's you and I take a big, deep breath and stretch before we keep playing.

            ◊ Displaced in play

            (The child has an action figure and a toy lion. He shows characters interacting, then suddenly begins slamming figures together, having lion growl, etc.)

            THERAPIST: Boy, that lion just got really mad all of a sudden. It seemed like they were playing calmly, and then the lion started growling. I wonder what's going on with him?

        ○ In interaction:

            (The adolescent comes in appearing angry and shut down, arms folded, no eye contact. When the therapist initially notices and comments on his appearance, the adolescent rejects it, stating, "Everything's fine." After several minutes of interaction, the adolescent starts to appear more relaxed.)

            THERAPIST: It looks like you're starting to calm down a little bit. I can see that your muscles aren't as tense, and you're looking at me more.

        ○ In statements:

            (The child talks about her relationship with her mother, which has always been a highly triggering subject. In previous conversations, the child's statements were accompanied by a high degree of distressed affect [loud tone of voice, fists clenching, arms crossed, etc.]. Today, the child still has apparent anger in her voice, but is less intense, and her body appears more relaxed [e.g., arms uncrossed].)

            THERAPIST: I'm noticing that when you talk about your mom today, you seem a little less angry.

    ◆ When observing your clients during various interactions, tune in to their attempts to modulate and their preferred strategies. For example, you may have clients who come into the office and immediately reach for a stress ball or other manipulative to squeeze, move, etc. Other clients may gently rock back and forth in their seat or begin tapping on their leg when their arousal starts to increase. Kids will often give us clues about which modulation activities are likely to be most successful for them.

✐ *Teach to Caregivers*

- *Reminder*: Teach the caregiver the Key Concepts.

- *Reminder*: Teach the caregiver relevant Developmental Considerations.

- In the Attunement section, we discussed the caregiver's important role in supporting child modulation and the steps toward doing so. We briefly revisit those here.

CAREGIVER ROLE IN CHILD AFFECT MODULATION

Teaching points	Caregivers play a key role in helping their children regulate emotional experience.
	Often, the best regulation is *coregulation*: in addition to verbal cuing, caregivers can engage in many of the exercises described above *with* their children. For instance, rather than cuing a child to stretch, teach the caregiver to stretch along with the child, take deep breaths together, etc.
	Teach caregivers to use their attunement skills to identify *variations* in their child's emotional experience and/or arousal level. What does the child look like when escalating? When shutting down? Develop a list of cues specific to the child.
	Teach caregivers the distinctions between *up-regulation* and *down-regulation*.
	Teach caregivers to support appropriate modulation strategies (i.e., down-regulation strategies when hyperaroused, up-regulation strategies when constricted). Develop a menu of strategies that caregivers are comfortable supporting.

Teach caregivers the following steps:

Caregiver steps to support affect modulation	1. Pay attention to signs that your child is having difficulty modulating emotional experience. Name what you see: • "It looks like your body is starting to have really high energy." • "Wow—you just started yelling—it seems like you're getting pretty upset." • "I'm not sure what happened, but it looks like you just kind of shut down." Be careful that the language used for labeling is not judgmental or blaming. It is important that the child is given permission for the feeling; caregivers' language should separate concern about modulation from concern about the emotion itself.
	2. Support the use of modulation techniques. Cue the child to use already learned skills, and/or practice the skills with the child: • "Let's try some breathing like you learned in therapy—then we can talk about what's upsetting you." • "Do you want to come cuddle for a moment to help calm down?" • "You just got really quiet and still when we were talking about school. I think it would help if we got up and shook it off, before we keep talking about this."
	3. Reinforce the use of modulation techniques: • "You just did a great job using your breathing to calm down." • "I'm really proud of you for trying to practice using your stress ball."
	4. Help your child identify and process what precipitated the difficult emotion. Use attunement skills and reflective listening skills.

⚒ *Tools:* **Affect Modulation Tools**

Skill #1: Understanding Degrees of Feeling

- An important step in modulation is to understand that feelings come in all sizes and to be able to tune in to those subtle differences.

- Modulation is often about gradation: Most children can tune in to extreme states more easily than subtle shifts.

- All of these techniques can be incorporated into opening and closing check-ins, as well as used during the session to help the child track changes in observable affect. Beyond formal exercises, use these concepts in the moment to help children build awareness of the range of feeling and arousal states.

- Although this skill is listed as "Degrees of *Feeling*," the same concept applies to energy and physiological regulation in general. Use this skill to help children identify energy or arousal level.

- Once children are able to use these techniques to identify their current feeling, the techniques can be used to:

  - *Link to past experience.* For example: "When that argument happened, how mad were you? If this circle was all the mad in the world, color in how much would be filled to show how mad you were."

  - *Help the child tune in to changes in affect.* For example: "What about 5 minutes later?"

  - *Compare across experiences.* For example: "I remember when we talked about how mad you were when your brother hit you. Do you think you're *more* mad this time, *less* mad, or about the same? How can you tell?"

  - *Link to specific modulation strategies.* For example: "Color this circle for how you were feeling when you first had that argument, then let's color this one for how you felt after you listened to your music for a little while."

  - *Generate ideas for modulation.* For example: "Right now you said you're at a 10. What would we need to do for you to go down to a 9?" *Note:* Do not try to reduce affect from a 10 to a 0; it is better for the child to successfully modulate small degrees of affect than to feel overwhelmed by the expectation of fully shifting an arousal state.

ACTIVITIES THAT BUILD UNDERSTANDING OF DEGREES OF FEELING

Activity	Description
Number scale	Have children identify current emotion on –1 to +10 or –10 to +100 scale. Use concrete markers to indicate what a –1, a 5, or a 10 might look like or feel like. Note the use of bidirectional number scales: For children who feel really frozen or shut down, it is important to have numbers or other markers that acknowledge that state.
Thermometer	Draw outline of thermometer. Have children color in how much of the identified feeling they are experiencing. Use concrete markers to indicate high, moderate, and low levels of feeling.
Circle	• Have children color in a portion of a circle to indicate how much of a single identified feeling they are experiencing. • Have children create a key of different feelings by using different colors. Color each in a circle, in proportion to how much children are currently feeling (in relation to identified event, last week, etc.).
Poker chips	Have children select a number of chips to indicate how strong their current emotion is (e.g., "If these chips were all the mad in the world, how mad are you right now?").
Clay	Identify chunk of clay as containing all the "[identified emotion]" in the world; have children tear off from the clay how much they are currently feeling.

Skill #2: Teach to Kids—Understanding Comfort Zone and Effective Modulation

- Building a language around, and an internal awareness of, energy or arousal level is a key foundation for doing modulation work with children.

- Developing a shared understanding of energy involves both an educational and an experiential component. Beyond just teaching the concepts below, consider, for instance, (1) mapping a child's energy onto a scale like those used in the "Degrees of Feeling" activities; (2) tossing a ball, jumping up and down, jogging in place, or dancing at different energy levels (low, medium, high); and (3) checking on energy level at various points during the session or before and after key activities.

- Educational points and sample activities (below) can be modified to meet the needs of children at different developmental levels. Keep in mind that distinctions for children at earlier stages of development will be broader (e.g., "low, medium, high"), whereas older children/ adolescents can often grasp more nuanced distinctions, such as those implicit in number scales.

MANAGING FEELINGS COMFORTABLY AND EFFECTIVELY

Target	Description

Normalizing and teaching the concept of energy	*Teaching point:* We all have different levels of energy in our bodies at different times.
	
	Sample language: "Everyone has energy in their bodies. Sometimes our energy is really low, like when we're sleepy; sometimes our energy is somewhere in the middle, like when we're feeling really focused and calm—such as doing homework or playing a board game; and sometimes our energy can be really high, like when we're running around with friends or playing sports.
	    "Energy helps us do what we need to do, and all kinds of energy are important. Low energy is important, because sometimes we need to sleep and rest, and high energy is important, because sometimes we need to be really active.
	    "A lot of things can affect our energy, like whether we've slept enough, or eaten enough, who we're with, where we are, and what time of day it is."
	
	Possible activities: Create an "energy scale" with the child (using numbers, high/ medium/low, etc.). Elicit from and list with the child different activities that need different energy levels, or different clues that show someone's energy is high, medium, or low. Cut out pictures of people engaged in different activities from magazines and label their energy. Use your created scale and engage in different activities—tossing a ball, dancing, jumping—at different levels of the scale: How does dancing at a 3, for instance, look and feel different from dancing at a 7?

Linking energy with feelings	*Teaching point:* How we feel has an impact on our energy/arousal. *Sample language:* "One of the really important things that can affect our energy level is how we feel. For example, being excited or angry or scared can make our energy get really high; being sad or lonely can make our energy get really low. "This is especially true for 'danger energy'; when our brain thinks that something is dangerous, our energy can change really quickly. *(Refer to Teach to Kids section on triggers, in "Affect Identification.")* Sometimes, having our energy change can be an important clue that something is going on with our feelings." *Possible activities:* Make a list of different feelings and have children label the feelings according to their own energy level: Do they have high or low energy when mad, sad, happy, etc.? Think about different kinds of energy levels within a feeling: "mad," for instance, comes in lots of sizes. Think of a range of feeling words that goes with a particular feeling (e.g., for *mad:* annoyed, irritated, frustrated, angry, enraged) and

Target	Description
	plot the words on an energy scale. Elicit the differences in situations that may lead to those feelings, ways they feel in the body (e.g., "Does *frustrated* feel different from *enraged*? How?"); how in control—or not—they feel when experiencing each feeling; different behaviors that might go with each feeling; etc. Have children act out the different feelings: "What does it look like when you walk into a room *annoyed* versus *enraged*?"
Understanding "comfort zone"	*Teaching point:* Some energy levels feel more comfortable than others. *Sample language:* "All of us have different bodies and different brains. That means that each of us feels most comfortable with different kinds of energy. Some people really, really like it when their energy is high, some people really like it when their energy stays low, and some people like their energy to stay somewhere in the middle. The place we like our energy to stay is our 'comfort zone.' If our energy gets too far out of our comfort zone—like if someone who likes low energy gets too heated up—it can feel really uncomfortable. Sometimes we try to do things to change our energy, to get it back where it's comfortable." *Possible activities:* Help children explore their comfort zones. Using your developed energy scale, have them plot what they think their most comfortable zone is. Pair this with the different modulation activities with which you experiment: Have children check in on their energy level (e.g., "Where is it? Did it go up or down from where it started?") and whether or not they like how their body feels.
Understanding the role of context	*Teaching point:* Context will affect how effective our energy level is. *Sample language:* "Where we are and what we are doing can make a difference in whether our energy level helps us or gets in our way, and in whether our energy is safe or not safe. Having really high energy may feel really good, but there are places that high energy can get in our way. *(Elicit examples from the child, e.g., the library, in class.)* When high energy starts to get out of control, like if we're really mad or really upset, it can get in the way of getting our needs met, or it can make us do things that aren't safe. "The same thing is true for low energy. Low energy can be really good when we're sleepy, but it can get in the way if we need to do something like chores or homework. Shutting down our energy when we're feeling scared or upset can sometimes feel safer, but doing that can also get in the way of asking for help or doing something that feels good." *Note:* It is important to use examples that are relevant to each child and to involve him or her in the discussion. *Possible activities:* Make a list of concrete activities relevant to the children. Include both relevant daily activities (e.g., sleeping, eating, playing football, doing homework) and relational activities (e.g., asking for help, telling someone they're angry). Explore what they think the "effective zone" is for each activity: At what energy level do they think engaging in that activity will be most effective? Why? Explore what might happen if energy were too low or too high.
Building a sense of agency over modulation	*Teaching point:* There are ways that we can shift our energy. *Sample language:* "There are a lot of different things we can do to change our energy when it doesn't feel comfortable or when it's getting in the way of something we want to do. We can think of these things as 'energy tools.' An energy tool helps us move our energy up or down. Not every tool works for every person, and not every tool works every time (just like sometimes you need a hammer, and sometimes you need a screwdriver). Because of that, we're going to practice different tools, and figure out which ones you like, which ones feel good in your body, and which ones feel like they might work." *Note:* Expanded education about this point appears in the next section, "Building a Feelings Toolbox." *Possible activities:* A wide range of activities is described later in this section.

Skill #3: Building a Feelings Toolbox

- The goal of this activity (or series of activities) is to identify, for specified emotions and energy states, safe skills children can use to cope with emotional experience. Because not every skill will work every time, it is important that children have a repertoire of available skills.

- Feelings Toolboxes are a concrete way to cue children in their use of identified skills; the toolboxes may be actual boxes or, for older children, lists or menus of skills.

- Pair this activity with experimentation in the modulation activities described later in this section. Although specific examples for the toolbox are listed below, ultimately, all modulation exercises are potential additions to the child's toolbox.

CREATING FEELINGS TOOLBOXES

How to build a toolbox	Suggested materials	*Box:* Shoebox or other container (e.g., lunchbox), materials to decorate box (e.g., magazines, stickers, construction paper), writing materials *Tools:* Possibilities are wide; may create symbolic tools with children using, for instance, clay, drawing, etc.; may also include actual tools (e.g., stress ball).

	Techniques	• Building a Feelings Toolbox is a technique that should be implemented only after children have an understanding of:
		  ♦ What feelings are and at least a basic language for them
		  ♦ The concept of energy and arousal
		  ♦ Current actions (safe and unsafe) when experiencing strong emotion
		• Frame the rationale for the Feelings Toolbox with children:
		  ♦ **Normalize feelings.** For example: "We've talked about how everyone has different kinds of feelings, and that no feeling is wrong."
		  ♦ **Differentiate safe versus unsafe expression.** For example: "Sometimes when people feel things really strongly, they do things that aren't all that helpful or safe." *(Give relevant examples from child's life, for example*: "Like, sometimes when kids are mad, they can get into fights and get in trouble at school, or when kids are really excited, it's hard for them to sit still and focus.")
		  ♦ **Highlight importance of feelings.** For example: "Feelings are important—they tell us a lot about what's going on and what we need. It's not healthy just to turn them off, because eventually they're going to build up or show up somewhere else."
		  ♦ **Provide rationale.** For example: "Since feelings are so important, we're going to build a toolbox [or, "create a menu"] of different things you can do when you're having different feelings."
		• Help children identify key emotions. Emotions addressed should include both (1) basic emotions (e.g., mad, sad, worried, happy) and (2) emotions that are difficult for children to cope with (e.g., embarrassment).
		• Alternatively (or in addition), identify different energy states. Again, pay attention to those that children find comfortable, as well as those that are more distressing or that interfere with their lives.
		• Work with children to create physical boxes. They can label their box, decorate it, etc., as desired. Older children can choose to keep a list in a journal, notebook, etc. It may be useful to have a separate page for each emotion, so that children can add new techniques as they are identified.

	Considerations	• When working to create a repertoire of skills, be wary of overdoing. Children should develop mastery over a small number of skills before adding new ones. • Keep in mind that creation of these boxes is a process. New techniques and skills can and should be added as they are identified. • It may be important to reevaluate identified techniques over time (e.g., as child enters a new developmental stage; with life transitions). What worked at one point in time may not work at another.

- In creating tools, consider the **energy of the emotion.** Often, anger, excitement, and fear are **externally directed "action" emotions,** and effective tools involve *releasing and focusing the energy.* In contrast, sadness and worry are often **"frozen" or internally directed emotions,** and effective tools involve self-soothing and reengaging.
- *Note:* The following are provided as examples; be creative and involve children in identifying helpful cues to include in their boxes.

Examples of tools for the toolbox	Excitement	• Small objects that children can manipulate in hands to channel energy (e.g., Wikki-Stix) • Small container of bubble liquid with wand • Doing specified number of jumping jacks (*cue for toolbox:* picture of child doing a jumping jack) • Butterfly hugs (folding arms across chest, and tapping shoulders like a butterfly flapping its wings) (*cue for toolbox:* picture of a butterfly)
	Anger	• Pushing against a wall or doorway (*cue for toolbox:* drawing of a doorway) • Stress ball to squeeze • Small ball of clay (to flatten)
	Sadness	• Picture of a favorite person or animal associated with comfort • Favorite or comforting object (e.g., teddy bear) • Soothing sensory object (e.g., piece of velvet) • Drawing materials or journal
	Worry	• Small box or container and pad of paper on which to write down worries and put them away • List of five distractions (i.e., activities child can engage in and/or positive things to think about) • Index card with stop sign on one side and positive statement on the other (e.g., "I can handle this") • Blank index cards and black marker; child can write down worry and then black it out.
	Fear	• Picture of a safe place • Picture of a strong person whom the child associates with safety • Small object from the therapy room or home (i.e., a transitional object) • Small tube of glitter cream or nice-smelling lotion for self-soothing (for younger children, can be "magic safety cream")

Skill #4: Exploring Arousal States—Exercises to Modulate Arousal

- Following is a series of exercises that may shift a child's arousal state. Work with the child to experiment with different activities. For each activity, notice and track with the child:

  ♦ Whether and the extent to which the activity changes the energy level to higher or lower, and how it affects the body (e.g., in terms of heart rate, breathing, temperature, muscles)

  ♦ Whether and the extent to which the activity feels comfortable or uncomfortable

- Techniques that are effective in shifting arousal and that feel comfortable to the child can then be added in to the child's toolbox.

- These charts provide examples of how to implement classic techniques with different age groups. Use your imagination to create new ones!

- It is often helpful to incorporate modulation activities into the session or daily routine. For instance, a modulation activity can be incorporated into the session opening and/or closing, start or end of classtime, before bedtime, and at other key points in a child's day.

- Work with caregivers to cue the child in the use of these skills outside of the therapy room. Consider incorporating caregivers into dyadic practice of these activities in the session, both to build attunement and to increase generalization.

- Beyond the caregiver role in *activities*, keep in mind that the act of engaging with another person (whether a primary caregiver, a helping adult, or a peer) is often a primary source of modulation (as well as, for some children, a source of dysregulation). Like any other activity described, dyadic engagement can be up-regulating or down-regulating. Work with children to identify modulation resources (see Chapter 10, "Affect Expression," for expanded information) and work with caregivers to tune in to the ways that interaction with their children increases, or decreases, arousal.

- When using formal exercises, it is often useful to modulate *toward* a child's extreme before modulating away (e.g., for a child who is already hyperaroused, "turn the volume up" before turning it down; this allows expression and engagement and normalizes affect).

- For exercises that involve cuing or guiding by the therapist, it may be useful to create an audiotape for the child to bring home.

- With all activities, keep in mind the role of the child's comfort zone: A highly aroused child may feel uncomfortable becoming too relaxed, and a highly constricted child may feel discomfort with too much arousal. Move slowly in shifting arousal states, emphasize the child's control, and check in often with the child.

- It is important to be particularly cautious when working with children who are in a constricted or numb state. Some children who become overwhelmed will shut down as a way of managing the affect. While in this "turned-off" state, children are able to tolerate, but unable to directly cope with, the immediate stressor or related affect, because the numbing effectively disconnects them from the situation. Initial modulation strategies are used to help children reengage with their own experience (both internal and external) and tolerate emotional and physical sensation. Once children are reengaged, they can then make use of more sophisticated coping mechanisms (e.g., modulation strategies to reduce affect, identification strategies to understand affect, and expression strategies to communicate experience). Keep in mind that constriction or numbing suggests the presence of underlying distress. Therefore, it is important to pace the use of these exercises and to be on the lookout for signs of distress.

DIAPHRAGMATIC BREATHING

- Diaphragmatic breathing is a particularly valuable skill for a child to gain, as breathing is the easiest and quickest way to have an impact on physiology. Use of deep, steady breathing will often need to be paired with other activities (e.g., learning to take three deep breaths before engaging in movement, muscle relaxation).

DIAPHRAGMATIC BREATHING

Developmental stage	Technique variation
Early childhood	• *Bubble breathing* (real or imaginary): Teach children to blow a very big bubble without letting it pop; to do this, they must blow slowly, evenly, and then release. • *Pillow breathing*: Have children lie on floor with pillow or stuffed animal on stomach. Teach them to breathe so that pillow/animal rises and falls with each breath.
Middle childhood	• *London Bridge:* Have children raise arms (like in game London Bridge). Breathe in as arms go up; breathe out as arms come down. See how slowly they can move their arms up and down. • *Imagery:* Have children imagine taking a deep breath and blowing out birthday candles; have them try to paint the opposite wall with their breath; have them smell the flowers and blow a dandelion puff.
Adolescence	• *Diaphragmatic breathing:* Teach adolescents principles of diaphragmatic breathing. Have them try to breathe in through their nose to a slow count of 3, pause, and then exhale slowly out through their mouth. Their abdomen should move out as they breathe in, and in as they breathe out. Their shoulders and chest should remain steady. Have them practice by placing a hand on their stomach and observing their hand rise and fall. • *Pair with visual imagery:* Have adolescents imagine calm/peace coming in as they breathe in through their nose, and the tension exiting as they breathe out through their mouth.

GROUNDING

- We have found adapted grounding techniques, as originally described by Marsha Linehan (1993), to be extremely useful for helping children and adolescents shift energy states.

- Grounding techniques can be used both for decreasing arousal (calming down from higher energy) and for increasing arousal, or reengaging from a constricted state. Keep in mind the following:

    ◆ When used for down-regulation, grounding may involve self-soothing and internal engagement (e.g., mental lists). When used for up-regulation, it is important that techniques focus children on reengaging with self and the environment.

    ◆ Once children have learned the techniques, external cuing may continue to be important.

    ◆ Verbal grounding techniques (e.g., lists, naming the days of the week, naming things in the office, "I Spy" for younger children) may be particularly useful for children who are disconnected.

    ◆ The shift from numb to embodied may be triggering for some children; to minimize this possibility, the grounding strategies should not overload the senses (e.g., use subtle vs. strong scents).

    ◆ As children become reembodied, it is often helpful to incorporate movement (next section).

GROUNDING

Developmental stage	Technique variation
	Grounding techniques appropriate for down-regulation
Early childhood	Have children tune into their senses, using concrete, easy-to-hold stimuli, such as: • Magic wands • Magic rocks • Worry stones • Piece of velvet cloth • Small stuffed animals • Glitter cream • Pleasurable smell
Middle childhood	Similar to early childhood. At this age, children like to have something they can carry with them and manipulate, such as: • Stress balls • Wikki Stix • Lanyard string • Grounding stone
Adolescence	Adolescents can use similar techniques as those above, but can also use more sophisticated and abstract techniques, such as: • Mentally listing simple information (e.g., days of the week, months of the year, favorite animals) • Listening to music • Writing or drawing • Noticing what they see, hear, and feel (physical sensation, not emotional)
	Grounding techniques appropriate for up-regulation
Early childhood	• Play "I Spy," tuning in to things in the immediate environment. • Have children describe a known (safe) environment. • Have children tune in to a feather being run up and down their arm (by self, therapist, or caregiver, as appropriate). • Have children rub hands with glitter cream. • Have children do butterfly self-hugs (arms crossed across chest). • Pretend the floor is sand and have children "dig a hole" with their toes.
Middle childhood	• Have children name 10 things they see in the office. • Have children describe their favorite (person, book, movie, television show, food, etc.). • Have children squeeze a stress ball.
Adolescence	• Ask adolescents to tune in to and describe physical sensations (e.g., body in the chair, feet on the floor). • Describe four, then three, then two, then one thing adolescent hears, sees, and feels (physical sensations) to gradually increase focal awareness of surroundings. • Have adolescents describe something step by step (e.g., what they did when they woke up that morning).

MOVEMENT

• Almost any kind of movement can be used to experiment with energy. In order to increase engagement, be creative, consider the child's interests and comfort level, and have fun. Examples are offered in the following table.

• Many activities can be tailored to different developmental stages. For instance, although "yoga poses" are listed in adolescence, many yoga activities are geared toward younger children as well (e.g., games such as Yoga Pretzels [Guber, Kalish, & Fatus, 2005] and Yoga Bingo [distributed by Spiraling Hearts, n.d.]).

MOVEMENT

Developmental stage	Technique variation
Early childhood	• Hop like frogs: Start slowly and gradually speed up. • Play (and sing) *head, shoulders, knees,* and *toes* (*knees and toes*). • Play the Hokey Pokey. • Play a follow-the-leader game using movement, "animal walks" (e.g., move like a horse or elephant), drumming, etc.
Middle childhood	• Challenge children to do as many jumping jacks as they can (or give a number: e.g., "I wonder if you can do 10 jumping jacks in a row"). • Put on music and have children dance; start with slower music and speed up. • Play Simon Says.
Adolescence	• Play door- or garbage-can basketball. • Toss a ball back and forth. • Turn on music and dance. • Drum or play another musical instrument. • Go for a walk. • Do yoga poses.

MUSCLE RELAXATION

- Muscle relaxation exercises are generally used to help children release stress or tension, either in the moment or as an ongoing relaxation strategy. Exercises that target muscle relaxation can help children feel a sense of control over their body, and are useful for exploring and recognizing the contrast between states of tension and relaxation. When using these exercises, help children tune in to and notice variations in muscular/physical experience before, during, and after engaging in the activity.

MUSCLE RELAXATION

Developmental stage	Technique variation
Early childhood	• *Robot/rag doll:* Teach children to walk stiffly like a robot, then melt into a rag doll. • *Spaghetti:* Have children move like uncooked spaghetti, then cooked spaghetti. • *Caterpillar/butterfly:* Have children move like a caterpillar still in the cocoon, then spread their wings like a butterfly. • *Turtle/giraffe:* Have children act like a turtle going into a shell, then turn into a giraffe stretching for a leaf.
Middle childhood	• *Curl and release:* Teach children to crouch and curl up like a football player getting ready for a play. After crouching for a moment, yell "Hike" and have children stretch up to catch a throw. Have them also do it in slow motion for instant replay. • *Doorway stretch:* Have children push with both arms against doorframe, hold for count of 7, then release. Have children notice the difference between pushing and releasing. Variations can include pushing against a wall or against the therapist's or caregiver's hands.
Adolescence	• *Tense and release:* Have adolescents move through different muscle groups in the body, tensing and then releasing. Have them tune in to and notice the difference between sensations when muscles are tensed versus relaxed. • *Pair with breathing:* Have adolescents tense muscles while breathing in, then relax while breathing out.

IMAGERY

- Visual imagery, whether self- or other-guided, can be useful for increasing felt safety, decreasing arousal, and (re)gaining control when feeling out of control. Techniques should be geared to children's developmental stage and personal preferences.

IMAGERY

Developmental stage	Technique variation
Early childhood	*Safe place:* Imagery is difficult for young children and therefore must utilize concrete cues. For instance, rather than imagining a safe place, have children draw it and/or have them and caregivers create a concrete safe place within the home that children can go to when distressed. Similarly, designate a section of the office as each child's "safe place."
Middle childhood	Use images and concepts that are relevant to children. For instance: • Have children identify favorite superhero or superpower (tuning in to strength, bravery, etc.); have them imagine being with that figure or having the power themselves. • Identify favorite television, movie, or book character that children associate with a sense of safety or admiration; have them visualize being friends with that character. • Have children draw a favorite place, real or imaginary, and guide them through imagining it (e.g., "What do you see? Hear? Feel? Taste?"). Have them practice this at home.
Adolescence	Adolescents can utilize imagery techniques independently or with cuing, depending on preference. Concrete cues become less important. For instance: • Have adolescents imagine a peaceful, healing light entering their body and erasing areas of tension. • Have adolescents imagine a protective force field surrounding their body to keep them safe; adolescents can choose the color of the force field, who is in the field with them, physical sensations they are experiencing, temperature, etc. • Have adolescents imagine a positive future self, including the qualities they might have, the feelings of calm and strength, etc. • Have adolescents create an imaginary safe, peaceful place. Teach them that they can use this image for brief visits (e.g., if feeling stressed in class) or for longer periods (e.g., to calm down before bed).

OTHER MODULATION STRATEGIES

- Many modulation strategies do not fit neatly into the above categories, and many more possibilities exist than can be described in this text. We salute the occupational therapists and other professionals from whom we have learned about myriad ways to support children in achieving physiological organization. Note how many of these strategies resemble the soothing techniques naturally used in earlier developmental periods; for many children, these techniques may continue to assist them with modulation. *An important note*: It is crucial that children remain in felt control of any modulation strategy; any strategy into which a child is forced or coerced will ultimately be retraumatizing. Given that important caveat, we offer the following as examples:

BLANKET WRAP. Some children may respond to the containment and organization provided by wrapping themselves in a blanket, whether weighted or standard. Blanket wraps offer a child a way to seek nurturance, soothing, and physiological organization without the arousing qualities of more relational soothing (e.g., a hug). Blanket wraps may be an alternative for children who are reluctant to accept physical affection in the face of distress or who struggle with appropriate boundaries.

DEEP PRESSURE. Some children will respond to sensations of deep pressure. Pressure can be self-applied (e.g., using a "self massager") or other-applied (e.g., with the child's consent, using pillows above and below the child to make a "child sandwich"). Application of pressure by others should be done carefully and at the child's direction.

TACTILE ENGAGEMENT. There is a range of tactile sensations that children may find naturally modulating. Rinsing hands, molding clay, sifting through marbles, and tossing bean bags may each appeal differently to children. Explore (and observe) the tactile sensations toward which a child is naturally drawn.

ACTIVITY ENGAGEMENT. Many of the natural activities of childhood can be modulating and organizing for children. Pay attention to the way a child's energy changes when engaging in crafts or artwork, listening to a story, playing a board game, or playing with peers. Any activity can be organizing for one child but disorganizing for another. Similarly, an activity that increases arousal for one child may decrease it for another. Explore and track each child's responses.

APPRAISAL AND CONTROL. A number of activities require children to harness focus and control. A popular one at our center is balancing peacock feathers (with a nod to the colleague who first shared this activity with us; Macy, personal communication). Other activities may include rolling Chinese Baoding balls (also known as medicine balls) without them clinking or chiming, balancing on one foot, or walking across a low balance beam or in a straight line. We have found these activities to be most effective when paired with breathing (e.g., teach the child to breathe deeply, three times, before engaging in the activity). We have also found it useful to frame these as a "challenge" for younger clients: "Let's see how many tries it takes to balance the peacock feather for 10 seconds." Remind children to take their breaths, then let them go . . . even if it takes seven (very active) tries; by the seventh, successful effort, the child will typically be more organized and calmer.

SOUND. For some clients, the use of sound may provide either up- or down-regulating experiences. Consider experimenting with different music, sounds, and so on, to elicit desired changes in physiological/emotional states.

Skill #5: Alternating-States Regulation Strategies

- *Alternating-states regulation* involves helping children learn how to flow through and tolerate increasing and decreasing levels of arousal.
- Many of the following techniques involve using fun activities to teach children how to tune in to and change arousal level on cue.
- These techniques are often particularly useful in dyadic work.
- Each technique can be adapted to be relevant to a particular client or age; some may be more appropriate for younger or older children.

ALTERNATING-STATES REGULATION

Technique	Technique description
Turn up the volume	This exercise uses music or a symbolic "knob," "controller," or "slide switch" to cue faster or slower movement. It may be helpful to allow the child to be the controller first, while the therapist models faster or slower movement.

Description:
1. Decide what will be used to control movement.
2. Agree on ranges (e.g., hands in the middle means medium movement, hands up in the air means fast, softer music means slow).
3. Designate who the first controller will be.
4. As the controller shifts (music level, hand position, etc.), the other person moves faster or slower.

Slo-Mo	This exercise uses slow-motion movement to teach children how to slow themselves down. Once children have gained skill in moving in slow motion, they can be cued to shift into it when in a hyperaroused state.

Description:
1. Teach children to move in slow motion by first modeling a typical movement (e.g., yawning, running):
   THERAPIST: Have you ever seen someone move in slow motion before? It's like moving through jello, or through really, really thick water. Moving in slow motion looks really funny, but it's really hard to do. Watch—what if I ran in slow motion? It might look like this . . . *(demonstrate moving in slow motion).*
2. Invite the child to join you in a slow-motion movement; the child can pick the action. If it is an older child (e.g., 10- to 14-year-old boy), it is often helpful to make this a challenge: "Let's see who can move the slowest from here to there."
3. Practice shifting to slow motion in response to cues; walk around the room normally with a child and take turns yelling, "Slo-mo." When the cue is given, each person has to immediately shift to slow motion until the "Slo-mo-off" cue is given or until a "freeze" cue is given.
4. If the child becomes practiced in this technique, the cue can be incorporated into daily routine by caregivers, teachers, etc. (e.g., if child is running through the halls, the teacher cues "Slo-mo."

Stop–start	These exercises involve games that shift children's actions from movement to immobility (e.g., freeze). Many classic children's games fall into this category (i.e., Red Light/Green Light, Musical Chairs).

Description:
Note: Use adapted versions of classic children's games. Example here is given for "Freeze Dance."
1. Frame the game for the child:
   THERAPIST: We're going to play a game that helps you practice being in control of your body. *(Elicit from child, "When is it okay to move and be silly?" For example, at recess. "When is it important to slow your body down?" For example, in class.)* This game is kind of like Musical Chairs. When the music plays, we can jump around and be as silly as we want. When the music stops, we have to freeze.
2. One person should be selected to be the controller (in a therapy group, the leader is typically the controller). In individual therapy, the controller should still move after turning on the music.
3. The controller should turn the music off without warning; everyone freezes. The therapist should provide reinforcement for the child's ability to freeze on cue.
Note: Variations can include verbal cues ("Freeze," "Go"), visual cues (red stop sign, green go sign), etc.

Technique	Technique description
Big–small	Big–small techniques are used to help children connect all the parts of self through movement (big, medium, small) and to identify appropriate situations for each style. This technique is useful for children who have difficulty with gross motor control and with awareness of self in space. *Description:* 1. Help children identify all the ways in which their body physically expresses itself (voice, movement, speed, posture, etc.). 2. Start with the child's preferred way of moving. For instance, for a child who typically runs instead of walks, shouts instead of talks, etc., start with "big." 3. Select a day to be "Big Day" in therapy (or a portion of the therapy session). On that day, select an array of ways to move *big*. For instance, do a body trace on a life-size piece of paper, run and jump, talk loudly, etc. *Note:* It is often useful to do "Big Day" outdoors or some other place where it is appropriate to talk or move loudly. 4. During or after Big Day, help children identify places where they usually are "big"—for instance, at a park, at a swimming pool, on the beach, with their friends at recess, etc. 5. Follow up Big Day with Small Day (this is typically much harder for children). Draw on teeny pieces of paper, talk in a whisper, tiptoe, etc. As with Big Day, identify places where children are typically "small"—for instance, in the library, in a classroom, at night, etc. 6. Integrate concepts of big, medium, and small into therapy. For instance, if a child typically runs down the hall, cue him or her to "Walk small"; in therapy, shift from moving "small" to "medium" to "big."
Drumming	Drumming (with actual drums or tapping on the knees, desk, etc.) and/or the use of other musical instruments may help children modulate through faster/louder and slower/softer movements. This technique is particularly useful for children who have difficulty slowing down. Drumming also is an excellent attunement exercise. *Description:* 1. Select the instrument. Actual hand drums can be used, or children can thump on their knees or a table. 2. Provide ground rules: For instance, drum sticks may not be used to hit anything other than the drum. 3. Both clinician and child should use the same instrument. 4. Possible variations: 　a. Follow-the-leader. Take turns tapping out a pattern. The second person must copy the pattern. Be conscious of incorporating faster and slower patterns. 　b. Simultaneous follow-the-leader. One person is designated as "leader"; the other person must match the first person's rhythm and/or pace. Take turns as leader and follower.

Special Topic: Self-Harming Behaviors

- Self-harm is a complex topic; safety should be prioritized in any treatment.

- A number of authors have developed interventions that include detailed modules for working with individuals who self-harm (e.g., Linehan, 1993; Miller, Rathus, & Linehan, 2006). Therapists are encouraged to familiarize themselves with the array of techniques for evaluating and intervening with self-harm. In the following table we offer some teaching points on self-harm as they relate to modulation work with children impacted by developmental trauma.

SELF-HARMING BEHAVIORS AND AFFECT MODULATION: KEY CONCEPTS

Self-harming behaviors generally represent the child's or adolescent's attempt to modulate emotional experience. Although it is not healthy, self-harm is used because it is—in the moment, at least—effective.

When intervening with self-harming behaviors, it is important to (1) understand the function of the behavior and (2) provide safer alternatives.

Be aware that, as with any modulation strategy, self-harm may serve dual functions. It may act as:
- A *down-regulation* strategy, helping the child turn off overwhelming affect.
- An *up-regulation* strategy, helping the child come back from a numb or constricted state.

Note that children may use self-harm to serve different functions at different times.

Replacement strategies should attempt to match the original function of the self-harming behavior.

Since trauma often occurs within a relational context, social support may not be a viable option for children and adolescents in times of significant distress. Therefore, to the degree possible, it is often useful for replacement strategies to include those that can be implemented independently.

It is important to provide psychoeducation about the function of self-harm. Help children and adolescents (and their caregivers) understand the role that self-harm has played in their attempts to modulate their own experience. Involve them in developing alternative strategies.

It is important that there be a balance between addressing imminent risk and providing a safe environment in which to discuss and address self-harming behavior. Self-harm often involves shame and secrecy, along with extreme reactions from caregivers (and, at times, clinicians). If every instance of self-harm is met with threats of hospitalization or extensive increase in services, the client's ability to actively participate in learning new skills will be reduced. Pay attention to your own emotional responses to a client's self-harm and work with caregivers to both understand and tolerate their own emotional reactions.

ᴪᴪᴪ DEVELOPMENTAL CONSIDERATIONS

Developmental stage	Affect modulation considerations
Early childhood	At this stage the role of the caregiver in affect modulation is crucial. Young children depend on caregivers for support and nurturing, and it would not be developmentally appropriate to expect them to modulate all on their own. Involve caregivers, as much as possible, in affect modulation work.
	Physiological regulation provided by caregivers (e.g., cuddling, rocking, back rubs) is often important for young children. However, keep in mind that some children may have built defenses against touch. It is important to normalize this response for caregivers and to help them find acceptable ways to interact physically with their children, while respecting the children's need for boundaries. Teach caregivers to ask even young children for permission to touch—allow some control.
	Younger children normatively view degrees of feeling in terms of extremes (e.g., big vs. small), rather than in nuanced increments. Match their level when teaching degrees of feeling and use concrete markers wherever possible. For instance: • Use of arms to show how big a feeling is • Use concrete anchors: for example, "feelings as big as this room," "feelings as small as a penny" • Coloring in (circles, thermometers, etc.)
Middle childhood	During this stage, children are increasingly able to identify degrees of emotion. Help children tune in to subtler variations of their own emotional experiences.
	Help children stop arousal *before* it hits crisis level. Children at this age can be taught to recognize internal cues of escalating arousal (e.g., changes in body state) as well as external cues (e.g., people saying, "Shhh"). Pair this recognition with modulation techniques.
	Increase child's involvement in modulation strategies at this stage. For instance, if a child identifies being "50 poker chips mad," ask, "What would it take to get you down to 45 poker chips?" Put children in the position of power/knowledge about their own affect state.

Developmental stage	Affect modulation considerations
Adolescence	Adolescents may be increasingly sophisticated in their capacity to understand changes in emotional experience. However, when triggered, adolescents may regress to earlier emotional stages and have difficulty making use of developed skills.
	Continue to provide external cuing and reinforcement, but be aware that adolescents may resist supports.
	Adolescents are at particular risk for use of risky modulation strategies, such as self-harm and/or substance use. It is particularly important that an adolescent have a repertoire of modulation skills that can be implemented independently.

🏠 APPLICATIONS

🏠 *Individual/Dyadic*

Modulation activities are often an important focus of individual therapy, as dysregulation in its various manifestations is a typical reason for referral. We view the building of modulation abilities as a process that involves many components, including the caregiver's own affect management, attunement, and support, as well as the child's awareness and understanding of his or her own physiological and emotional states and a slow building of skill in managing these.

An essential foundation of this work is developing a common language with a child and caregiver to serve as a cue for future attempts at modulation (e.g., "I see that your energy is getting really big . . . ") as well as in depathologizing child behaviors and responses. Similarly, engaging the caregiver and child in the building and using of feeling and energy "tools" supports agency on both sides and creates an expectation that the child and caregiver are collaborators in observing and managing arousal.

We have found it useful to build modulation practice into our session routine; for instance, children who typically enter the session with a great deal of energy may need a quick up-regulation activity to meet them where they are at, and then a focusing or down-regulation activity to help them engage. Many modulation activities are perceived by younger children as games; by adding a reflective or curious layer to the game (e.g., noticing the child's energy shift or asking about the child's experience), the clinician can help the child build awareness of his or her body's energy and control.

Many modulation activities can be applied in the moment to help a child navigate difficult moments like session transitions. For instance, an older child can be cued to walk up the hall at an energy level of 3 instead of 7; a younger child can be cued to walk up the hall as a turtle or in slow motion. Modulation strategies for adolescents can be practiced and planned for negotiating anticipated challenges. For instance, prior to inviting a caregiver into a session for a difficult conversation, explore and practice with the adolescent strategies (e.g., holding a grounding stone, squeezing a stress ball, doing deep breathing) that will help him or her maintain an effective level of modulation. Any attempts at modulation (whether successful or not) should be noticed and reinforced by the clinician and (ideally) by the caregiver. Effective tools should be shared with caregivers, so that they can be practiced and reinforced in the home setting.

Beyond session tools, work with caregivers to notice and incorporate into daily life activities that naturally modulate and organize a child (e.g., drawing, cuddling, listening to music, singing) as well as to pay attention to the events and activities that seem to disorganize a child.

When these events/activities are unavoidable (e.g., transitions), consider ways to build modulation exercises into the routine. For many children, adjunctive activities such as participating in sports, martial arts, yoga, or the performing and expressive arts provide natural forums for learning how to control, manage, and express arousal and emotion.

🏠 Group

Many of the skills, exercises, and psychoeducation described in this chapter can be incorporated into group activities. As in individual therapy, modulation activities can be incorporated into group session routine (e.g., a starting "warm-up," opening "energy check," closing "cool down"). Consider paying attention to group modulation as well as individual modulation: For instance, at the start of a group, plot all members' energy levels on a magnetic or paper thermometer. Notice differences in group dynamics when all group members are at high energy versus low or diffuse energy levels.

Many modulation activities work particularly well in a group format. For instance, drumming, turn-up-the-volume games, and follow-the-leader activities all work well in groups, and can be adapted to apply to younger children as well as adolescents.

🏠 Milieu

Building an awareness of and support for modulation is essential to supporting the experience of children and adolescents who struggle with management of arousal and emotion within a milieu environment. A primary first step for many milieus (schools, residential programs, hospital settings, etc.) is learning to differentiate the need for limits from the need for modulation. Note that these are not mutually exclusive; however, it is often helpful to consider these a two-step process: When a child or adolescent is dysregulated, noncompliant, overly shut down, etc., the *first step* is to support the child in modulating him- or herself (including ensuring physical safety); the *second step* is to apply limits and consequences, when appropriate. It is our experience that for many milieu programs, application of consequences in moments of significant arousal leads inevitably to escalation, as the child or adolescent feels increasingly helpless and triggered; ultimately, this arousal and mutual escalation may lead to a need for physical restraint. In programs in which we worked to build an increased awareness of modulation strategies, along with support for staff members and awareness of their own affect management needs, restraints dropped to almost zero, *despite a complete lack of focus on restraint reduction as a target.*

Modulation can be supported via daily routines. Consider, for instance, use of focusing activities at the start of the school day; relaxation and yoga groups as youth are making significant transitions or schedule shifts; energizing activities such as sports to help youth express energy after lengthy periods of focused time; and down-regulating activities in the evening. It is particularly important to pay attention to decreasing highly arousing activities in the evening, given the particular difficulty of traumatized children in navigating the transition from wakefulness to sleep.

Many modulation tools can be made available throughout a milieu. We have worked with programs that have (1) incorporated baskets of hand-held manipulatives into the classroom (allowing children to squeeze stress balls, twist Wikki Stix, etc., to manage arousal); (2) built and filled Feelings Toolboxes for each child to keep in his or her room; and (3) added blankets, pillows, and other self-soothing materials into classic time-out rooms. Our favorite example is the "Sensory Room" built by one program to replace one of their time-out rooms. The room is lit softly, lined with blankets and pillows, and contains baskets of materials designed to appeal to the five senses (e.g., a range of tactile objects, various lotions, pictures of peaceful scenes, different kinds of music). Rather than simply being placed in a time-out area, adolescents in this program are given the option of requesting time in the sensory room.

Addressing modulation is one of the domains in which programs can be the most creative, given the "buy-in" and understanding of the staff. Psychoeducation and support for staff—and the parallel active practice of modulation by team members at all levels—are essential for successful change in this area.

🌐 REAL-WORLD THERAPY

🌐 **Practice, but be realistic.** Children will not be able to apply modulation skills in the moment immediately; it takes time for these to translate from the intervention setting to the real world. Help kids stick with it. Allow time each week for children to practice these skills.

🌐 **Why should I?** Admit it—sometimes it feels good to feel angry, or sad, or over-the-top excited. Don't be too quick to modulate—a child may need time to engage in a feeling or energy state before working to change it. As long as a child is safe, don't rush the state shift.

Affect Expression

★ KEY CONCEPTS

★ *Why Target Affect Expression?*

- Sharing emotional experience is a key aspect of human relationships. An inability to effectively communicate affect prevents children from being able to form and maintain ongoing healthy attachments and subsequently from mastering developmental tasks that rely heavily on this skill. There are several reasons why expression may be impacted in children who have experienced trauma:

  ♦ *Early attachment.* In a healthy attachment relationship, children's emotional experiences are validated by reflection, mirroring, and appropriate response by caregivers to shared information. When children's attempts to communicate emotion are met with anger, rejection, and/or indifference, they learn two things:

    1. **Shame.** "My emotions are wrong, bad, or unimportant."

    2. **Need for secrecy.** "If I share my emotions, something bad will happen."

  ♦ *Vulnerability.* Emotions are an aspect of human existence associated, in many ways, with vulnerability. Sharing emotions allows others a window into the internal self. Acknowledging fear, sadness, anger, or joy involves risk for everyone, but particularly for a child who has experienced harm. In the mindset of a child who has been exposed to family violence, for instance, acknowledging joy raises the possibility of it being taken away; expressing anger may increase the potential of threat. For children whose lives have been organized around survival, minimization of risk is often a primary adaptation. Learning to hide emotional experience may help children feel more in control or less vulnerable.

★ *How Does Trauma Impact Affect Expression?*

- In the face of shame and a need for secrecy, children may *fail to share emotional experience* with others. They may:
    - ◆ Put on a "false front" (e.g., "Everything's fine").
    - ◆ Isolate themselves.
    - ◆ Substitute acceptable emotions for unacceptable ones, or powerful emotions for less powerful ones.
    - ◆ Minimize emotional experience.
- Emotions that are not expressed in healthy ways may emerge in other forms, such as:
    - ◆ *Somatic expression:* for example, headaches, stomachaches, fatigue
    - ◆ *Behavioral expression:* for example, disorganization, agitation, withdrawal
- Children may also *attempt to communicate emotion in ineffective ways*; for instance, they may:
    - ◆ Substitute actions for verbal communication (e.g., punching instead of telling someone they are angry).
    - ◆ Externalize emotions by projecting them onto others (e.g., "I think my mom is really sad about this").
- Some children *overcommunicate*—that is, they share information indiscriminately, without awareness of appropriate boundaries. This may occur for different reasons:
    - ◆ **Inability to contain intrusive traumatic material.** Children may experience recurrent, intrusive memories that are triggered by thoughts, feelings, interactions, etc. In the face of this *reexperiencing*, indiscriminate sharing (i.e., detailed retelling of traumatic experiences) may be an attempt to gain mastery over overwhelming internal material. However, in the absence of modulation strategies, this attempt at mastery may actually be retraumatizing. Furthermore, an inability to discriminate appropriate contexts for sharing this material may have negative social and emotional consequences.
    - ◆ **Poor relational awareness.** Children may also overcommunicate about nontraumatic material. In an attempt to connect, form relationships, or meet emotional needs, children may share overly personal information with individuals with whom they have not yet developed relational intimacy. This ineffective attempt to share emotional experience often ends up backfiring, as others may distance themselves in an attempt to reattain appropriate boundaries.

🧰 THERAPIST TOOLBOX

🎬 *Behind the Scenes*

- The goal of affect expression work is to support children in learning to effectively share emotional experience with others, in order to meet emotional or practical needs.
- Because affect expression may be impacted in a number of ways, different skills may need to

be targeted. Assess whether children's difficulties include knowledge of with *whom* to share, knowledge of *how* to communicate, and/or knowledge of *what* to communicate.

- Because the goal is *effective* communication, it is often important to pair modulation skills with affect expression work. For instance, a child who is in a calm state will be more effective in communicating frustration to a teacher or caregiver than one who is angry or hyperaroused.

- Effective communication is largely governed by context. What is effective and appropriate in one setting (e.g., with peers) may be ineffective in another (e.g., with grandparents). Clinicians should explore the nuances of effective communication, including issues such as language choice, boundaries, style of interacting, etc., in building affect expression skills.

⊏ The ways in which humans express emotions are strongly influenced by culture. The use of language (or not), the role of nonverbal cues, the nuances of interaction, and even choosing with whom to share with are all impacted by culture. Consider the following example:

> In certain native Alaskan tribal cultures, direct eye contact by a child toward an adult may be considered disrespectful. Facial expressions, to an outside observer, may appear constricted and flat. A clinician began treatment with a 12-year-old boy of native Alaskan background who had been terminated from three prior therapies due to therapists' belief that he could not "do the work." In building a forum for therapeutic communication with this child, the clinician learned that the most comfortable expression for him occurred when he was engaged in parallel, nonverbal activities.

In this example, had the clinician failed to take into account the role of culture in this child's interaction, he might have misinterpreted the child's behaviors as avoidant or resistant. In working with this child, pushing him to make eye contact (as described later in this section) would have run counter to his cultural norms and would be likely to cause distress. When working with children and families, it is important to understand the role of cultural norms in typical emotional expression, as well as the ways these intersect with the dominant culture.

- Affect expression work frequently happens in the moment. Tune in to signs or statements that reflect emotional experience. Ask questions to expand children's communication. Reinforce attempts to share experience. Work with caregivers to model effective strategies.

⌂ *Teach to Caregivers*

- *Reminder:* Teach the caregiver the Key Concepts.

- *Reminder:* Teach the caregiver relevant Developmental Considerations.

- *Reminder:* Review trauma response and triggers. Because children will be less able to access language when triggered, the caregiver(s) will often need to practice modulation support strategies prior to eliciting the child's expression of affect.

- Attunement work with caregivers will help support children's emotional expression. As appropriate, integrate caregivers into sessions so that communication about emotional experience can be practiced in the moment. Treatment often provides a safe forum for familial communication. Have caregivers reframe the child's somatic and behavioral expressions by linking them with possible "I" statements.

- Help caregivers apply reflective listening skills, as taught in Attunement.

- Teach caregivers to model "I" statements when communicating their own experience to the child.

- Help caregivers develop routine forums in the home to encourage familial communication. Forums can be informal or formal. For instance, informal forums include eating a meal together, bedtime rituals, family meetings, etc. Formal strategies can also be used. With younger children, concrete methods, such as a family feelings chart, can be helpful (e.g., a whiteboard with each member's name, on which all family members draw or select a feelings face each day to show how they are feeling or how their day went). For adolescents, communication logs can be used to share experience. Set up family expectations around how the logs will be used (e.g., each person must write one entry in the log each day, such as how they felt about one thing that happened that day).

⫽ *Tools:* **Affect Expression Tools**

Skill #1: Identifying Resources for Emotional Expression

Goal   Building children's awareness of safe people with whom to share emotional experience

Materials   Paper, crayons or markers, photographs of safe people (optional)

Description

- **Teach importance of expressing feelings:** Why do people need to share emotional experience with others?
  - ◆ *Point 1:* "**When kids keep feelings all to themselves, they may come out in lots of other ways, like stomachaches, headaches, and behavior.**" Check in with child: How does he or she think feelings come out? Query about different types of feelings.
  - ◆ *Point 2:* "**Talking to other people about feelings can sometimes help kids get what they want or need.**" Give an example (e.g., if mad about something a family member is doing, the child cannot tell anyone, and things probably won't change . . . or the child can communicate how he or she feels and work toward a resolution).
  - ◆ *Point 3:* "**Letting other people know how we feel can help us feel better. Sometimes, we can't change what's going on, but people who know how we're feeling can help us deal with it.**" Query: Can child think of a time when other people supported him or her in a hard situation?

- **Help the child identify safe people in his or her life.** If the child has difficulty doing this, make suggestions. Consider caregivers, teachers, friends, other relatives, therapist, etc. Note that different people may be safe for different things. Help children differentiate who can help when they are angry, sad, scared, happy, etc.

- **Make it concrete.** Create lists (or drawings, pictures, book, etc.) of safe resources.

- *Circles of Trust:* On a blank piece of paper, write the child's name in the center (or draw a picture). Draw a series of circles around the child. Teach the child: "**We all have different people in our life. Some of them we're really close to, and we can tell them anything. Other people we're kind of close to, and we can tell them some things, and still other people we know just to say 'hi,' or talk about little things like schoolwork, sports, or TV shows.**" With the child's help, write names in each circle, showing increasing intimacy as the circles become closer to the child. Help the child identify different types of information he or she feels comfortable sharing with people in each circle. Explore differences in communication style with different resources and across contexts. (*Note:* A sample form appears in Appendix D.)

- **Circles of Trust expansion:** Expand on this or similar exercises to explore the child's interpersonal relationships further. For instance, explore *roles* that different individuals play. Have the child circle, in different colors, people to whom the child can talk about important things, people with whom the child has fun, people who comfort the child, etc. Any individual can be circled more than once. Use this technique to explore types of relationships the child has, and/or the types of relationships the child may want to build. Use arrows to indicate the child's satisfaction with level of intimacy: An arrow pointed inward may indicate someone with whom the child wants to become closer; one pointed outward may indicate someone from whom the child wants distance.

Effectively Using Resources

- Even with awareness of social resources, children who have experienced trauma may have difficulty effectively communicating emotional experience. Given a history of failed or rejected attempts at self-expression, and/or a lack of modeling and early "practice" in sharing experience, these children may have failed to develop key skills.

- The activities in the following table target several areas of vulnerability that may interfere with a child's ability to effectively communicate with identified resources. These vulnerable areas include initiating communication, using effective nonverbal communication, and using effective verbal communication.

- The overarching goal of these activities is to support children in effectively communicating their feelings to identified resources. However, be aware that failure to share experience is often due only in part to skills deficits; difficulty with trust and lack of perceived safety in relationships also play a key role. It is therefore important to pair this work with the previous skill (building awareness of key safe resources).

Skill #2: Initiating Communication

Picking your moment	*Rationale:* It is important for children with trauma histories to be successful in sharing their emotional experiences with others, because past communication has often been met with rejection, punishment, or indifference. Teaching children how to identify appropriate moments to initiate support can help with successful interaction.
	Steps: Consider the following steps: • Teach children that communication is more effective if the other person is ready to hear them. Ask children to consider when they might not want to listen to someone else. (If a child has a hard time, give examples: when busy, when in a hurry, when talking to someone else, when mad or grumpy, etc.) • Help children identify "good times" and "not-so-good times" to share their feelings with people in general. • Select the safest (most talked to, most liked, etc.) people on the child's list of identified resources. Help the child identify specific "good" and "not-so-good" times for each of those people. Help the child describe specific cues (e.g., "How do you know when your mother is busy?"). • Ask the child, "Have there ever been times when you tried to communicate with one of those safe people, and it didn't work?" Problem-solve together about why the interaction might not have gone well. • If appropriate, invite the child's caregiver(s) or other safe communication resources to do a portion of this work dyadically. Have the child and the caregiver problem-solve together about good ways to initiate communication.
Initiating conversation	*Rationale:* Often, children who have experienced trauma have historically attempted to communicate through indirect means. The goal of this skill is to teach them to directly communicate a need to share experience.

	Steps: Consider the following steps:
	• Teach children that the first step in effective communication is letting someone know you want to communicate. Ask the child, "How do you know when different people in your life want to talk to you?"
	• Teach children how to let other people know they want to talk. Consider multiple modalities:
	  ♦ *Verbal:* "I'd like to talk to you."
	  ♦ *Gestural:* Secret hand signal (that both parties know in advance).
	  ♦ *Written:* Leaving a note for caregiver.
	  ♦ *Symbolic:* Door sign or other symbol requesting communication.

- Differentiate *immediate* versus *delayed* responses to communication bids. Sometimes a caregiver will be able to respond immediately to a child's request for communication, but other times this response will necessarily be delayed.
  - Discuss reasons why it may sometimes be necessary to delay communication.
  - Set up rules or expectations with the identified communication resource. For instance, if the child leaves the caregiver a note or hangs a door sign, by when will the caregiver respond (e.g., before bedtime? by dinner?)?
  - Help children identify modulation strategies to help with tolerating delays in communication.

Skill #3: Building Nonverbal Communication Skills

⌂ When working with children on nonverbal communication skills, keep in mind that there is significant variation in what is considered normative and appropriate. Family norms, culture, and other contextual variables all impact acceptable nonverbal signals. For instance, in some families, a child looking directly at his or her parents may be considered a sign of disrespect; in others, *not* looking directly may be considered disrespectful. Take the time to assess, with both the child and the family, their understanding of the meaning of nonverbal cues such as those discussed in the following table.

NONVERBAL COMMUNICATION SKILLS

Rationale	One of the contributors to traumatized children's difficulty with effective emotional expression is difficulty using nonverbal cues to communicate effectively.
Teaching point	• Teach children that communication involves more than words or language. Often, nonverbal cues (eye contact, tone of voice, etc.) are important clues that help other people read or understand what we are trying to communicate. • *Ask:* **"Have you ever thought someone was angry at you, even if they didn't say anything? How could you tell? If someone is yelling at you, does that make it easier or harder for you to talk to them? Learning about nonverbal cues—what we do with our voice and body—helps us communicate more effectively."**

Target the following specific skills:

Tone of voice	**Goal:** Teach children to speak in a conversational tone of voice (not too loud, not too soft) when communicating their feelings to others. **Possible activities:** • Select an emotion and a situation. Role-play a conversation between two people. Have one conversation in an overly loud (or overly soft) tone of voice. Repeat the role play in a conversational tone. 　　◆ Afterward discuss what the conversation felt like to the child. Was it different, using different tones of voice? 　　◆ Play out different possible endings. Be realistic—how might someone respond if the other person is yelling? Speaking calmly? Whispering? • Refer back to feelings detective work (in Chapter 8, "Affect Identification"). Have children create a list of their own "emotion clues." • Work with both child and caregiver to develop a list of nonverbal clues (one for caregiver, one for child) connected to different emotions. • Work with both child and caregiver to pick a topic and practice communicating in a calm tone. Start with a neutral topic and work toward more difficult topics. Provide lots of reinforcement for successful communication! • Have caregiver and child create a list together of "communication rules"—how do they respectfully communicate? Pay attention to respectful communication by the caregiver as well as the child.

Physical
space

Goal: Teach children how to maintain comfortable/appropriate physical boundaries when communicating, and how to read other people's "physical space" cues.

Possible activities:
- **Teach child:**
  - ♦ "We all have a 'comfort zone': an invisible area around our body that is ours alone, and other people should not enter that space without permission."
  - ♦ "Our comfort zone can grow bigger or smaller, depending on who the other person is, what kind of mood we're in, what kind of mood the other person is in, etc."
  - ♦ "Our comfort zone helps us to feel safe."
  - ♦ "When we're talking to other people, we have to pay attention to their comfort zone, too. If we're too close or too far, it's hard for them to listen to us, because their brain will be too focused on not having enough space or having too much."
- **Own your zone:** The child stands still, and the therapist (or caregiver, other child) should stand across the room. When the child gives permission, the second person should begin walking toward the child. When the child decides the other person is "comfortably close," child says, "Stop." Once the second person stops, the child can make adjustments, as needed (e.g., take a small step back) until comfortable. Possible additions:
  - ♦ Use a measuring tape to measure child's preferred space.
  - ♦ Pretend that the second person represents different people (e.g., child's mother, teacher, best friend, biggest enemy). Repeat exercise and make note of different space requirements.
  - ♦ Have second person convey different emotional states while walking toward child (e.g., very angry, very excited). Make note of different space requirements.
  - ♦ With child's permission, enter his or her comfort zone. Have child (1) notice what she feels and (2) notice what she does (e.g., leans back, steps back). Teach child that these are cues others may give if she enters their comfort zone.
  - ♦ Reverse roles. Have child walk toward second person; repeat exercise and/or variations.
- **Personal bubble:** Have the child create a circle with his arms, or use a piece of string to create a circle around the child. Teach him that everything enclosed by the circle is his personal space, and that other people have the same amount of space. Practice (and model) asking permission to enter the other person's space.
- **Coping with space violations:** Although it is important to know our spatial needs, sometimes we are unable to control our boundary as much as we would like (e.g., on a crowded train, in a busy line in the school cafeteria). Work with children to identify strategies for coping with inadvertent spatial violations.

Eye
contact

Goal: Teach children that eye contact can help other people know that we are listening and paying attention to what they are saying, that we are interested in the conversation, and that what they (or we) are saying is important.

Possible activities:
- **Messages we send:** Pick a scenario that involves interaction between two people. Consider scenarios such as asking to have a need met, asking for support, giving advice or support, etc. Act out the scenario two times (at least). The first time, do not make eye contact; the second time, do. Play out possible different scenarios: How interested is the second person? How available is he or she to the conversation or to the request? Discuss afterward.
- **Active listener:** Have child tell a story to you (or to caregiver, other child, etc.). Second person may *not* speak. For the first minute, have the second person sit with face turned away; for the second minute, allow the second person to make eye contact while listening. Explore what it feels like when someone is looking, versus not, while listening. Reverse roles.
- **Ball toss (group activity):** Have group sit in a circle. Toss a ball around. Each child must throw to the same person each time, and everyone must be thrown to within the pattern. Before tossing the ball, child must say the person's name and make eye contact. Tell children, "See how fast you can get!" Discuss tuning into how eye contact helps make throwing more accurate.

Skill #4: Building Verbal Communication Skills

VERBAL COMMUNICATION: "I" STATEMENTS

Rationale	Language is the most direct means of communication: Before anything else, people listen to the words we say. Using appropriate, direct language is often the best way for children to get their emotional needs met and to share experience. "I" statements are a specific way to let people know how we feel, what we want, and what we need.
"I" statements	**Possible activities:**

          • Teach child that "I" statements are ways to let other people know how we feel. There are a lot of different ways we can start a sentence:
               ♦ I feel _____ (or, When _____ happened, I felt _____).
               ♦ I want _____.
               ♦ I would like _____.
               ♦ I need _____ etc.
               ♦ It makes me feel _____ when you _____.
          • Have children practice using above statements to describe past and/or current experiences.
          • **What I Need:** Help children develop a list of what helps when they are trying to share emotional experience (e.g., a hug, silence, brainstorming, help thinking of ways to feel better). Keep in mind that the list may differ for different people or different feelings. Help child practice using "I statements" to ask for those. If possible, bring caregiver into session and do this exercise interactively.
          • Use this technique in the moment and connect it with affect identification skills. When a child describes an experience that involves emotions, prompt him or her to use "I" statements to describe the emotional experience (e.g., "When your aunt did that, how did that make you feel?").

Skill #5: Self-Expression

- Expressing emotional experience is not always about communicating to others; sometimes *self*-expression is equally important.

- The goal of these activities is to help children build a repertoire for symbolically and/or directly expressing their inner experience.

- Often, children may choose to share the product of suggested activities with others; however, the primary goal here is to build expression resources that are (1) *not* dependent on others and (2) go beyond a verbal exchange.

- Keep in mind that many expressive strategies may lead to an increase in children's arousal. Teach children to pair expression with previously learned modulation strategies.

- Possibilities here are almost endless. Different possible modalities for self-expression are suggested in the following table. Help children identify and refine their own preferred means of self-expression.

EMOTIONAL SELF-EXPRESSION

Play	As one of the most important ways young children share their experience, play in any form—with puppets, dollhouse characters, animals, and other figures—can be used to help children express emotions in a displaced manner. Clinicians (and caregivers) can introduce effective communication strategies, emotional support, and possible resolutions into the play whenever possible.

        Example:
          • The child has previously witnessed domestic violence. In the child's play, the child character is hitting the mother character. The therapist might:
               ♦ *Observe:* "Wow, that boy looks really angry."
               ♦ *Query about communication:* "How can that boy tell his mom that he's mad without hitting?"

♦ *Take on a role in the play:* [Therapist enters as "neighbor."] "I heard lots of yelling. Is everyone okay? Can I help?"
♦ *Suggest communication:* "What if that boy tried telling his mom that he needed to talk? What do you think might happen?"

Art	Use drawing, painting, clay, etc., to help children express themselves. With young children, structure is often helpful; however, create a balance between structured and unstructured time to allow for children's creativity. • In addition to general activities, consider incorporating art into familial (or other) communication. For instance, use strategies such as "picture of the day" to allow children to use a drawing to communicate experience with their families. • *Collages* are a wonderful group project for self-expression, but also useful one on one. • *Outside–Inside:* Masks, boxes, two-sided faces, etc., can be used to help children express what they think people see on the *outside* (labels, masks, "fake fronts," etc.), and how they feel on the *inside*.
Writing	Support children in the use of writing for self-expression. Forms of writing might include poetry, journaling, fiction/stories, lyrics/raps, etc. Consider providing a journal for each child (and/or creating one in session through use of construction paper, blank paper, etc.). Invite children to share some of their writing, if comfortable, with one of the safe resources identified in "Identifying Resources" work (Skill #1, this chapter).
Movement	Movement includes dance as well as more focused expressive movements. For instance, a child who wishes to express anger at an individual who is not present (e.g., an absent father) can develop a strategy of "symbolically" expressing (e.g., throwing clay at a target on the wall, modeling and then punching down clay). Keep in mind: This type of activity may increase arousal and should be paired with modulation strategies.
Drama	Acting is a way for children to express feelings, experiences, etc., in a displaced way. Acting techniques can be incorporated into sessions, and/or children can be encouraged to take part in adjunctive, theatre-based programs.
Music	Music provides a powerful nonverbal expression strategy. Even children who do not have an immediate interest in, or talent for, a musical instrument can effectively express themselves on drums or other simple musical instruments. In addition, the process of sharing music (e.g., having a child bring a favorite CD or song to the therapy session) can act as a vehicle for communication of internal experience.

👪 DEVELOPMENTAL CONSIDERATIONS

Developmental stage	Affect expression considerations
Early childhood	Caregivers are generally the primary resource for shared communication for young children. It is particularly important to include caregivers in sessions for this age group. Young children's communication is generally more concrete and less sophisticated than that of older children or adolescents. Often, their sharing of experience will simply let important adults know how they feel. It is important that adults take greater responsibility for noticing and eliciting communication and identifying child needs. Because early childhood is an egocentric stage, young children will have greater difficulty considering others' perspectives, reading cues, etc., and expectations for these skills should be limited.
Middle childhood	Peers, teachers, and other adults may become important resources for communication in addition to primary caregivers. Because children's social worlds are expanding during this time period, understanding of appropriate boundaries and social resources becomes particularly important. Help children learn to differentiate with whom they can share different kinds of experience.

Developmental stage	Affect expression considerations
Adolescence	The peer group becomes a primary resource for communication during adolescence, and a desire for increased privacy from caregivers is a normative developmental shift.
	Work with caregivers to tolerate decreased detailed communication and to tolerate the adolescent's increased need for independence. However, help caregivers and adolescents strike a balance. For instance, it may be important for an adolescent to communicate to a caregiver, "I'm angry and need some space," but the details of the emotion or precipitating events may not necessarily need to be shared immediately.
	Avoid all-or-nothing interactions. It is important that (1) caregivers remain available for communication, (2) adolescents continue to view them as a resource, and (3) certain lines of communication remain open. Help adolescents define material that may be important to share with caregivers.

 ## APPLICATIONS

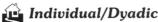 ### *Individual/Dyadic*

Work with the child on the skills identified in the section titled "Therapist Toolbox." Because affect expression generally involves expression *to* someone, whenever possible, integrate caregivers or other appropriate adults directly into this work. It is particularly important to work with caregivers when building communication strategies. Help caregivers and children develop communication routines together. Consider the following example:

> An adoptive mother of five children had a busy schedule and many demands on her time. However, it was important to her that each of her children have the opportunity for "special" one-on-one time. In addition to routinely scheduled time together, she took each of her children to the store to pick out a special blanket, in different colors. The blanket acted as a tool for comfort and security, but also served a different purpose. When one of her children was having a particularly hard day or needed to talk about something, he or she hung the blanket on her doorknob. The mother's promise was that, if she saw the child's blanket on her door, she would find time to sit with that child and talk before the child went to bed that night.

Beyond primary caregivers, work with the child and the surrounding systems (e.g., school, day care) to develop communication plans and resources for when the child is not at home. Develop concrete plans for how a child could access safe communication resources when needed (e.g., at school, while at friends' homes). Consider working with collaterals on appropriate ways to cue the child to use communication resources, when needed.

In addition to the specific skills listed, this target involves an exploration of the meaning and understanding of interpersonal relationships, both present and historical, and the impact of making oneself vulnerable in relationship. For older children and adolescents in particular, it will be important to take the time to explore these ideas and to process any thoughts and feelings that may emerge.

🏠 Group

Many affect expression exercises lend themselves well to a group format. Consider using role play or other improvisational theatre techniques as a way to have group members practice appropriate communication or identify inappropriate communication (often, a more fun exercise for kids!). "Own your zone" (boundaries) and the ball toss exercises (eye contact) are all great group activities and good forums for eliciting discussion of individual differences and similarities in nonverbal communication cues. Exercises targeting identification of resources also translate easily to group format, but be cautious about the need for privacy, particularly with adolescent clients; allow clients to use initials or other symbolic markings to keep their information private.

🏠 Milieu

Integrate group activities described above into milieu clinical programs. Within the milieu, work with individual clients to identify communication resources. Troubleshoot communication plans: for instance, a child might identify a particular staff member as his or her "safest" resource, but what will the child do on a day when that staff member is unavailable? Build strategies that allow all to communicate feelings, needs, and thoughts both verbally and nonverbally. For example, in residential programs, we have found door signs and door magnets to be useful communication techniques. Door signs can be decorated by the resident so that one side reflects a positive mood, or a desire for interaction, while the other side reflects harder feelings, a desire for comfort, or a desire to be left alone. A magnet on the door can be used to request one-on-one time with a staff member. It is crucial that all staff members receive training about the rationale behind the use of these strategies and the importance of consistent follow-through with the established response.

When working with staff members to support youth expression, it is important to differentiate the *goal* of expression from the *method* and the *message*. In other words, support staff in reinforcing youth attempts to communicate, even if the communication itself is less than ideal. Consider the following example:

> A 15-year-old girl in a residential program walks out of a group session. When a staff member follows her and asks her what is going on, she yells, "This group sucks—I'm sick of it. You all must think I'm some kind of *** to sit and talk about this stuff."

In her own way, this adolescent is attempting to communicate. What are the possible responses? One possibility is to respond to her *method* of communicating: "You're being really inappropriate, and you've just lost 5 points for swearing." A second possibility is to respond to her *message:* "It seems like everyone else is getting something from this group, you just need to try harder." A third possibility is to respond to her *attempt at communication:* "I can see that you have pretty strong feelings about this group, and I'd really like to hear them. It's hard for me to do that when you're this upset. Can we try to find a way to calm down first and then talk about this?" *Note:* Although the third option is, from our perspective, a more therapeutic response to the adolescent's attempt to communicate, we do not negate that within a program, the first two options may be equally valid responses. In selecting a response, we urge staff to consider timing: first support expression, along with appropriate modulation, before addressing limits or other consequences for behavior.

🌐 REAL-WORLD THERAPY

🌐 **Practice, practice, practice.** Communication is difficult, particularly for children and adults who are not used to doing it. Ability to do it in session does not always translate to ability to do it in the midst of a crisis. However, the more practice there has been, the more likely that effective communication will eventually occur (particularly if practice takes place in a dyadic and/or familial context).

🌐 **Be realistic, patient, and respectful.** Sharing internal experience brings vulnerability. Children, like adults, will be better at (and more open to) sharing certain emotions and experiences than others. Praise any attempts at communicating internal experience, and *slooooooooowly* support expanded risk in communication.

PART IV

COMPETENCY

WHY TARGET DEVELOPMENTAL COMPETENCY?

- Development is a dynamic process, and each developmental stage is associated with key tasks that children must negotiate, drawing on emergent assets such as growth in cognitive functioning, as well as on past successes.

- Tasks at each stage build on tasks from previous stages. So, for instance, successful establishment of peer relationships in middle childhood builds in part on the early childhood success in developing secure attachment relationships.

- Throughout childhood, competencies emerge across domains: cognitive, interpersonal, intrapersonal, emotional, and physical/motor.

- Many developmental competencies are, in themselves, associated with resilient outcome in future life stages. It is therefore important that treatment go beyond symptom reduction to target achievement of key developmental tasks as a primary goal. Given the impact of trauma on developmental course, targeting developmental competency should be considered an integral component of, rather than an adjunct to, "trauma-focused therapy."

HOW DOES TRAUMA IMPACT ACHIEVEMENT OF DEVELOPMENT TASKS?

- As detailed in previous sections' Key Concepts, there is extensive evidence that trauma has the potential to derail developmental competencies across domains of functioning and across developmental stages.

- Exposure to trauma is implicated in the impaired development of:

  - *Interpersonal competencies*, such as building early secure attachment relationships, positive peer relationships, and mature relationships in adulthood.

  - *Intrapersonal competencies*, such as positive self-concept, awareness of internal states, realistic assessment of self-competencies, and capacity to integrate self-states.

  - *Cognitive competencies*, such as language development, school performance and achieve-

169

ment, and growth of executive function skills, including problem solving, frustration tolerance, sustained attention, and abstract reasoning.

♦ *Regulatory competencies*, such as the ability to identify emotional states; realistically interpret others' cues and expression; regulate physiological and emotional arousal; manage, organize, and coordinate physical/motor responses; and share emotional experience.

A THREE-PART MODEL, REVISITED

- In Chapter 2 of this text, we highlighted a three-part model for understanding child behaviors through the lens of (1) impacted systems of meaning, including a prominent assumption of danger; (2) activation of functional danger-avoidance and need-fulfillment strategies in the face of relevant cues, leading to dysregulation of emotion, behavior, and physiology; and (3) interference from developmental challenges, with reliance on alternative adaptations to regain equilibrium.

  ♦ In the *Attachment* section of this framework, we target the first level of this model by seeking to build safe-enough surrounding systems and to strengthen or repair child–caregiver relationships.

  ♦ In the *Self-Regulation* section of this framework, we target the second level of the model by working with children and their caregivers to foster a healthy understanding of internal experience, the acquisition and use of strategies for managing and shifting emotional and physiological states, and the acquisition and use of strategies for sharing those experiences with others.

  ♦ In this, the *Competency* section, we highlight the importance of targeting the third level: the range of additional developmental competencies relevant to successful navigation of life experiences.

- Given the number of key developmental tasks, we focus more intensively on two key domains identified as particularly relevant to resilient outcome among highly stress-impacted youth: the ability to engage executive functions in the service of making active choices, and the healthy development of personal identity. In this introductory section, we briefly highlight additional domains that may be important to target in work with trauma-impacted youth.

- In assessing and selecting relevant developmental tasks to target, keep in mind the importance of considering *developmental stage* rather than *chronological age*. Children vary in level of developmental competency across domains (e.g., consider a cognitively advanced child with earlier developmental interpersonal competencies) and across time or setting (e.g., consider a child whose emotional competencies vary by level of stressor, or a child who regresses when placed in a new home).

Early Childhood

A primary task of early childhood is the establishment of a secure attachment and development of basic self-regulation skills. In addition, consider addressing the following target domains:

Social Skills

- Work with caregivers to build children's ability to interact with others in appropriate ways. Teach and model cooperative play. Set limits around negative behaviors in interaction.

- Involve children in natural forums for social interaction. Consider the use of play dates, preschool, Head Start, community centers, playrooms, etc. Caregivers should remain present and involved in these contexts with young children.

- Balance structured with unstructured activities. It is important that children develop the ability to follow the rules as well as use their imaginations. It is also important that children be able to play both cooperatively and independently.

- Help children develop an early understanding of empathy. Teach that different people have different feelings. Encourage children to respond to others' emotions in appropriate ways. It is important to differentiate between taking undue *responsibility* for others' feelings and *caring* about those feelings.

Motor Skills

- Involve children in activities that build gross and fine motor skills.

- For gross motor, consider the use of sports, dance, martial arts, gymboree, etc. Focus on cooperative rather than competitive play during this period.

- For fine motor, consider the use of arts and crafts projects, puzzles, tracing objects and letters, etc.

- When possible, caregivers should be involved in activities with their children; doing so fosters positive dyadic experience along with motor skill development.

Learning Readiness

- Work with caregivers to facilitate and motivate children's interest in learning. Primary at this stage is an interest in exploring the surrounding environment.

- Encourage caregivers to explore *with* their children. Tap into natural forums: Take a walk, go to the park, read a book, go to the library, etc. Pay attention to asking and wondering together.

- Work with caregivers to help their children apply new information. For instance, if the child has developed interest in how spaghetti is made, suggest that child and caregiver cook a dish together. If a child is learning a new game, play it together at home or in the session.

- Work with caregivers to challenge children. Encourage children to try tasks just above their comfort zone. Normalize the reality that some tasks are more difficult than others. Use regulation strategies to help children build frustration tolerance. Identify/articulate frustrations when they happen and encourage continued effort. Help children achieve cooperatively what would be just above their grasp individually.

Elementary School/Middle Childhood

Industry is increasingly important in middle childhood, as children explore the world outside of their homes. At this stage it is important to target both individual achievements and connections to others and to the larger world.

Social Skills

- Peer relationships become increasingly important throughout the elementary school years. To be successful, children need to accurately read others' intentions, negotiate interactions, experience empathy, and tolerate delay, disappointment, and frustration. Ability to work cooperatively and tolerate compromise is particularly important. Pay attention to deficits in these areas and work with children to build appropriate skills.

- Help children become increasingly involved in adjunctive activities. Encourage participation in sports, clubs, arts activities, after-school programming, etc. As children become involved in competitive activities, emotion regulation skills become increasingly important.

- Many other skills highlighted in this framework, such as problem-solving and affect regulation skills, are often important to successful peer interaction. Pair those skills when helping a child navigate real-life interactions.

- Traumatic triggers are often prominent in social interactions. Help children identify when "old" feelings get in the way of new relationships.

School Connection/Achievement

- School is a primary domain of competency in middle childhood. It is more important that children be invested in and feel positive about school involvement than that they be academically successful.

- Work with school systems to support children in experiencing success. Create a team. Identify school personnel who can serve as resources for the child in the school setting. Collaborate in treatment planning.

- Work with caregivers to reinforce effort and to show interest in children's school accomplishments. Build lines of communication with the school setting. Balance encouragement and praise with limit setting.

- Work with caregivers to provide a structure that accommodates changes in routine. Pay attention to transitions and create appropriate routines, as needed. Help structure the home setting in a way that supports children as they strive to accomplish school goals (e.g., homework).

- Help caregivers balance prioritization of goal accomplishment with unstructured time. It is important that children have opportunities for rest and play in addition to work.

Personal Responsibility

- It is important for children to have clear and reasonable expectations. They need to know what the rules are, what the expectations are, and to know that people believe that they can accomplish their relevant goals. Children will often live up—or down—to our expectations of them.

- Children are increasingly able to understand the rationale for rules. Help them differentiate rules in different locations (e.g., home vs. school) and the reasons for those rules. Involve them, to some degree, in setting household rules.

- Encourage children to take increasing responsibility. Work with caregivers to build age-appropriate chores in the home setting. Because it is important that children experience success in completing chores, work with caregivers to designate appropriate tasks and to monitor and reinforce task completion. Caregivers should provide support, as needed, with an ultimate goal of independent task mastery.

Adolescence

Primary tasks of adolescence include exploration and establishment of a coherent identity, beginning stages of separation and individuation from caregivers, and building a foundation for independent functioning. Many of these skills are discussed in other sections of this framework; additional considerations are highlighted here.

Social Skills

- Adolescents must increasingly be able to negotiate a variety of social interactions independently. These include peer interactions but also interactions with teachers, potential employers, community members, etc.
- Create opportunities for adolescents to come into contact with a range of people in different contexts and work with them to practice effective communication skills.
- Work with caregivers to balance involvement with the adolescent need for privacy. Caregiver involvement may shift toward expressing interest, rather than knowledge, per se.
- Work with adolescents to maintain individual opinions, thoughts, and goals even in the midst of peer influence. Pair social skills with identity work.
- For teens who have experienced harm in interpersonal relationships, social connections can trigger fear as well as either premature intimacy or rejection of intimacy. Help adolescents define positive relationships and then develop them.
- Help adolescents develop effective conflict resolution skills. Note that this area involves many of the same skills previously addressed in affect identification, modulation, and expression, as well as problem solving. Work with adolescents to use the following steps in addressing conflicts:
    - *Know your own cues* (tune in to cues of self-distress: **Affect Identification**).
    - *Choose your moments* (calm down before approaching a difficult situation: **Affect Modulation**).
    - *Identify goals* (what does adolescent want to accomplish?: **Problem Solving**).
    - *Take perspective* (what might the other person be experiencing?: **Affect Identification— Other**).
    - *Evaluate outcomes* (be flexible—what has/has not worked? Generate alternatives: **Problem Solving**).

Community Connection

- Work with adolescents to expand their involvement in the world outside of the home. This may include extracurricular activities, participation in community programs, employment, etc.
- There are many ways for adolescents to contribute to the larger community. Community involve-

ment develops agency, efficacy, and social connection. Keep in mind that community involvement can be formal or informal. Help adolescents define the ways in which they currently make a difference, and/or how they want to make a difference.

- It is normative for adolescents to develop relationships with people from an expanded social circle, including other adults. Work with caregivers to tolerate these connections; although caregivers should stay aware of those with whom their child is interacting, it is important to allow some latitude as adolescents struggle to gain independence in their interactions.

- Community connections are a key forum for exploring interests as well as building or expanding individual skills and attributes.

Independent Functioning

- Throughout this developmental stage, adolescents are moving toward increasingly independent functioning. It is important that tasks and activities begin to reflect this independence.

- School accomplishments are increasingly important to future functioning. Work with adolescents to connect current achievements with current and future goals.

- Work with caregivers to involve adolescents in discussion about and establishment of household rules, roles, and structure.

- Jobs can be an important forum for building self-efficacy, self-reliance, and responsibility. However, help adolescents establish realistic expectations and goals. It is important that jobs not interfere with adolescents' ability to continue to participate in other important domains of their lives.

- Personal responsibility is an essential value for adolescents, and it is strongly associated with resiliency. Help adolescents explore their own actions and the natural consequences of those actions. Bring the language of "choice" into conversations.

- Pay attention to fostering the range of life skills relevant to future independent functioning. Work with adolescents to learn to open bank accounts and budget money, navigate appropriate interaction in a range of settings, manage basic household tasks, identify and access external resources, etc. A focus on these key areas is particularly important for those adolescents who will have less of a caregiving "buffer" as they transition into young adulthood (e.g., adolescents who will be "aging out of" substitute care). Whenever possible, work to connect adolescents with individuals and other social resources who will be able to provide support through and beyond this transition.

Each core domain of this framework emphasizes key developmental competencies for trauma-impacted youth and their caregiving systems. Given the dynamic nature of development and the impact that trauma has on developmental processes, it is essential that the treatment of chronic trauma include assessment and intervention focused on the myriad of developmental strengths and challenges. As we move forward in this section and the next, we focus on helping children move beyond survival so that they are consciously *acting*, rather than reacting; establish a sense of self that is coherent, strengths-based, and future-oriented; and understand and transform early traumatic experiences so that they are able to establish a coherent life narrative.

CHAPTER 11

Strengthening Executive Functions

THE MAIN IDEA

Work with children to act, instead of react, by using higher-order cognitive processes to solve problems and make active choices in the service of reaching identified goals.

★ KEY CONCEPTS

★ *What Are "Executive Functions"?*

- Executive functions can be thought of as the "captain of the cognitive ship." They help human beings navigate through the world in a goal-directed, thoughtful way.

- Many skills are classified as executive functions. Among them are the following:

  - ◆ Delaying or inhibiting response
  - ◆ Active decision making
  - ◆ Anticipating consequences
  - ◆ Evaluating outcomes
  - ◆ Generating alternative solutions

★ *Why Build Executive Function Skills?*

How Does Trauma Impact Executive Functions?

- Development of executive functions parallels development of the **prefrontal cortex**. Normatively, executive functions develop over the course of childhood and adolescence, allowing children to become increasingly sophisticated in their cognitive meaning making and problem solving. Goal-directed human behavior is guided by this part of the brain much of the time.

- Along with many other brain systems, the prefrontal cortex is implicated in the traumatic stress response. When stress overwhelms normal coping mechanisms and the danger response is activated, key survival systems (e.g., the **limbic system**) take charge, and "nonessential" systems are deactivated. In the moment of significant danger, higher cognitive processes are considered nonessential! (Think about it—if you are in the middle of the jungle, and a lion is speeding toward you, do you want to be thinking, or do you want to be running?)

- The limbic system and the prefrontal cortex are mutually inhibitory: As one increases in activation, the other decreases, and vice versa. Consider the way in which frustration, for instance, interferes with your ability to remain focused on a difficult task and continue to work toward a solution: As arousal goes up, cognitive processes begin to fragment. Conversely, consider the ways in which using your "thinking brain" (e.g., focusing on logic, breaking tasks into step-by-step solutions) can help decrease feelings of being overwhelmed: That is, the act of harnessing higher-order cognition can serve to regulate arousal levels.

- For children who experience chronic trauma, the ongoing exposure to danger (both real and perceived) takes a toll on the development of higher cognitive abilities. With increased sensitization to danger signals, the brains of chronically traumatized youth are frequently readying the body to run from the lion, and therefore prioritizing limbic over prefrontal activation. Because there are many potential triggers of danger, these children may be as likely to be in limbic control in the midst of math class as they would be in the midst of the jungle.

- Research indicates that children who have experienced trauma lag behind their peers over time in development of age-appropriate executive function skills. They do less well on tasks requiring several distinct abilities: to inhibit responses, to plan and make active choices, and to sustain attention.

Why Target Executive Functions?

- Executive functions allow us to participate actively in our own lives. They provide a sense of control and agency. In the absence of higher cognitive control, we are caught in stimulus–response mode: Life throws something at us, and we react. Executive functions bring *conscious thought* to our actions; rather than simply reacting, we consider our actions in context.

- Research on resilience highlights the importance of these executive abilities. In study after study, the ability to problem-solve, make active choices, and function independently predicts resilient outcome among high-risk youth.

🧰 THERAPIST TOOLBOX

📋 *Teach to Caregivers*

- *Reminder:* Teach caregivers the Key Concepts.

- *Reminder:* Teach caregivers relevant Developmental Considerations.

- Teach caregivers the problem-solving steps. As appropriate, involve caregivers in active attempts to help children problem-solve and generate and implement solutions. The ultimate goal is for children to be able to use problem-solving skills in the moment, rather than just in the context of treatment. The likelihood of this generalization will significantly increase if members of children's caregiving systems are able to recognize, cue, and support their attempts to make active choices.

- Work with caregivers to notice and name choices and related outcomes and teach them to reinforce positive choices. When setting limits, work with caregivers to avoid power struggles and instead to focus on choices and outcomes.

▶ *Behind the Scenes*

- Although executive functions encompass many different areas, this section specifically targets three key skills: active evaluation of situations, inhibition of response, and decision making. All of these are encompassed in problem-solving skills. As originally outlined by D'Zurilla and Goldfried (1971), problem-solving skills have been integrated into a wide array of cognitive-behavioral and social skills treatments for both children and adults (e.g., D'Zurilla & Nezu, 2007; Kazdin, 1985; Kazdin, Esveldt-Dawson, French, & Unis, 1987; Kazdin, Siegel, & Bass, 1992; Matthews, 1999). Below we describe a variation on these steps that encompasses a recognition of the role of the danger response in the problem-solving capacities of children and adolescents who have experienced traumatic stress.

- For children to engage in and practice these skills effectively, they must be in a regulated state of arousal. Teach children to pair the use of modulation strategies with these skills.

- A primary goal of this work is to increase children's recognition of their ability to actively make *choices*. Understanding the concept of choice increases the child's sense of empowerment and fosters several key competencies: **agency**, or the self-knowledge that child actions can impact their world; **personal responsibility**, or ownership of decision making and consequences; and **mastery**, or the ability to implement, evaluate, practice, and own personal actions and decisions.

- Often, children (and adults) are presented with two less-than-ideal choices, rather than a clearly positive and clearly negative one. At times, our choice may be between doing *something* and doing *nothing*. The process of reflecting and actively choosing remains important: There is a clear difference in internal experience between *choosing* to do nothing (when acting will invariably bring negative consequences) and *feeling or thinking that you can't do anything*. It is the difference between agency and helplessness. It is important to teach children that problem solving will sometimes involve choosing among solutions that don't necessarily feel good, but that ultimately remain the best choice toward meeting our goals.

- Although the problem-solving steps are taught in sequence below, we can apply them from any point. For instance, in some situations, we might start at Step 3 (identifying the problem) and work our way through understanding our goals, generating possible solutions, and anticipating outcomes. In other situations, we might start at the end: That is, for what outcome are we looking? Given that outcome, we can work our way back to possible actions, behaviors, or coping strategies and the situations or problems that may interfere. Or, we can work with an outcome (whether positive or negative) that has already occurred and track back to identify the precipitating factors and the behaviors and coping strategies employed that led to the given outcome. In the instance of a negative outcome, we might also work to identify the desired outcome and alternatives that would help clients succeed.

- It is crucial to notice and name choices when they occur, particularly with children who struggle with them. Consider the following example:

An adolescent girl who recently started a part-time job is talking about her frustration with the assistant manager at the store. "She keeps getting in my face, telling me what to do and how to do it, and how I need to be working faster." When the therapist asks how the teen is handling this, she says, "What am I supposed to do? I just keep my mouth shut and do what she says." When the therapist comments that the adolescent has sometimes struggled with managing her temper in the past, the teen states, "Well, I don't want to lose this job—I need the money." The therapist responds, "I'm so impressed. You know that you want to keep this job, and it's helping you make a choice to manage your feelings and not jump into arguing or yelling back, even though you're feeling frustrated and upset."

In this situation, it is important that the therapist notice, name, and reinforce the active choice the adolescent is making (to control her behavior, because of her goal of keeping the job). It is equally important that the therapist then work with the adolescent on possible solutions for addressing any resulting problems (e.g., how to manage the challenging feelings and arousal resulting from these interactions).

- Below, we list the key steps involved in making active choices. Following these, we highlight strategies for "catching" and applying these skills in the moment.

🔧 Tools: Tools to Build Executive Functions

Problem-Solving Skills

- Problem-solving skills can be used formally or informally, in conversation or in structured writing or drawing tasks, and can be used to think about an upcoming challenge or to explore a situation that has already occurred.

- For many people, the problem-solving steps are an unconscious, rapid process used to assess situations and make various choices. For children exposed to trauma, however, these steps are skipped as they move straight to reaction. The goal of this work, then, is to make this unconscious process *conscious*.

- The steps in the following table address each of the primary skills identified above. Each step can be targeted in isolation and should be practiced separately until some level of comfort is achieved. Over time, however, the goal is to build a child's ability to apply all of the relevant steps in a given situation.

Step	Description
Step 1: Notice there is a problem.	**Teach to Kids:** • **Connect to previous skill building.** "Lots of situations can bring up feelings. We've talked a lot about ways to recognize feelings and how to deal with them." • **Feelings provide useful information.** "Sometimes feelings are hard, and we want to get rid of them. But—feelings give us important information. They let us know that something is going on that we like, or don't like, or are worried about, etc." • **Use "feelings detective" work to recognize problems.** "We've talked about recognizing feelings so that you can cope with them, share them with other people, and understand them. Now we're going to talk about how to use feelings to help you make good choices." • **Emphasize building child control.** "We're going to work on using all the skills you've learned to recognize feelings and then to stop and think before you act. This helps *you, not your feelings*, be in charge of what you do."

Step	Description

Goal: For children to be able to *recognize* "problem situations" (e.g., moments in which they are upset or triggered).

How to:

- Build children's ability to notice *internal* cues and link this to **Affect Identification** work. As a feelings detective, children learn cues that indicate when they are sad, mad, worried, etc. Identify the most prominent cues, such as energy level, body sensations, thoughts, behaviors, etc., and help children practice noticing when they happen. Include caregivers, as appropriate, to help.
- Help children tune in to *external* cues indicating that other people think there is a problem. Review signs of affect in *others* learned during affect identification exercises. Help children tune in to key cues, such as tone of voice, facial expressions, body language, etc. How does the child know when other people are upset, angry, worried, etc.?

Step 2: Establish basic safety and inhibit instinctive danger response.

Teach to Kids:

- **Teach about the brain and normalize the rapid danger response.** "One of the things feelings do is send a message to our brain that there's something going on. Different parts of our brain control different things. One part of our brain is really good at *doing*, or *action*—like, if we touch a stove, pain is a message to the action brain that we need to move our hand away quickly. Another part of our brain is really good at *thinking*, but sometimes we don't want that part to be in charge—like, if you're touching a hot stove, do you really want to spend time *thinking* before you move your hand?"
- **Provide rationale for skill.**
  - "Sometimes, though, it is important for the *thinking brain* to be involved. When we have physical feelings, like pain, it can be important to react quickly. But other types of feelings, like being afraid, angry, excited, or frustrated, can make us act *too* quickly. This is good when we're really in danger, but not so good if we're not."
  - "Kids who have been in danger before get really good at reacting quickly when situations, thoughts, or feelings come up that seem to signal danger. Most of the time, though, it's important to know what is going on before we react."
    (Query: "Has there ever been a time when feelings made you react too quickly? Give examples—for example, yelling at a teacher or punching a sibling. What was the consequence of reacting too quickly?")
- **Engage children in assessing real versus perceived danger.** "When you have strong feelings, the first thing that it's important to do is to figure out if you're safe or in danger. We've already talked about how our brains learn to pay attention to clues that tell us that something *might* be dangerous. Sometimes there is real danger, but other times, the clues are things that remind us of something that *was* dangerous in the past. Do you remember what those are called? [Reteach concept of triggers, if needed.] Triggers activate the body's alarm system. What we're going to work on is figuring out when it's a real alarm and when it's a false alarm—like a fire drill at school."

Goal: For children to establish a basic sense of safety and then to *inhibit* initial survival reactions until they are able to make an active choice.

How to:

- *Step 2.1:* Before anything else happens, the child must establish a basic sense of safety. Pair a child's ability to recognize that he or she is upset with the ability to scan the environment immediately and assess: **"Am I actually in danger?"**
  - *Assess for physical danger:* "Is there something in my environment that could hurt me? Is there someone *physically* threatening me? If not . . . "
  - *Assess for triggers:* If not previously taught, work with children to identify their own triggers. What things elicit strong emotions or make them feel unsafe? Help children find their own words to describe situations (e.g., "People giving me a hard time" vs. "Injustice"). Pay attention to multiple types of triggers:
    - Internal (e.g., feeling lonely or vulnerable/powerless)
    - Relational (e.g., exertion of authority, intimacy)
    - Sensory (e.g., smells, sounds, facial expressions, touch)
- Help children identify cues that go along with being triggered. Link fight–flight–freeze response to triggers. What have they identified as their own behaviors or feelings when they are in the fight response? Flight response? Freeze response? Keep in mind that different reactions may go with different types of triggers.

Step	Description
	• **The goal here is for children to become proficient at recognizing when they are triggered (vs. actually in danger) and delaying their response until they can make an active choice.** • *Step 2.2:* Inhibition of response ♦ Help children build tools to delay immediate response. Once children recognize that a situation is "a problem," it is important that they be able to delay further response until they have had time to manage their affect and actively make choices. ♦ This is an incredibly hard step for many children, and significant practice is often needed. ♦ Consider multiple possible tools (including many of those discussed in Chapter 9, "**Modulation**"). For example: ○ Focused breathing ○ Cognitive tools (e.g., self-statement: "Stop and think") ○ Visual tools (e.g., small stop sign or stop light) ○ Social resources (e.g., caregiver or teacher cue) ○ Grounding tools (e.g., teach child to focus on hand-held manipulatives) • As in affect modulation, pair regulatory skill with state of arousal. • Work with caregivers and other adults to support and reinforce this skill.
Step 3: Identify and understand the problem.	**Teach to Kids:** • **Getting to the root of the problem.** "Once you know you're not really in danger, you can take the time to figure out what is *really* going on. Emotions come from somewhere." **Goal**: For a child to *consciously evaluate a situation* to understand the origins of his or her own and others' emotions. **How to** (*or* **learn to be a problem detective**): Take the time to understand what *is* going on. • Once children can recognize that they are feeling something, teach them to *concretely* identify what, exactly, the problem is. • A situation is generally "a problem" because the *child* is unhappy about something, because someone *else* is unhappy with the child, or both. • Help children with prompts. Use the *wh-* questions to **backtrack**, as described in the next section, "Recognizing Opportunities to Apply Problem-Solving Skills": ♦ "When did you start noticing that funny feeling in your stomach?" ♦ "Who were you with?" ♦ "What were you doing?" ♦ "Where were you doing it?" *or* ♦ "What made you think your dad was upset?" ♦ "What were you doing?" ♦ "What was he doing?" • It is important that children, to the degree possible, are the ones who identify the problem (as well as possible solutions). Help them with cues, but let them figure out what they can.
Step 4: Brainstorm: Identify possible solutions. Don't throw out anything yet!	**Teach to Kids:** • **The point of knowing that there is a problem is to be able to actively deal with it.** "Once you know something is a problem, you can make an active choice, instead of just reacting." • **There is *always* more than one choice.** "A lot of times, kids feel like they don't have a choice when things feel hard. But—almost all the time, there *are* choices, even if the choice is to not do anything." • **Sometimes, the choice is about what happens inside of us, instead of about action.** "There may be times when the choice we make is to work on how we feel and think about something, rather than about taking action to address a situation. For instance, if we are in a situation we cannot change, our choices may be (a) to feel angry and resentful, or (b) to work on accepting the situation, to think about something that makes us happy, to think forward to a time when the situation will be over." **Goal**: To help children identify many possible solutions, so that they can make an active choice. **How to**: • *Step 4.1:* Name and validate current choice. ♦ If a choice has already been made (e.g., work is being done in the aftermath of a situation), it is important to first *name* the choice the child has already made and *validate* it.

Step	Description

- *Step 4.2:* Identify the goal.
  - ♦ Every situation has many possible goals. The choices we make in a hard situation will depend on what our goal is (e.g., if a child is in trouble at school for fighting, the goal may be to teach the child how to calm down from being mad, to think of ways to resolve the problem, or to think of a different solution for next time).
  - ♦ Help child concretely identify what he or she is trying to accomplish. Consider expressing feelings, seeking support, avoiding a consequence, gaining a reward or privilege, fixing a difficult situation, etc.
  - ♦ If the goal the child picks is not a realistic one, help him or her to examine that, and, when necessary, to identify an alternative goal. For instance, consider a child who is having difficult visits with a biological parent due to conflict with a sibling; the child's goal may be, "To make my brother disappear." While understandable (and important to validate), help the child consider alternative goals (e.g., "How to deal with my brother so I can still see Mom").
- *Step 4.3:* Generate ideas about possible choices.
  - ♦ Help children generate as many ideas as possible. It is crucial at this point to refrain from commenting on any of the potential choices. For instance, if you ask a child all the different ways he or she could handle a confrontation at school, and the child lists punching someone, throwing a brick through a window, running off, etc., then all of these go on the list.
  - ♦ Keep in mind at this stage, you're not trying to get to the *best* solution. You're trying to highlight that there *are* solutions, and that—even when it doesn't seem like it—children are making choices. For instance, choosing to punch someone is a solution, but there are almost always alternatives.
  - ♦ If a child is unable to generate any positive solutions, the clinician has two choices: Continue with the steps below, evaluating consequences, and then come back and look for alternatives, *or* try to generate a few more with the child in the moment (e.g., "I wonder if we can think of a few ideas that don't involve hitting someone").

Step	Description

Step 5: Evaluate all the possible consequences (good and bad) of each solution, and then make a choice.

Teach to Kids:
- **All choices have consequences, good and bad.** "Every choice we make has consequences—sometimes they're good, sometimes they're not so good, and sometimes they're both. Like—if you help out your mom, it might make you (and her) feel good, but you might not have time to watch your favorite show that day. Or—if you decide to hit someone, it might make you feel better, but you'd probably get in trouble."
- **Make a choice.** "Sometimes there's no perfect choice. Usually, though, we can figure out what some *good* choices are, based on what you want to happen, or what you don't want to happen."

Goal: To support children in evaluating outcomes so that they are able to select solutions in service of meeting goals.

How to:
- *Step 5.1:* Evaluate possible consequences for each idea generated.
  - ♦ Work with the child to evaluate each idea on the list. It is important to acknowledge that most choices potentially have both positive and negative outcomes.
  - ♦ Pay attention to immediate and delayed outcomes. Help the child to think through not just what will happen in the moment, but what may happen later on as a result of the choice.
  - ♦ Go through this process for every solution the child has generated.
- *Step 5.2:* Based on potential consequences, help the child make a choice.
  - ♦ *Help the child actively examine all choices.* "Given the situation, the goal, the possible rewards, and the possible consequences, what seems like the best choice for you now?"
  - ♦ *Help child to examine combinations:* "Sometimes the best choice involves doing a few different things. For instance, one of the goals may be to express your feelings, and another is to seek support. Does it make more sense to pick choices that help you do both, or does one need to have priority over the other?"
  - ♦ *Name consequences of negative choices, but don't engage in a power struggle.* Be aware that children may select a negative choice, even after having gone through this process. Acknowledge that this may be the choice they would really like to make, but highlight that making the choice will mean that they need to accept the consequences. Emphasizing consequences increases awareness of responsibility and personal control.

Step	Description
	♦ *Help children be realistic in their assessment.* Some choices sound good but will be difficult to implement. For instance, in choosing a solution for dealing with peer conflict, a child decides that the best choice is to "Just not get mad." The clinician may: ○ *Normalize emotion:* "Well, I think it would be really hard to have someone yell at you and not feel a little bit mad. Remember how we've talked about how it's okay to have all feelings, it's just important to make safe choices? And trying to turn off your feelings isn't really good for you, because your feelings will come out in other ways." ○ *Identify a safe way to cope with the emotion and still reach goal.* For situations involving difficult affect, integrate self-regulation strategies into potential choices. For instance, a child might choose to calm down by squeezing a stress ball and then try talking to an adult.
Step 6: Implement and evaluate solutions and revise as needed.	**Teach to Kids:** • **Try it out.** "We don't always know what the best choice is, and we don't always know what is going to happen when we make a choice. Sometimes we have to experiment—that means picking what we *think* is the best solution and trying it out." • **Evaluate outcomes.** "Once we've tried out something, we can decide if we made the right choice. We can always go back and try something else or choose a different solution the next time." **Goal**: To support children in actively engaging in choices, and then reflecting upon them. **How to**: • *Step 6.1:* Act on the choice. ♦ The goal here is for children to implement the choice they have made. This is, in many ways, the hardest step. It can be difficult for children to generalize from the therapy room to their daily lives. ♦ *Anticipate:* Work with the child to identify factors that will increase the possibility of success, as well as any possible barriers. Help the child think of ways to increase positive factors and decrease or cope with barriers. ♦ *Role-play:* Help the child practice carrying out the chosen solution. Use role play to act out different scenarios and outcomes. ♦ *Build a team:* Help the child achieve success by drawing in other resources. Elicit suggestions from the child: "Who will it be okay to talk to about helping you with this?" To the degree possible, involve caregivers, teachers, etc., in supporting implementation. Teach the child's team to cue the child in using target skills. ♦ *Experiment:* Frame the attempt at implementation as an experiment. Teach the child that no one can completely predict the results of a new action or behavior. Have the child actively observe outcomes, and report back. • *Step 6.2:* Evaluate outcomes and revise as needed. ♦ In situations where the child is going to attempt a new solution, it is important to take a look at what happened. Celebrate successes. ♦ Even if the solution did not work, reinforce any *attempt* the child has made to implement a positive solution. ♦ If the implemented choice was not successful, work with the child to critically identify and evaluate possible barriers. Was it that the solution wasn't the right one? Was it the timing? Was it the other person? Was it that other feelings got so strong that the child couldn't remember the choice in the moment? Help find solutions that address the barriers to implementation, going back through the above steps.

Recognizing Opportunities to Apply Problem-Solving Skills

• Often, the best place to apply problem-solving skills is in the moment, in response to child statements, or in situations in which a choice should be—or has been—made. In the above table, each step of the problem-solving process is detailed, with key teaching points and goals. Here, suggestions are given for ways to recognize opportunities to use and apply this skill.

"I DON'T KNOW WHY EVERYONE'S SO MAD."

- *Entry point:* Listen for moments when children are confused about why a situation happened or show a lack of awareness that something was a problem.

- *Goal:* To increase children's awareness of internal and external cues that signify a "problem situation" and to help them evaluate and understand what the problem was/is (**Steps 1–3**).

- *Note:* When applied in the aftermath of a situation, *backtracking* can be used to help children learn to track and tune in to subtle cues in their body and in the environment:

    ◆ Help children ***concretely define the situation*** about which they are confused (e.g., "Suddenly everyone was mad").

    ◆ ***Track backward.*** What was happening 5 minutes before "everyone was mad"? Assess the situation, child's body state, feelings, thoughts, etc.

    ◆ ***Continue to move backward to the earliest cues available.*** Help children notice clues that there is "a problem"—for example, that their feelings were getting out of control, or that other people were upset. Tie in to Affect Identification skills.

- *Example:*

    (The child comes into session appearing sad and shut down.)

    THERAPIST: You look kind of down today. What's going on?

    CHILD: Everyone hates me, and I don't know why. [**Language of confusion about situation**]

    THERAPIST: Everyone hates you? What makes you think that?

    CHILD: I don't know, I was just trying to play and everyone told me to go away. [**Defining the situation**]

    THERAPIST: Wow—I can see why you're down. Let's try to figure out what was happening. What happened right before everyone told you to go away? [**Backtrack**]

    CHILD: I don't know. It was recess, and some kids were playing, and I wanted to play, and then they got mad.

    THERAPIST: How did you know they were mad? [**Tuning in to clues of "a problem"**]

    CHILD: 'Cause they were yelling, and they said I was stupid.

    THERAPIST: Okay, sounds like they were mad. What happened right before they yelled? [**Backtrack**]

- *Note:* This process can continue until child and therapist have identified early clues indicating that there was "a problem," define/understand the situation, and then continue through the problem-solving steps (i.e., alternatives for next time).

"BUT I HAD TO . . . "

- *Entry point:* Listen for moments when children identify a situation, either past or future, in which they did not or do not feel as if they have a choice.

- *Goal:* Increase awareness of choices (**Step 4**).

- *Example:*

    (The child is on program restriction for shoving another resident in their group home.)

    CHILD: I don't get what the big deal is. He started it, so I *had to.* [**Language of "no choice"**]

    MILIEU COUNSELOR: Sounds like it really felt like you didn't have a choice.

    CHILD: Well, I didn't. He was getting in my face.

    MILIEU COUNSELOR: Okay, Manuel was getting in your face, so you chose to shove him. [**Language of choice**] Because of that, you got put on restriction. [**Language of consequences**] Let's think of why it might have happened so quickly. [**Acknowledgment of the role of triggers or dysregulated response**] and whether there was anything else you could have done.

"I'M GONNA . . . [INSERT BAD CHOICE HERE]."

- *Entry point:* Listen for moments when children name a potentially negative choice that they plan on making.

- *Goal:* Increase understanding of consequences for actions (**Step 5**).

- *Example:*

    (The adolescent has had an argument with her parents and comes into session very angry.)

    ADOLESCENT: I hate my parents. I'm sick of this, I'm taking off. [**Potentially negative choice**] I've got friends in New York—I can always go there.

    THERAPIST: Okay, sounds like things are really heating up. I can understand why you would want to take off. Can we take a couple of minutes to think about it?

    ADOLESCENT: Fine, but I'm not changing my mind.

    THERAPIST: Okay, well that's your choice. [**Don't power struggle; reiterate choice**] It sounds like you're feeling like you need a break. Can we think of some different choices you might have, including taking off [**don't leave anything out when brainstorming**], and then think about what's going to work best for you? [**Generate alternative solutions, then evaluate them**]

    Note: In a situation in which a child/adolescent continues to reiterate intent to make negative or unsafe choices, despite support in problem solving, the adult may be in the position of needing to address those actions. Continue to use the language of choice, as follows:

    ADOLESCENT: This is stupid! I'm serious—I'm leaving.

    THERAPIST: I can understand that you want to leave, but you know that part of my job is helping you to stay safe. If this is really the choice that you want to make, then the choice I'm going to have to make is to do something to help keep you safe, like speaking with your mom about this.

"IT'S ALL [MY MOTHER'S, MY FRIEND'S, THE TEACHER'S, MY DOG'S, ETC.] FAULT!"

- *Entry point:* Listen for moments when children externalize responsibility for a choice they have made.

- *Goal:* Increase understanding of consequences for actions (**Step 5**).

- *Example:*

   (*The adolescent comes into session angry because his parents have taken away his PlaySta-tion.*)

   ADOLESCENT: I hate my parents! I'm sick of this, they're always taking stuff away for the stupidest little things. They do it just to piss me off. [**Externalizing responsibility**]

   THERAPIST: Okay, sounds like you're pretty mad. What happened?

   ADOLESCENT: I told you, they're trying to piss me off, so they took away my PS2.

   THERAPIST: Wow—they just took it away out of the blue? What was going on before it hap-pened?

   ADOLESCENT: Nothing—I was just playing, and I was gonna do my homework after I fin-ished the game, and they came in out of nowhere and started yelling.

   THERAPIST: Is this something you guys had talked about before?

   ADOLESCENT: Yeah, I guess so, but I was gonna do it in a minute. I don't see what the big deal is.

   THERAPIST: Can I make sure I understand? So you and your folks had talked about doing homework—did they tell you that you needed to do it before playing?

   ADOLESCENT: Yeah.

   THERAPIST: Did they tell you you'd lose the PS2 if you didn't do your homework?

   ADOLESCENT: Yeah, but I was planning on doing it—I was just gonna finish my game.

   THERAPIST: Okay, this is making more sense. It sounds like your folks asked you to do something, and you made a choice to use the PS2 instead of doing your homework when they asked. [**Highlight choice made by adolescent**] Do you think there's any other choices you could have made, that wouldn't have gotten the PS2 taken away? [**Generate future alternative choices**]

👪 DEVELOPMENTAL CONSIDERATIONS

Developmental stage	Executive function considerations
Early childhood	Executive function skills develop over the course of childhood, into adolescence and young adulthood. Young children are not able—and should not be expected—to independently implement problem solving.
	However, young children are able to learn basic if–then relationships. The goal with this age group is to establish a basic understanding of choice, or action, and consequence (both good and bad).

Developmental stage	Executive function considerations
	Agency is a key developmental task in early childhood. Work with caregivers to actively notice and name child choices and actions and link them to outcomes. For example: The child builds a tower, then knocks it down: "Look at that! You hit that tower, and it went boom! That was really neat!"
Middle childhood	Normatively, there should be a progression in children's ability to control and reflect on actions and choices. Cognitive abilities can begin to be used in the service of goal-directed activities.
	With this developmental stage, increase focus on support in anticipating, planning, and evaluating possible choices and outcomes. Involve caregivers and other adults in increasing the language of choice. For example: "You have soccer today, and I know sometimes you feel frustrated at practice. What choices do you think you could make to help with that today?"
	At this stage, mastery becomes increasingly important. Work with caregivers and other adults to actively identify how choices children made have led to successful outcomes. Keep in mind that "success" should be defined in a child-specific way, and may be about effort as much as outcome.
Adolescence	Normatively, adolescents have developed the cognitive capacity for critical thinking and independent problem solving. For traumatized adolescents, however, this area continues to remain a challenge. Several factors are important to consider: • Because adolescents often wish to keep their inner lives private, shared problem solving may feel like an invasion. Allow adolescents some degree of autonomy in selecting problem situations to share. • Foster adolescents' ability to generate solutions independently and to take responsibility for the consequences. Emphasis is often on teaching and supporting the problem-solving skills, rather than judging choices.
	Keep in mind that adolescents' interpretation of situations (and possible outcomes) is often idiosyncratic. Clinician and/or caregiver goals likely differ from those of adolescents. It is important to try to understand their perspective and individual goals.

APPLICATIONS

Individual/Dyadic

It is likely that, to some degree, strengthening executive functions in the form of addressing problem-solving skills will come into most individual sessions with a child or adolescent. The problem-solving steps are often taught formally (i.e., step by step), but are most often applied less formally, by "catching the moment." Identifying difficult situations, exploring and defining "problems," exploring and defining goals, examining and generating choices, and linking actions to consequences are all an important part of ongoing therapeutic work. The more this process is made explicit, the more likely it is that a child will be able to internalize this set of skills over time.

The process of solving problems and making active choices will link, in some way, to every target encapsulated within this framework. A child will use **Affect Identification** skills to support identification of problem situations and his or her own responses; **Modulation** skills are vital to remaining regulated enough to harness higher-order cognitive processes; and **Affect Expression** skills may be a key component of generated solutions (e.g., in expressing feelings or seeking support). **Self and Identity** work, as described in the next chapter, often intertwines with choices: A child's future goals, for instance, may help in identifying situational goals; values may help in considering the benefits and consequences of various choices. **Attachment** targets are vital to supporting child problem solving: The caregiver's capacity to stay regulated and to tune in to the child's thoughts, feelings, challenges, and strengths will help in identifying the problem and cuing and supporting the child in the use of these skills. Eliciting the child's understanding of choices can assist in the application of **Consistent Response** (e.g., by proactively helping a child make positive choices, rather than relying on limits and consequences). The clinician can help the child and caregiver understand the important links among the skills and goals they have worked to develop.

Pay attention to recognizing "choice" situations, either in anticipation (e.g., an anticipated problem or upcoming challenge) or in the aftermath. Notice, name, and reinforce positive choices as well as attempts toward making choices, even when less positive. Whenever appropriate, involve caregivers (parents, teachers, other helping adults) in supporting child choices or in jointly generating potential solutions. It is particularly important to involve key adults whenever a child will be attempting to implement a new skill (e.g., making a choice to seek an adult's support instead of getting in a fight). Teach children's caregivers the problem-solving steps and actively practice and reinforce their support of these skills.

In addition to supporting the child/adolescent's own problem-solving abilities, it may be valuable to use transparency around decision-making processes, particularly as these decisions apply to the child's own life. Transparency helps both in modeling the skill and in decreasing a child's perception of the "randomness" of life decisions. For instance, consider the child who is being moved to a different classroom due to behavioral dysregulation. The clinician or caregiver might describe the decision-making process:

> "Like we had talked about, Mom, Mrs. Jones, Mr. Rivera, and I all met to talk about what would help you the most to be successful in school. We thought about different possibilities, like having someone sit with you in class, or having you leave the class for part of the day. We thought the best solution was _____. The reasons we thought _____ might not work so well were _____. So here's what we're going to try. . . . "

Explanations should be developmentally appropriate and solution-focused.

Group

There are many ways to apply problem-solving skills in a group format. Consider, when developing activities, the ultimate goal: increasing child awareness of choices and the capacity to actively make them in the service of reaching a goal. In group situations the process of collaborative problem solving is often a more valuable teaching tool than simply providing explicit instruction in the steps, so long as there is a follow-up process. Consider, for instance, engaging the group in a collaborative process in which members must actively generate solutions to solve a problem (examples are provided in Appendix C). Following the activity, explore the process (e.g., "What was it like to work together? What helped you to be successful? What got in the way?"), the decisions (e.g., "What was it that made you pick x instead of y?"), and the outcomes (e.g., "How well do you think you did? Can you think of anything that would have made this turn out better? What about something that would have made this turn out worse?"). When appropriate, redo the activity, this time inviting group members to use their experiences to anticipate challenges/obstacles as well as successful solutions. In follow-up discussion, link these processes to "real-world" decisions: the process of making choices, the obstacles that get in the way, the supports that can help, the ways in which our choices affect outcomes, and the ways that anticipating outcomes (and practical experience) can help in making increasingly positive choices.

Similar work can be done by engaging group members in a discussion of situations relevant to their lives through use of prompt scenarios; consider the use of appropriate movie clips, books, and current events. Most useful in this work is examining ambiguous situations—that is, those in which there is no clear "right" solution. Invite the group to identify what the problematic issues are; to discuss and generate possible goals, choices, and outcomes; and to consider the ways in which potential obstacles and resources will intertwine with choices. It is important that group leaders not steer the group toward a "correct" choice; in this work, the process is more important than the decisions made.

Milieu

Supporting the child or adolescent in active problem solving, in combination with the use of modulation strategies, should be a key goal of milieu programs. Often, it is the demonstrated capacity to independently implement these skills that is seen as indicating the child's readiness for less restrictive levels of care.

Train staff, across levels, in the problem-solving skills and in ways to recognize, cue, and support children in making active, healthy choices. Training should highlight the role of timing: Modulation skills are the necessary first step to successful engagement of higher-order cognitive processes. Offering choice often has the power to reduce power struggles, escalation, and the need for limits.

In milieu settings staff members have many opportunities to support children in the application of problem-solving skills. The approach will vary depending on the entry point. For example, when problem situations have been identified in advance by both staff members and children—for example, common triggers such as visits or phone calls with family, unstructured social situations, transitions, and changes in schedule—it is particularly helpful to create a "problem-solving plan." Work with each child to plan for challenging situations and to identify strategies for effectively coping and achieving a desired outcome (e.g., earning rewards or avoiding consequences, using Steps 3–6 as a guide). Involve youth in planning for these situations in advance; as with all skills, the skill of actively making positive choices is most successful when it has been practiced.

Problem-solving skills can also be applied when an outcome has already occurred. Formal processing of events that led to negative outcomes, such as restriction or therapeutic holds, can include each step outlined above. It may be helpful, when processing, to provide visual cues of different affective states (feelings faces), energy levels (high, medium, low), etc. Additionally, if the outcome is related to peer conflict, consider formally implementing problem-solving steps in the approach to conflict resolution. Each resident involved in the conflict can have the opportunity to reflect on the situation individually, share his or her perspective, and then to jointly engage in problem solving based on a mutually agreed-upon goal/outcome. Milieus often have external structures for dealing with conflict-related problems such as boundary breaches. When possible, involve youth in the process of evaluating the situation and selecting appropriate solutions, including reparation with peers or staff, as well as potential programmatic consequences.

Problem-solving steps are most often applied in the moment with residents. In this case, use staff forums for communication to develop plans for implementing problem solving in the moment. Consider a meeting structure that draws on staff attunement to each client and includes discussion of client triggers; cues indicating distress, behaviors associated with fight, flight, and freeze responses; and current modulation strategies being used by client, both positive and negative (e.g., asking for space, cutting). Use that information to develop a menu of modulation strategies from which each resident can choose when a problem situation appears to be occurring. For example, a staff member may observe that a resident is experiencing distress, as indicated by noncompliance. That staff member could reflect cues to the client and offer choices such as "Would you like a break? Would you like to blow bubbles or try something else from your toolbox?"

In summary, consider the entry point when developing programming that emphasizes this skill and incorporate both formal and informal approaches.

🌎 REAL-WORLD THERAPY

🌎 **Practice makes . . . well, not quite perfect.** These skills are hard. Children will be much better at using them in the office than in the "real world," particularly in moments of emotional arousal. Expect that it will take some time for children to gain any mastery over these skills, especially with difficult problem situations. Don't throw out a skill because it doesn't work the first time, or the second time, or the tenth time. Repetition will eventually increase children's sense of control; even if they are unable to make the desired choice in the moment, over time they will be increasingly aware that they *have* choices. This, in itself, is a success.

CHAPTER 12

Self-Development and Identity

THE MAIN IDEA

Support children in exploring and building an understanding of self and personal identity, including identification of unique and positive qualities, development of a sense of coherence across time and experience, and support in the capacity to imagine and work toward a range of future possibilities.

★ KEY CONCEPTS

★ *Why Target Self-Development and Identity?*

- A key developmental process is the growth of a sense of self, an understanding of individuality, and eventually the formation of a coherent identity.

- Establishment of a coherent self advances across developmental stages:

  - **In infancy and early childhood, identity formation begins as a basic awareness of self as separate from, but related to, others.** This basic self-concept grows as others—primarily immediate caregivers—respond in predictable ways to child actions, behaviors, and interactions. Children internalize the typical response of others: A child who receives frequent praise and affection, for instance, internalizes an understanding of self as positive and worthy of love. A child who is routinely rejected, in contrast, may internalize an understanding of self as unworthy. These internalized messages are incorporated into the child's burgeoning understanding of self.

  - **In middle childhood, understanding of self expands to incorporate the experiences from multiple domains of a child's life.** Children focus in part on concrete attributes and outcomes: "I am a girl [or a boy]," "I am strong [or weak]," "I am smart [or dumb]." Attributes are often understood in dichotomies, with shades of gray developing over the course of this stage. Interactions with caregivers continue to be important to self-concept; however, the responses of peers, teachers, and other key figures are factored in as well. Over time, a sense of self grows to encompass personal attributes, likes and dislikes, and individual values.

♦ **During adolescence, early understanding of self grows into a more coherent identity encompassing abstract attributes, an integration of multiple aspects of experience, and future possibilities.** Normatively, this is an active process, as adolescents explore their own likes/dislikes, goals, values, and needs. Adolescents may "try on" different attributes in an attempt to crystallize a sense of self. Integrated into this sense of self are current and past experiences as well as future goals.

• *Growth of personal identity is an ongoing process that rarely ends in adolescence.*

★ *How Does Trauma Impact Self-Development and Identity?*

• Impaired establishment of a positive, coherent sense of self is a primary consequence of early trauma and attachment disruption. Empirical studies indicate impaired self-concept beginning in early childhood, and continuing through adolescence and adulthood.

• There are several reasons why trauma may impact development of a coherent, positive identity and sense of self.

Internalization of Negative Experiences

Like all children, traumatized children internalize and incorporate experiences into their sense of self. Children who are routinely rejected, harmed, or ignored internalize an understanding of self as unlovable, unworthy, helpless, or damaged.

⌑ Keep in mind that broader societal messages have the potential to play a role in development of self-concept, both positive and negative. Media and other forums send messages about gender roles, body image, ethnic and culturally based expectations, language use, etc. Any member of a group who is marginalized in some way by media or other societal messages may be vulnerable to the impact of those messages on self-concept and identity. Children who have experienced trauma may be particularly vulnerable to internalization of negative attributions.

Fragmentation of Experience

The development of identity requires the ability to integrate experiences and aspects of self into a coherent whole. Traumatized children often rely on dissociative coping methods involving fragmentation and disconnection from their experiences. As such, traumatized children may have multiple "senses of self": the frightened self, the angry self, the invisible self, and the okay self. Often, these *state-dependent self-concepts* emerge in response to specific experiences and emotions. As such, children have difficulty integrating a coherent sense of self across experiences and affective states.

Lack of Exploration

Normatively, secure attachments provide the safety that allows children to explore their worlds, and, by extension, different aspects of themselves. Children learn whether they can accomplish goals, experiment with novelty, explore likes and dislikes, etc. Traumatized children often curtail exploration in the service of safety, instead relying on rigid control and repetition. Without exploration, children are limited to what immediately *is*, rather than the possibilities of what *could be*. This limitation on imagination cuts off potential facets of self, both in the present and in the future.

THERAPIST TOOLBOX

Behind the Scenes

- There are multiple facets involved in development of a coherent sense of self and identity. These include:

  ♦ *Unique self:* An understanding of individual characteristics, including concrete attributes, likes/dislikes, opinions, values, strengths and vulnerabilities, familial and cultural influences, spiritual beliefs, etc.

  ♦ *Positive self:* Ability to tune in to, identify, and own positive attributes of self.

  ♦ *Coherent self:* Ability to integrate multiple aspects of self, both strengths and vulnerabilities, across experiences (i.e., past and present) and across affective states.

  ♦ *Future self:* Ability to envision possibilities, to imagine the self in the future, and to imagine ways to become that self, incorporating both short- and long-term goals.

- For all of the above, sense of identity may encompass self alone as well as **self in relation to others** and **self in context** (e.g., within the context of family, of culture, of school). It is important to explore each of these facets of self on multiple levels.

- Each of these facets of self progresses over the course of development. A 5-year-old's understanding of his or her unique self will differ from an adolescent's, but the concept remains important across developmental stages. See Developmental Considerations.

- A number of techniques that may be useful for exploration of self and identity are offered in this chapter. However, when working with children to build self-concept and positive identity, it is crucial to extend the work beyond the therapy room. It is important that children not just talk about who they are, but find ways to explore and express what they identify as self attributes in their daily lives.

- Problem-solve with child and caregivers about potential barriers to exploring areas of interest. For instance, if a child has an interest in the theater but is shy, can the caregiver support the child in going to the activity with a friend? Provide a safety object for the child to carry?

- When engaging in the techniques described below, as well as in "real-world" applications and explorations of self-interests, it is important to include the use of modulation strategies. Many children struggle with sense of self, so activities related to self and identity may elicit a range of affect and arousal.

🗂 *Teach to Caregivers*

- *Reminder:* Teach caregivers the Key Concepts.
- *Reminder:* Teach caregivers relevant Developmental Considerations.
- Incorporate caregivers, as appropriate, into treatment. Many of the tasks described below can be completed dyadically, and, in fact, may be more powerful if done so.
- Teach caregivers—whether in the home, milieu, or other settings—about the four specific identity targets, as described below. The moments that will contribute most strongly to identity formation are likely to occur in daily life rather than in the treatment room. Work with caregivers to observe, reflect, reinforce, and support a child's exploration of self. This may involve:
  - ♦ Noticing and reinforcing key concepts in the home setting (e.g., "I knew right away that this was your school book cover, because I can see all the symbols that you like decorating it").
  - ♦ Using key language across settings (e.g., the language of mixed emotions: "I wonder if you might be feeling more than one thing right now—I know I'm kind of nervous and kind of excited").
  - ♦ Incorporating therapeutic activities in the home setting (e.g., creating a "pride wall" at home).
  - ♦ Creating unique activities specific to the home setting (e.g., a family photo album, family trees, family collage).
- In group caregiving settings (e.g., residential programs, schools) pay attention to *group* as well as *individual* identity. This may involve both a celebration of diversity (e.g., the unique characteristics of all the individuals who make up the group) and a celebration of coherence (e.g., those characteristics that unite group members). As with primary caregivers, milieu and other group caregiving systems can tune in to each of the primary targets of identity:
  - ♦ *Unique self*
    - ○ *Individual:* What characteristics does *this* child contribute to the setting? In what ways does the child stand out? Use basic reflection and attunement to notice, name, and highlight unique child attributes.
    - ○ *Group:* What makes individuals within this (program, school, classroom) unique? What are the group values? Goals? Name and explore these. For instance, a classroom might identify and create signs to highlight class values (e.g., respect, safety); a residential program might create bulletin boards highlighting group member "favorites" (e.g., animals, colors), etc.
  - ♦ *Positive self*
    - ○ *Individual:* What successes has the child had (both relative and absolute)? Work with staff to notice and name achievements. Highlight these concretely, when possible.
    - ○ *Group:* Establish "community pride"; work with group members toward collaborative successes. For instance, set a group goal—perhaps earning a total of x points across group members—and celebrate the achievement as a group success.

♦ *Coherent self*

 ○ *Individual:* Pay attention to ways in which a child's experience may be fragmented (e.g., across affective states, across placements, across peer groups) and name/reflect observed patterns (e.g., "It seems that you feel like you need to be a little tougher when you're hanging out with Lisa and Janice than when you're just with one of the adults"). Normalize differences in experience while working to help children create coherence (e.g., "It makes sense that the toughest part of you has to show up when you're talking with girls who you know have been in gangs, and that you can let that part of you relax when you're with staff").

 ○ *Group:* Where is there coherence and/or fragmentation across group members? Tune in to the ways that group members' behavior changes when most members are excited, for instance, versus frustrated. Notice times when "factions" of group members splinter off from others and explore the group identity of this faction while also supporting each individual in honoring unique aspects of self.

♦ *Future self*

 ○ *Individual:* As in individual treatment or in family settings, work with children to imagine themselves in the future, to set concrete goals, and to work toward those goals, considering immediate, short-term, and long-term goals. Within programs, it is particularly important to shift the work eventually beyond the tomorrow/next-week goals and to pay attention to "life-outside-the-program" goals.

 ○ *Group:* Work with group members to set programmatic, future-oriented goals. For instance, help group members identify a program-relevant goal (e.g., creating a comfortable group space in a common room, putting on a play, working as a team in a competition) and work with them to identify steps toward reaching it.

✂ Tools: Self-Development and Identity

- Self-development involves a number of different skills; the following table highlights key aspects of identity and sample tasks.

- As with other skills highlighted in this framework, the best tasks are often individually targeted; use the following as a guideline, but be creative.

- Techniques should, to the degree possible, be interactive. Use them to generate discussion between the child and clinician/caregiver.

Target #1: Individuality—The Unique Self

- **Overarching goal:** *Help children identify personal attributes. These include likes and dislikes, values, talents, preferences, opinions, family and cultural influences, spiritual beliefs, etc.*

- In addition to formal techniques, tune in to child statements in daily life that represent this concept. Help children expand on these.

INDIVIDUALITY

Sample activity	Description	
"All about Me" books	Suggested materials	Paper, construction paper (for covers), markers/crayons/writing and drawing materials, materials to decorate book, clips or ribbon to bind book, pictures of child or others, as desired
	Techniques	• Introduce activity to children. Highlight that they will be creating a book that is all about them. • "All-about-Me" books are generally created over time. Often, clinicians will choose to do one page per session with the child. • Content of "All-about-Me" books varies in accordance with child needs and developmental stage. • Content often shifts over time when working in a longer-term therapeutic relationship. It may be important to complete a book and then begin another as a child enters a new developmental stage or life phase, rather than continuing the same book. Creating a new book highlights the theme of change and growth. • Provide structure for young children. For instance, create a page listing the child's favorite colors, names of pets, favorite foods, etc. The focus is generally on concrete attributes. Drawings can be used in lieu of words. • Consider using more abstract concepts with older children. Incorporate affect. For instance, list or draw exciting or frightening experiences that the child has had. • Pay attention to including *personal values*: What is important to this particular child? Keep in mind ways that developmental stage will impact these values (e.g., for a 5-year-old, "Be nice" is a value; for a 15-year-old, "It's important not to pick on people who are weaker than me" is a value). • Tailor entries to child milestones, achievements, and current experiences. Listen for opportunities in the session. For instance, if a child is describing an experience that seems important, suggest writing or drawing about it, and including it in the "All-about-Me" book.
Personal collage	Suggested materials	Posterboard or sturdy construction paper, glue, magazines, pictures, drawings, stickers, letters, etc.
	Techniques	• Collage is a way for children to represent aspects of the self without a need for words or verbal explanation. • Introduce the technique to children; highlight that they will be creating a collage, using provided materials, to represent different aspects of the self. • Invite children to find materials that either represent something about who they are or that appeal to them. They do not need to be able to explain *why* they are choosing the picture, material, etc. • Collages can be *general* (e.g., "All about you") or they can target *specific ideas* (e.g., "the you no one else sees"; "who you are at school"; "things you enjoy").
Artistic self-expression	Suggested materials	Dependent on modality; may include clay, paints, drawing materials, music, pen/paper/journal, etc.
	Techniques	• Use array of fine and expressive arts to help children express aspects of identity. Consider drawing, writing, poetry, rapping, sculpture, movement, etc. • Artistic self-expression can be done in a structured or informal way. For instance, clinician may provide a prompt and have child generate a poem or rap; *or* clinician may encourage child to engage in artistic self-expression, which child may (or may not) choose to share in the session. • Consider incorporating caregivers; have caregivers work with children on artistic projects (this is particularly important with younger children). Encourage older children and adolescents to share the results of their projects with caregivers; if appropriate, invite caregivers into session.

Sample activity	Description	
Try it out	Suggested materials	Varies
	Techniques	Exploring identity only goes so far if it is restricted to the office. Help children identify an interest (e.g., hobby, sport, extracurricular activity) and encourage them to "try it out." Incorporate caregivers as allies.

Target #2: Esteem and Efficacy—The Positive Self

- **Overarching goal:** *Build internal resources and identification of positive aspects of self.*

- In working on self-esteem and efficacy, it is important to take note of both *absolute* strengths (e.g., a child's skill at math or athletics) and *relative successes* (e.g., working hard at a difficult task or recognizing an area of vulnerability and choosing to address it). Help children and the system reframe the concept of success.

ESTEEM AND EFFICACY

Sample Activity	Description	
Power book	Suggested materials	Paper, construction paper (for covers), markers/crayons/writing and drawing materials, materials to decorate book, clips or ribbon to bind book, pictures of child or others, as desired
	Techniques	<ul><li>Introduce activity to children. Highlight that they will be creating a book about things that make them feel powerful.</li><li>Like "All-about-Me" books, power books are generally created over time. Often clinicians choose to do one page per session with a child.</li><li>Help children create a cover for the power book. The only rule is that the cover must embody strength or individual power in some way; encourage children to use their imagination.</li><li>The goal of a power book is to highlight children's (real and potential) strengths, successes, positive experiences, and internal and external resources. Note that resources do not need to be reality-based; encourage children to use their imaginations to picture *possibilities*. For instance, children might imagine qualities that would make them feel powerful and then picture themselves as an animal, superhero, athlete, etc., who has that quality.</li><li>There are two primary ways to complete power books:<ul><li>◆ *Provide structured prompts* to elicit drawings or writing. For instance, ask children to list their five best qualities; to draw themselves as a superhero; to draw themselves doing something at which they are good.</li><li>◆ *Include spontaneous success.* Tune in to moments when children display strength, success, or power. Note that definitions of success should include effort as well as relative successes (e.g., the child who is able to get through the day without fighting). When spontaneous successes occur, write or draw about them and include them in the power book.</li></ul>(*Note* that the above two are not mutually exclusive and that most power books will contain a combination.)<ul><li>◆ Review power books regularly; include them while reviewing treatment plans and goals with child and family. Power books provide a concrete way to track child and family successes.</li></ul></li></ul>

Sample Activity	Description	
Pride wall	Suggested materials	Bulletin board or blank wall; index cards or award cards; pen or marker (or other writing utensil); tape or thumbtacks
	Techniques	• A pride wall is similar to a power book in that the goal is to notice and reinforce moments of success. There are several ways to implement a pride wall, depending in part on the setting. Examples are given here.

Techniques (continued):

• *Therapy office:*
  ♦ Designate a wall or area of the office as a "Pride Wall" (or "Power Wall"). Create a sign or lettering to mark it as such.
  ♦ Place near the pride wall a basket or other container with index cards, award cards, etc., as well as pens or markers.
  ♦ Invite children (or families) to add things of which they are proud to the wall. Children should write a statement about what they are proud of (e.g., "I cleaned my room when Mom asked") and place it on the wall. Note that children should *not* include their name (for reasons of confidentiality).
  ♦ Invite caregivers to also add pride statements about their child to the wall.
• *Home:*
  ♦ Pride walls at home are an excellent way to help caregivers "catch their children being good." Invite a family to designate a wall or other area (e.g., large bulletin board) as the pride wall. Again, have index cards and other materials available nearby.
  ♦ Pair the pride wall creations with attachment work. Work with caregivers to notice and reinforce positive child effort and behavior as well as accomplishments.
  ♦ For families who have difficulty providing positive forms of attention, create structure (e.g., the family must place one item on the pride wall every day).
  ♦ A family pride wall should include not just individual successes but family successes and accomplishments.
• *School or milieu:*
  ♦ If treatment is provided in a school or milieu setting, work with staff to create a program pride wall. The wall can be classroom- or group-specific, or in a hallway or other public area.
  ♦ Create rules about who may add to the pride wall, and when. It may be helpful to designate a time when people may add to the wall. Encourage self-nominations, peer nominations, staff nominations, etc.
  ♦ Celebrate success whenever it happens.

Superhero self	Suggested materials	Drawing materials (e.g., paper, markers/crayons); writing materials; clay or other sculpture materials; other arts materials (e.g., popsicle sticks, felt, pipe cleaners)
	Techniques	• The goal of this activity is to help the child imagine him- or herself as a superhero.

Techniques (continued):

• Help children define qualities that make a true superhero. Note that these qualities should go beyond simple muscular strength. Have a conversation about what it means to be "strong." Consider that there are many kinds of strength. Help children think of examples of strength they have witnessed, heard about, felt, or learned of via movies or books. Provide examples, if necessary (e.g., the strength to raise a child by yourself, the strength to be kind to someone when others are not, the strength to stand up to a bully, the strength to walk away from a fight).
• Help children create a list of superhero qualities: What qualities do the children admire? What qualities are shared by their (real and imaginary) heroes? By people they know and like?

Sample Activity	Description

- *Trauma note:* Many children who have been harmed at the hands of a primary caregiver may retain an idealized version of that caregiver, particularly if they have been removed/separated from that caregiver. It is not uncommon, then, for children to name that person as someone who has qualities they admire. If this happens, consider the following steps:
  - ◆ Validate the child's feelings. It may be important for the child to retain a positive sense of that caregiver.
  - ◆ Normalize that all people have both positive and not-so-positive qualities.
  - ◆ Name the qualities (or help the child name the qualities) that the child still admires about that person and/or feelings the child has. This may be as simple as "He's my Dad," or "I love him."
  - ◆ Reinforce for the child that it is okay to have more than one feeling about a person, and that the child can love someone (for instance) and still be angry at that person or sad about things that have happened. (*Note:* Don't push this part of the conversation; some children may not want to go there. The goal is simply to acknowledge the possibility of feeling more than one way.)
- Once a list of qualities has been created, help children imagine themselves as a superhero with all of those qualities. What would they look like? What would their powers be? They might make up a new superhero or choose to imagine themselves as an already existing one—either is fine.
- Go beyond drawing or writing; act out with the child the role of superhero, or have doll or action figure characters take on the role. Imagine dealing with a problem situation as the superhero—how would the superhero use his or her special qualities? How might those qualities help with difficult situations? Play it all out.
- Build on this project; be creative. For instance, children can create a small "secret symbol" of their superhero self and carry it with them, or they can build a model of their superhero self and place it in their room to remind them of strength.

Other tasks	Be creative in choosing tasks to build a child's sense of personal esteem and efficacy. Use drawings, writing, etc., to capture moments when the child succeeds. Make it concrete, so that over time each child has physical representations of moments of success. Incorporate caregivers and other adults into this work.

Target #3: The Coherent Self

- **Overarching goal:** *Help children build a sense of self that integrates past and present experiences and incorporates multiple aspects of self.*

- A primary contributor to the fragmented self of traumatized children is a difficulty with integrating emotional states. The tasks below focus on helping children incorporate an understanding and normalization of multiple affective states and reactions, including ways that feelings flow and change over time.

- Many children with whom we work have lived in different homes, with different caregivers, different schools, different neighborhoods, different peers, and different surrounding environments. As children move across contexts, they must enter and adjust to often vastly different cultures. They may be conscious of differences in spoken language or skin color; they may be confronted with new rules, values, food choices, customs, and rituals. These shifts involve numerous challenges. Children may feel they have to abandon the old and create a new self in each new context; they may struggle to integrate different aspects of their environment; and/or they may reject the offerings of new home environments, often leading to further placement disruption. Work with the child to explore the ways in which all of their experiences have contributed to who they are and how they see themselves. In addition, work with caregivers to acknowledge, explore, and understand similarities and differences in their child's experience.

- Caregivers are often the bearers of children's histories: They hold the memories of "firsts" and other early experiences, of familial history, and of patterns and rhythms of the child's life over time and the ways these weave into a larger narrative. Often, caregivers are the owners of the concrete markers of children's lives, such as photographs, report cards, drawings, and writings. Work with caregivers to support their children in the development of a coherent narrative. For children who have transitioned (and who continue to transition) among caregiving systems, it is particularly important to work with caregivers to concretely document and capture moments of the child's history, as it is developing.

- An understanding of coherent self includes an awareness of the ways that experiences (emotional, behavioral, relational) relate to one another. Observe and help children tune in to patterns. Help children notice similarities and differences in their experiences over time and across contexts.

THE COHERENT SELF

Sample activity	Description	
Life books	Suggested materials	Paper, construction paper (for covers), markers/crayons/writing and drawing materials, materials to decorate book, clips or ribbon to bind book, pictures of child and significant others (including pets), etc.
	Techniques	<ul><li>The goal of a life book is to help the child create and "own" a coherent narrative of who she is, where he comes from, and significant life events.</li><li>Life books can be particularly useful for children who have been in multiple or disrupted placements, those who have not yet attained permanency in placement, and those who have been adopted or placed into a family that is not their family of origin. Life books are also often helpful for adolescents who are working to understand, make meaning of, and create a narrative about their life experiences and current identity.</li></ul>
		<ul><li>For younger children, life books should ideally be done with the assistance of a primary caregiver and/or someone who has known the child over time (e.g., an ongoing social services caseworker, a school staff member).</li><li>There is no single best way to do a life book, and there are many existing models for their construction. In working with a child to construct a life book, consider the following:</li><li>*Timeline:*<ul><li>Begin with the basics: What happened, when, and who was involved?</li><li>Help children create a timeline of significant life events. For example: Where were they born? How old were they when they started school? Who was their teacher then? What was their house like?</li><li>For children who have experienced multiple placements, help them name the different homes in which they have lived and what they did and did not like about each of those homes.</li><li>Is there a significant object (e.g., toy, blanket, piece of clothing) that a child has carried over time? If so, draw it or write about it.</li><li>Fill in significant events that the child designates—for instance, the child's favorite memory, a birthday party, visits with caregivers or siblings, etc.</li><li>Help the child fill in missing information. Elicit help from current caregivers, teachers (with consent), caseworkers, etc.</li><li>Once significant life events are identified, place them in roughly chronological order.</li></ul></li></ul>

Sample activity	Description	

		• *Thoughts and feelings:*
		  ◆ Go back through the book with the child. Slowly (be aware of pacing) help the child add information about his or her thoughts and feelings in connection with specific events. Incorporate pictures, words, etc., into relevant places in the book.
		  (*Note:* It is very important that children have ready access to basic affect regulation skills learned prior to beginning this task. These exercises may elicit strong feelings, and children must have a basic repertoire of coping skills.)
		  ◆ For children who are able to do so, help them consider any changes in their feelings: Is how a child feels *now* about the event the same or different from how he or she felt *then*? Write or draw about both.
		• *Meaning and connections:*
		  ◆ Primarily with older children and adolescents, a next step is to look at past events and experiences in connection with the present. Consider examining the following:
		  ◆ How has each event impacted the present? Pay attention to both positive and negative impacts.
		  ◆ How did the child or adolescent cope with or manage the events? What skills were used to survive or get through? How do these skills connect to skills the child or adolescent continues to use? How have these skills changed?
		  ◆ Upon whom was the child or adolescent able to rely when those events happened? Are those people still in the child's life? If not, are there other people who fill similar roles? For people who are no longer present, are there ways for the child to concretely remember them or incorporate their qualities into present life?
		  ◆ In what ways is the child or adolescent still similar to who they were when the events happened? In what ways has he or she changed?

Aspects of self	Suggested materials	Drawing supplies, paints, felt, popsicle sticks, magazines, masks, shoebox, posterboard, heavy cardboard, white T-shirts, papier-mâché materials, etc. (*Note:* Match materials to selected project.)

	Techniques	The goal of these techniques is to help the child concretely symbolize multiple aspects of self, and to create a single project that integrates the techniques. Note that many different projects could be used for this purpose; suggestions follow.
		
		• Each of these projects is generally nonverbal; however, it is important that the clinician provide some context for the selected activity. Consider the following teaching point to introduce the project: "We all have many different parts that make up who we are. In this project, we will explore some of those parts."
		  ◆ *Personal crest:* Look up (in books, online, etc.) personal crests or shields so that children have a model. Help children create their own crest. (For younger children or those who have difficulty with unstructured tasks, it is often helpful to provide an outline of a crest as a starting point; see sample crests in Appendix D.) The crest should include several sections (this can be as simple as drawing a crosshatch to break the crest into four parts). Help children generate symbols that represent different aspects of self; incorporate these into each child's personal crest. Note that this activity can be as simple or complex as a child wishes.
		  ◆ *Masks:* Create (or purchase) blank white masks and decorate according to selected goal. Many different variations on this task are possible, and clinician and child may choose to do more than one. For instance:
		    ○ How the child feels on the inside (inside of mask) versus what he or she shows on the outside (outside of mask)
		    ○ Different facets of the child on different sections of mask
		    ○ Different emotions: Where the child shows emotion; how often (or how much of) that emotion the child shows; how much of that emotion the child feels, etc.
		    ○ How different people see the child versus how the child sees him- or herself
		    ○ The child in different contexts

Sample activity	Description
	♦ *Ingredients of self:* Use a shoebox or other container to help the child symbolically represent the multiple aspects of self. Place in the shoebox pictures, objects, words, etc., that symbolize different qualities that the child selects to represent him- or herself. Child may choose to decorate the outside of the box or leave it blank. ♦ *Building blocks:* On thick posterboard trace a flattened three-dimensional block or have available ready-made foam blocks. Help the child decorate each block with symbols, pictures, or words that represent one facet of him- or herself. Put the blocks together. ♦ *Personal puzzles:* Prior to working with the child, cut a puzzle out from thick posterboard. Provide the child with individual puzzle pieces and ask him or her to decorate each piece with symbols, pictures, or words that represent one facet of him- or herself. Put the puzzle together and look at the different ways the parts intersect.

Target #4: Future Orientation

- **Overarching goal:** *Build children's ability to imagine self in the future and to build connections between current actions and future outcomes.*

- Keep in mind that "future" will be a different concept at different developmental stages; for young children, the future may be a week from now; for adolescents, the future may be 20 years from now.

- In addition to formal exercises, pay attention in the session to connecting current actions and experiences to future goals.

FUTURE ORIENTATION

Sample activity	Description	
Future self drawing	Suggested materials	Paper, drawing materials
	Techniques	• The future self drawing is a concrete tool to help children begin to imagine themselves in the future. The technique can be more or less sophisticated, depending on each child's developmental stage. • Prompt children to imagine themselves in the future. Where will they be? What will they look like? Who else might be with them? What will they be doing? For children who have difficulty imagining a future self, prompts should be as concrete as possible (e.g., "What do you think you might want to be when you grow up?"). • Have children draw a picture of their imagined future self. • This technique is often helpful to repeat over the course of treatment. Note differences in children's ability to imagine a future self. • Older children may prefer to describe the future self in words rather than drawing a picture.
5 years, 10 years, 20 years in the future	Suggested materials	Paper, drawing materials
	Techniques	• This technique is similar to the above future self drawing, but expands the concept to help children imagine the steps needed in reaching their future self. This technique is primarily geared toward older children and adolescents. • Separate a piece of paper into three sections (or use three sheets of paper). Sections represent increments of time (e.g., 5 years, 10 years, and 20 years in the future).

Sample activity	Description	
		• Prompt children to imagine future goals: Where would they like to be 20 years from now? Based on response, what goals would children want to accomplish in 5 and 10 years as steps toward achieving that goal. For instance: If a child states that he wants to be a professional baseball player in 20 years, what would help him get there in the immediate future? In 5 years? In 10 years? • Incorporate, to the degree possible, external sources of support. For instance, who in the child's life can help him reach his goal? What kind of person (or people) might the child want to have in his life in the future? • Draw (or write about) each of these stages. • Note that this task involves both anticipating and imagining the future, as well as goal-oriented planning and understanding the concept of goal-related steps.
Life book addendum	Suggested materials	Previously created life book, drawing and/or writing materials
	Techniques	• This task is an addendum to the already created life book by adding "future" into previously examined "past" and "present." • Work with the child to imagine him- or herself in the future (note that this can be done via the previous exercise). • Review the life book. What qualities has the child already developed that will help him or her reach the goal? What experiences has the child had that will prepare him or her for the future? What qualities or skills does child still want to build for the future?

👪 DEVELOPMENTAL CONSIDERATIONS

Developmental stage	Self-development and identity considerations
Early childhood	Early childhood understanding of the unique self is basic and often concrete. Help children build an understanding of individual qualities and unique attributes. Ask children's opinions: What flavor do they like best? What color shirt would they like to wear today? Work with caregivers to encourage children to have unique likes and dislikes and to express themselves (even if their clothing doesn't match).
	Children can start developing a sense of personal values from an early age. Work with children and caregivers to understand and build child and family values. Again, keep it simple. Work with caregivers to use age-appropriate language to explain personal choices (e.g., why the family goes to church), rationale for rules (e.g., why it is not okay to hit someone), etc.
	Help children begin to track changes in self over time. Concrete markers are useful. For instance, have a family designate a doorway on which to measure a child's growth at regular intervals, create a collage of school pictures from year to year, etc.
	Future orientation at this age is often fantasy- rather than reality-based. Encourage this; it is important for young children to have multiple possible futures and to engage their imaginations.
Middle childhood	Individuality becomes more nuanced as children become more independent. Work with caregivers to tolerate children's expression of independent preferences (e.g., decorating their bedrooms, hairstyle, clothing).
	Middle childhood is an age of vulnerability to peer influence. Help children identify unique qualities that make them stand out from other children, as well as ways in which they are similar to their peers.

Developmental stage	Self-development and identity considerations
	Understanding of values begins to be more sophisticated at this stage. Work with caregivers and children to identify personal values, familial values, and cultural values. Encourage children to act on their values. Work with caregivers to find forums in which children can concretely express personal and familial values (e.g., volunteer opportunities).
	Children in this stage are able to develop a basic understanding of short- and long-term goals and ways in which present choices impact the future. Work with children to identify goals and the steps with which to achieve them. Keep in mind that long-term goals often continue to be fantasy-oriented at this age (e.g., the child may still want to be a major league baseball player or a rock star), but short-term goals begin to be more grounded in day-to-day experience.
Adolescence	Identity is a primary task of adolescence. Keep in mind that adolescence is an age of extremes and exploration. Adolescents try on, experiment with, and discard various aspects of self. Help them do this in a meaningful way: What appeals to them about the people with whom they associate? The activities they are trying? What do these activities help them know about themselves? Continue to build coherence in sense of self.
	Adolescents are often self-conscious; as they focus on exploration of their own identity, there is a belief that others are similarly focused on them. For teens who have experienced trauma, this self-consciousness can exacerbate feelings of damage, difference, and disconnection. This may be particularly true for teens who identify as being separate from the mainstream in some way (e.g., teens exploring sexual identity). Because of these additional challenges, it may be particularly important to work with adolescents to identify and celebrate aspects of the unique self.
	Adolescents with trauma histories often disconnect from their physical self, particularly as the developing body begins to change. It is particularly important at this stage to incorporate the physical self into identity development tasks. Help adolescents (re)connect to their body and tune in to their physical self. Pay attention to self-care, physiological expression, and sexual identity. Psychoeducation and open discussion are essential.
	Adolescent values often grow beyond those of their family to encompass peer, iconic/cultural, and personal/independent values. Help adolescents explore and delineate values that are separate from those of their family.
	In normative development, adolescents are able to envision the future self in an abstract way while setting realistic goals. It is important to work with adolescent clients to build this ability as a primary developmental task.

APPLICATIONS

Individual/Dyadic

Self/identity activities are often integrated in different ways at different stages of therapy. Early in treatment, the self may be an area of focus as the therapist learns about the child. Particularly in trauma-focused treatment, it is essential that clinicians communicate an interest in the whole child, rather than in just the trauma experience. Over time, exploration of the self generally becomes deeper. Self and identity book activities, as described in this chapter, are good exercises to incorporate into routine check-ins (e.g., consider adding a weekly experience to the child's book). Self activities can be used to help the child build a coherent narrative about the trauma experience as well as other life stories. Often, the focus on self and identity happens "in the moment": Listen for opportunities relevant to the targets of unique self, positive self, coherent self, and future self, and build on these with conversation and activities. When possible and appropriate, integrate caregivers for a portion of this work. For instance, caregivers may be able to (1) provide additional information for a child's life story, (2) name and reinforce their child's strengths, and (3) help in building "action plans" for trying out new skills and interests.

Group

Group activities can easily be designed around and incorporate self and identity activities, particularly with adolescents. Activities can be both overt and subtle. For instance, consider incorporating questions relevant to identity into routine group "icebreakers" (e.g., all group members name their favorite car, the animal they would be). Group identity activities should generally start by focusing on the external self and more concrete attributes before moving to the internal self, in order to allow group safety to build. Examples of group activities that incorporate identity concepts include paired interviews (e.g., children interview each other about individual attributes and report back to the group); creation of collages, masks, and identity shields; creation of physical value lines (e.g., group members identify a range of values; for each value, children physically place themselves between two points to indicate how important that value is to them); and creation of family sculptures (e.g., physical placement of group members in a frozen table to represent family dynamics). Examples of group activities relevant to this construct appear in Appendix C.

Milieu

A milieu system offers an excellent way to tap into and celebrate individual client identity as well as system identity. Consider incorporating visual displays that celebrate diversity, positive child accomplishments, and systemic philosophy and values. Build forums that tap into children's positive self, such as talent shows, as well as unique self, such as special holiday celebrations. Help clients concretely work toward their future self by supporting goal setting and by teaching and supporting tasks relevant to success beyond the particular milieu program. Teach staff about the four facets of self and work with staff to recognize, explore, and reinforce key identity issues in day-to-day conversation.

REAL-WORLD THERAPY

- **Give it time.** Many (if not all) of the children with whom we work with have developed a strongly damaged sense of self. Tuning in to the positives is not only foreign but may be triggering, because the positive self is ego-dystonic. Be aware of pacing, and don't force something on children that they are not yet ready to accept. Be flexible—if a child cannot name any current positive qualities, for instance, can he or she imagine one he or she might someday have? Can you or the caregiver name one? Work *around* and *with* children's defenses.

- **Risks are scary.** Much of the work described above involves not just naming aspects of self but also exploring and trying them on. However . . . new exploration involves risks, and traumatized children have learned to minimize those. Go slowly and build internal and external resources that will help children manage the anxiety that comes with taking risks.

❧ **Whose business is it?** Identity and self are, at core, often private domains. Sharing the self with another can create vulnerability. Be aware that clients may choose not to share aspects of self (particularly those they have learned to routinely hide from others) and/or may err on the side of sharing only "pleasing" aspects of self. It is important to validate the need for privacy and to acknowledge that we all have parts of self that we are more or less comfortable sharing. Look for ways to do this work that increase children's sense of safety. For instance, allow children to write or draw in a journal that only they see, create symbols without using words; allow children to choose which of the symbols/drawings/etc. they wish to share.

PART V

INTEGRATION

CHAPTER 13

Trauma Experience Integration

THE MAIN IDEA

Work with children to actively explore, process, and integrate historical experiences into a coherent and comprehensive understanding of self in order to enhance their capacity to effectively engage in present life.

★ KEY CONCEPTS

★ *Why Target Trauma Experience Integration?*

- From our perspective, the ultimate goal of treatment for children who have been exposed to chronic, complex early traumatic experiences is to build their capacity to harness internal and external resources in service of effective and fulfilling navigation of their life, across domains of functioning, as they define and meet self-identified personal goals.

- Past experiences often interfere with and override children's capacity to engage purposely in present life. Their current reactions are primarily driven by the overwhelming biological mandate of safety seeking, elicited by perceptions of harm and lack of need fulfillment in their environment.

- Present moments may elicit intense, fragmented self-states that are linked to past experience and may include affects, cognitions, sensory experiences, actions or inaction, sense of self, and relational style, and which serve some function for the child. Although these are frequently disconnected from previous experience in the child's conscious awareness, they are often driven by that experience.

★ *What Is Trauma Experience Integration?*

- Many thoughtful models of trauma-focused treatment address "trauma processing," or the exploration and integration of traumatic memories and associated affects, cognitions, sensory experiences, and behavioral responses within the larger narrative of self.

- The definition of trauma processing is a more challenging one for children who have experienced multiple, prolonged stressful exposures, than for those who have experienced single or well-defined events. For a child whose life has involved, for instance, chronic early neglect, unpredictable caregiving associated with parental mental illness or substance abuse, repeated acts of violence, separation from a biological parent, multiple out-of-home placements and attachment disruptions, and revictimization due to difficulty negotiating relationships, it is difficult to define the starting and end points for focal trauma processing.

- A term that many use, and that feels to us more fitting for children who have experienced complex trauma, is "trauma experience integration"; this term is intended to encompass the range of ways that children exposed to more complex trauma may process traumatic experiences.

- For purposes of this framework, we define two related but distinct types of trauma experience integration that may be relevant for children who have experienced more chronic trauma exposures, each of which will be explored in more detail in the sections below. In describing these, consider the accompanying examples.

1. *The Integration of Thematic, or Fragmented, Self-States and Associated Early Experiences.* Identifying and reflecting upon current fragmented aspects of self-functioning (including emotions, actions or inability to act, interpersonal relational styles, cognition, physiological states, and embedded models of self and other) and linking these to the subjective themes (e.g., shame, helplessness, rage, attachment loss, vulnerability) relevant to the repeated experiences of early childhood.

> Emma's aunt, who is her legal guardian, has picked her up from school and is driving her to an appointment. Emma, 13, begins to tell her aunt a story about something that happened at school that day. Her aunt is focused on the road, and midway through the story, fails to respond to a question Emma asked. Emma becomes enraged, yelling and calling her aunt an expletive. When the aunt begins to set a limit ("Calm down! I'm trying to drive") Emma shouts, "Stop yelling at me!" She then unlocks the car door and begins to open it, threatening to jump out even though the car is still in motion.

In the above example, Emma's behavior clearly stems from more than the present moment. Without needing to explicate her history, we can see the impacts of themes of perceived rejection, associated shame, loss of control, and potential danger. In the face of these cues, Emma shifts self-states: From being relatively in control and sharing a positive experience, she shifts into rage, increased arousal, danger avoidance, and preemptive rejection. These reactions are elicited by the present moment, but they are driven by the past.

2. *Processing of Specific Events.* Building a narrative around the emotions, actions or inability to act, interpersonal relational styles, cognitions, and physiological states, along with embedded models of self and other, evoked in relation to specific past memories of trauma or overwhelming stress, and incorporating or shifting these into a more coherent, realistic, and broader narrative of self and other.

> Emma's memories of her biological father are hazy. Although she knows he sexually abused her when she was young, her explicit memories feel "foggy" and mixed up. She has a hard

time distinguishing one memory from the next, but when she thinks about him, she always pictures the tattoo on the right side of his chest, remembers the feel of his stubble against her stomach, and begins to feel panicky and out of breath. She tries really hard not to think about him, but on a recent date a boy tried to kiss her, and she suddenly felt like she couldn't breathe and her body had turned cold, as if she were frozen. Before she could stop it, she saw the image of her dad's tattoo, and felt like she couldn't move.

Emma's memories of her mother are clearer, and she feels angry and confused when she thinks about their relationship. Her mother was unpredictable. Most of the time it felt like she was checked out, just not really available, but sometimes she got really emotional, either violent and rageful or weepy and dramatic, and on rare occasions she was affectionate. Emma likes to think about her mother only in small pieces and finds it easier to remember the things she's mad about than the things she misses.

For the many children who are like Emma, past experiences influence present reactions in a way that is not fully contextualized in the present moment. By continuing to be guided by fragmented self-states that emerge in response to feelings of danger, shame, rage, helplessness, and loss, and to be impacted by specific memories and associated intense experiences, these children are unable to engage in their lives in purposeful, goal-oriented, and fulfilling ways.

THERAPIST TOOLBOX

Behind the Scenes

- Given the complexity of this topic and the range of treatment models that have thoughtfully and carefully addressed this area, we will primarily focus in this text on our understanding of the broader goals, targets, and steps of trauma experience integration, particularly for the integration of fragmented/thematic self-states, rather than on specific techniques.

- We view trauma experience integration as a process, and one that incorporates all other building blocks, or treatment targets, referenced in this framework. Particularly when addressing the exploration and integration of fragmented self-states, this work is layered, complex, and builds on the range of internal and external resources that this framework has previously addressed.

- **Reflection** and **attunement** play a key role in both thematic and specific trauma experience integration. For many children, their lives have involved a *lack* of reflection or a *misreflection*. As children act out distress with often apparently contradictory behaviors, there continues to be both internal and external misattunement. Integration of traumatic experiences requires the capacity to observe and be curious about actions, thoughts, feelings, physiological states, and embedded models of self and other that play out in the present in relation to historical experiences. The holder of the "reflective lens" (i.e., the curious observer) is likely to shift developmentally: For younger children, and for all clients early in this process, it is likely that the initial holder of this lens will be external: a caregiver, whether professional or primary. Over time, particularly for older children and adolescents, the goal is to increasingly build the capacity for self-reflective processes and for accurate self-attunement. As such, we view trauma experience integration as a process that is embedded within the caregiving/attachment system.

The Role of Caregiver Affect Management

- Trauma experience integration in the children with whom we work and for whom we care requires that the caregiver bear witness. Whether the techniques we use are verbal or nonverbal; focus on narrative, expressive strategies, movement, or play; whether we are in the role of therapist, counselor, case manager, or primary caregiver—accurate reflection and attunement necessitate our witnessing of often unbearable pain and the recognition that humans are capable of terribly distressing acts.

- Bearing witness is rarely a completely disconnected process. Although most professionals learn the skills to maintain a reasonably comfortable objectivity and distance, empathic work requires, to some degree, the capacity to resonate with and respond to the affect, relational dynamics, thoughts, systems of meaning, and physiological energy of our clients. Just as attachment is a dyadic, rather than a one-sided, process, therapeutic work happens in the context of a relationship, and these relational connections have an impact on both the child client and the helping professional.

- The understandable affect of the clinician can misdirect us in this work. It can lead us to prematurely close topic areas that the child needs to explore, because of our own anxiety or discomfort with material; to open up other topic areas for which the child is not yet ready because of our own "need to know"; and to carry our work (and its associated sequelae) with us beyond our treatment space. These possibilities make it particularly important for clinicians to monitor, modulate, and seek support for their own affective responses. A number of written resources on this topic may be useful (e.g., Pearlman & Saakvitne, 1995; Saakvitne, Gamble, Pearlman, & Lev, 2000).

Target #1: The Integration of Thematic, or Fragmented, Self-States and Associated Early Experiences

ORIGINS OF THEMATICALLY DRIVEN OR FRAGMENTED SELF-STATES

- As described in the early chapters of this text, children who have experienced complex developmental trauma have been exposed to recurring, chronic stressors that activate the parts of their brain responsible for survival. As with any recurring pattern, when children experience repeated and similar sources of stressful input over time, their brains develop increasingly efficient patterns of response to help them cope with and manage these stressors. These patterns of response can be behavioral (e.g., action or stilling), affective (e.g., surges of rage, shame, and/or fear), cognitive (e.g., shifts in cognitive focus, specific meaning making around cues or experiences), physiological (e.g., increase or decrease in arousal, muscular tension), and/or relational (e.g., shifts in patterns of approach or avoidance). Embedded within those patterns of response that have their origins in interpersonal trauma, and therefore in relationship, is a system of meaning regarding *self, other,* and *self-in-relation-to-other*—that is, distinct attachment patterns and meaning making about self and relationships. These often include dichotomous beliefs about other people that may be grounded in themes such as safety, trust, and acceptance (e.g., safe vs. unsafe, accepting vs. rejecting, trustworthy vs. likely to betray). These beliefs are often associated with meaning making about the self and involve feelings of self-worth versus feelings of shame and damage.

These patterns of response have developed to serve some function—in the brain of the child, at essence, the function is survival—and as such they are often rigid and largely automatic when elicited by pertinent cues. Furthermore, these patterns may be encapsulated and fragmented, or dissociated, from other self-states, such that many different functional patterns are elicited in the child by the range of cues, or themes, related to past experience.

- Prominent *themes* associated with developmental trauma, referred to in previous sections as "triggers" or cues of potential danger, include (but are certainly not limited to) shame, loss, vulnerability, deprivation, helplessness/loss of control, isolation, mistrust/betrayal, injustice, attachment disruption, and invasion/violation of boundaries (emotional, relational, and physical). As described in Chapter 2, detection of and response to these themes does not require their actual presence, merely the *perception* of their presence. In other words, if a child's brain decides that rejection exists, then the pattern of self that developed for self-protection in the face of rejection will emerge—regardless of whether the rejection was objectively present and intended, or not.

WORKING WITH THEMATICALLY DRIVEN OR FRAGMENTED SELF-STATES

- Integration of fragmented self-states requires the building of a reflective process that includes an observation of and curiosity about the patterns of behavior, self- and other-perception, thoughts, feelings, and physiological states that emerge in daily life and that may be driven by past experience. As noted above, this reflective process frequently begins as an externally directed one, with a goal, as developmentally appropriate, of building the child's own curiosity and self-reflective process.

- Engaging in this work involves the integration of many different skills and resources, both internal and external, and much of this work is a process that builds over time.

- An important caution: Although pieces of this work can be done with children who continue to live in chaotic or stressed environments, it is crucial to be careful. An important goal of this work is to help children to shift from "danger response" mode; this goal may not be fully realistic, or safe, for children whose lives continue to be impacted by potential danger, particularly at the hands of their primary caregivers.

- Below we describe 10 steps involved in the process of integrating fragmented self-states; at each step we reference the relevant skills previously taught in this framework. Note that these steps are often cyclical, rather than sequential, and that professionals and clients will find themselves revisiting these steps many different times, regarding different patterns, during different developmental stages, and at different stages of treatment. Because we view this work as a process rather than a specific technique, we include these steps in this "Behind the Scenes" section rather than in the "Tools" section.

- We link each step back to the case example provided at the beginning of this chapter (p. 210).

**STEPS TOWARD ADDRESSING INTEGRATION OF THEMATIC
OR FRAGMENTED SELF-STATES**

- *Step 1:* **Develop a good formulation.**

→ ATTUNEMENT

♦ *Overarching point.* The starting point is always to work to understand the child within the context of his or her life, and the necessary adaptations that have developed in response.

♦ *The main idea.* Identify themes and current cued coping patterns relevant to your client. Go beyond diagnosis to build a trauma-informed conceptualization of behaviors and responses. For instance, imagine that you are working in a residential program with an adolescent boy who has an extensive history of physical abuse by an adult male caregiver. We could imagine that themes involving issues of trust, respect, and control versus mistrust, disrespect, helplessness, and vulnerability would be relevant. Keeping these themes in mind, observe the child within the milieu. The child's history suggests that he may be particularly triggered by, and leery of, authority figures, especially males. In what way do the child's behaviors and interactions with adults and with peers suggest adaptations that make sense? For instance, is the child reactive to limit setting? Quick to engage in a power struggle? Withdrawn when challenged by authority? Identify key patterns and themes, along with functional associated patterns of self, so that rather than focusing purely on diagnostic presentation (e.g., "This child has oppositional defiant disorder"), the response to difficult behaviors is, "Yes, that makes sense."

> Emma's history includes neglect and inadequate attention to her needs, physical abuse, sexual abuse, and attachment losses and disruptions. Although we have minimal information about her adaptations from this case example, we might imagine that triggers, or areas of sensitivity, would include perceived rejection and deprivation, loss of control, boundary invasions, and perceived cues of physical danger. In the face of these "themes," Emma is likely to engage in patterns of behavior that hold as a function, on some level, safety seeking, danger avoidance, or need fulfillment.

- *Step 2:* **Tune in to and observe specific patterns as they occur.**

→ ATTUNEMENT

♦ *Overarching point.* Catch the patterns in the moment: Tune in to and observe patterns of behavior as they occur.

♦ *The main idea.* Work to observe and understand, as they occur, a child's specific patterns of recurring behavior that (1) resonate with the predominant themes associated with developmental trauma, (2) appear linked to previous experience, and (3) serve some current functional purpose (e.g., danger avoidance, need fulfillment). If there is an external caregiver or a team of professionals working with this child, help them to understand the behavior(s) in the context of the function they are serving. At this stage, the goal is for the professional(s) and caregiver(s) to tune in to and observe these patterns; it will be important to engage in Steps 3 and 4 before reflecting on these with the child.

> Emma has a history that includes neglect/inadequate attention to needs as well as physical assault by her mother. In the face of perceived rejection (her aunt not paying atten-

tion), Emma's initial danger signal goes off; when the aunt sets a limit, Emma's "danger signal" escalates and she seeks to escape. Just as the clinician or other professional observes this pattern, it will be important to support Emma's aunt in understanding the various themes and patterns related to Emma's past.

- *Step 3:* **Validate the child's current perceived experience.**

→ ATTUNEMENT, Support of AFFECT IDENTIFICATION, AFFECT EXPRESSION

- ♦ *Overarching point.* Reflect and validate the child's experience in the present moment.

- ♦ *The main idea.* Although we work with clients to observe and reflect on patterns of self-response in the context of *past* experience, it is crucial to first validate their experience *in the present moment.* In other words, no matter how much we may be aware of and recognize larger themes of helplessness, loss of control, rejection, etc., along with functional responses, the child's experience in that moment is as simple—and meaningful— as "Someone did something that felt really upsetting, and now I feel really lousy." If we do not acknowledge the "lousy" feeling, we are not going to get very much further. Use attunement skills to support children in identifying and expressing their experience in the moment. Note that some children may be more readily able to accept validation and reflection than others: For some children, feeling "seen" or observed may in itself be triggering or lead to feelings of vulnerability. As discussed in the Attunement and Affect Identification chapters, it is important, when offering reflections, to allow the child to "own" his or her experience.

    Emma's experience was that she attempted to tell a story, and her aunt refused to listen. Before we can go to observation of this moment in the context of past experiences, it is important to first reflect and validate, "I can see how upsetting it was that your aunt didn't listen when you tried to speak to her. It's really hard when we have something to say, and it feels like people aren't listening."

- *Step 4:* **Support the child in use of modulation strategies.**

→ MODULATION

- ♦ *Overarching point.* Support children in accessing modulation strategies that will allow them to engage meaningfully in the work.

- ♦ *The main idea.* The process of reflecting on patterns of behavior, particularly as they relate to past experiences, has the potential to elicit a range of affective, physiological, and cognitive responses. Among these is a perception of danger *in the present moment.* In other words, in the process of addressing traumatic material within the therapeutic setting, even when the stage has been set to engage in this work on an *explicit* level, on an internal/ instinctive level, children's "danger signals" may still be activated, leading them to engage in self-protective patterns of behavior (e.g., avoidance, numbing, arousal, defense). Children who comply with the therapy process despite these signals of danger may feel revictimized by the process itself, even when they have given apparent consent to discuss or explore their experience. Given that, it is important that children have sufficient awareness of their own internal state and access to a range of skills to support comfortable and effective modulation. When engaging a child in this work, use the skills described in Chapter 9, "Modulation." Invite a child to do a self-check: "What do you notice happening in your body as we're talking about this?" Partner with the child in identifying the effective/comfortable state in which to do this work: "Where is your energy now, and where do you think it needs to go for us to have this conversation?" Acknowledge the difficulty in addressing this material, and normalize the activation of the child's "danger brain" and associated protective behaviors. Work with the child to engage in appropriate skills; ideally, this work will take place *after* a child has had an opportunity to add a range of modulation strategies to his or her "feelings toolbox," along with some practice in observing and identifying internal states. This step will often need to be repeated many times, within and across sessions.

> Emma's clinician checks in with her as they begin to talk about the event in the car. "Emma, can you do a quick self-check and let me know where your energy is at right now?" Emma responds that she's feeling kind of spacy and that she's hovering in the "minuses" (on a –1 to +10 scale). The clinician states, "It makes sense to me that you might be feeling kind of shut down; you had some really big feelings this week, and even talking about them may make your danger brain want to protect you." She suggests that they toss a beanbag back and forth to each other as they talk—a strategy that Emma has previously identified as helping her to stay present and connected. Once Emma agrees, the clinician states, "I think it's important that we talk about this, so we can figure out some of what happened. But you're in charge of how much we talk about it, and if your feelings start to get too big or too shut down, we can take a break or do something to help get your energy back at a place that feels comfortable. We'll keep checking in as we go, okay?"

- *Step 5:* **Observe/reflect on patterns and identify the theme(s).**

→ AFFECT IDENTIFICATION, AFFECT EXPRESSION supported by ATTUNEMENT, CAREGIVER AFFECT MANAGEMENT

   ◆ *Overarching point.* Observe and/or invite the child to observe and reflect on the ways in which the current event or experience may link to previous experiences.

   ◆ *The main idea.* In this step we reflect, and/or invite the child to reflect, on the ways that the current behavior or experience may resonate with previous experiences. Try to identify the relevant theme(s) using the child's language. The holder of the "reflective lens" is likely to vary, depending on the child's developmental stage. For instance, when working with a younger child, the primary observer may be the clinician: "I know there were lots of times when kids got yelled at in your house, and that it was kind of scary. It seems like when the teacher got mad, that felt kind of scary, too." If the child agrees, the clinician might observe, "It seems like something that feels pretty hard is people being mad."

   This can be done outside of the context of individual therapy—for example, after an adolescent reacts to a perceived space invasion in a residential program, the staff member might say, "I'm sorry, I think I just got in your space—I know you've had people get in your space before and that you don't like it"—although caregivers should use caution in addressing vulnerable areas in a less protected context.

   For an older child or a child with more experience in self-reflection, it is important to invite him or her to be the observer. For example: "From what you're describing, you started to feel this funny pit-of-your-stomach kind of feeling, and then got really down, really fast, and that it happened when your friend sent you that e-mail. We've talked about different kinds of triggers, or things that push your buttons. I'm wondering if you think any of them were going on for you here."

Support children in engaging in this reflective process not just in the aftermath of experiences but, ideally, in the moment. For instance, as a child demonstrates a shift in states during a therapy session or other interaction, the clinician might observe, "I'm noticing that as we're talking about this, your fists are clenching but your face is going kind of blank. What do you notice going on inside of you?"

The more experience the caregiver (clinician or otherwise) has with the child, the easier it will be to jointly identify patterns. For example: "This kind of reminds me of the time you got upset when your brother came into your room without permission, and we were able to figure out that you felt like your space was really invaded. Does this feel similar to that?"

CLINICIAN: *(Reflects back what Emma has identified.)* Okay, so you were excited when you got in the car, because of the A– on your math test, and you knew your aunt had been waiting to hear about it. But then, when you went to tell her, she wasn't looking at you, and you felt like she was brushing you off, and you just got really mad all of a sudden. Then it felt like she got really upset, and then you just felt more upset and scared and like you had to get away, is that right?

EMMA: *(Nods her agreement.)* Yeah, that's all right. It's like she wasn't even interested, even though she's been riding me about studying, and then she freaked out when I got mad.

CLINICIAN: So she got upset, and you got upset. But it was a pretty big upset—big enough that you almost jumped out of the car when it was moving. You weren't really feeling upset when you got in the car, were you?" *(Emma shakes her head no.)* "Do you remember how we talked about the danger brain—how its job is to kick in really quickly whenever it thinks something is dangerous?

EMMA: Yeah, I actually thought that was kind of cool. Kind of like, "Super-brain." *(She sings.)*

CLINICIAN: *(Laughs.)* Yeah, well, I'm wondering if maybe your danger brain might have gone off, because you kind of went from 0 to 60 pretty quickly.

EMMA: *(Shrugs.)* Yeah, maybe, I guess.

CLINICIAN: Okay. So we've talked about some of your big push buttons of things that remind you of the things that happened in your house when you were younger, like people being aggressive and getting in your face, people being condescending, and people not paying attention. Do you think one of those might have been going on, or maybe something else that we haven't talked about yet?

EMMA: I don't know. I guess maybe the not paying attention part, and then she got all angry. I just reacted really fast, you know? I just wanted to tell her about the test, and then everything just flipped out.

- *Step 6:* Identify the function of the current response.

→ SELF-ATTUNEMENT

- ♦ *Overarching point.* Support the child in identifying the function of the current response in relation to the theme.

- ♦ *The main idea.* The primary goal of this step is to support the child in understanding the function of his or her behavior in relation to the cues that elicited it. At essence, this step is about building the child's *self-attunement*, just as we work with caregivers to build attunement toward the child.

  Work to identify the behaviors in which the child engages and link these to the cue (i.e., the relevant theme or trigger) and the need for the behaviors in the context of previous experiences.

  Emma's clinician observes, "So when your aunt didn't listen, you got upset, which makes sense to me, because there were times when you had really important things to say to your mom, and she didn't listen. The only way you could get her attention back then was to get really big, and it seems like you tried to do that with your aunt. But then she got upset, because she was driving, and it seems like when she yelled, it hit your danger buttons in a big way, and your first instinct was to get out. And that makes total sense, because when your mom used to yell, things got really dangerous, really quickly. So even though you almost got hurt this time, your brain really was doing its best to take care of you."

- *Step 7:* Differentiate past and present.

→ EXECUTIVE FUNCTIONS

- ♦ *Overarching point.* Support the child in distinguishing between past and present.

- ♦ *The main idea.* Work with the child to realistically distinguish the context in which the current functional behavior arose from the current context. An important factor here is the differentiation of both the stakes and the need. For instance, in the past, having someone appear angry might mean imminent physical threat—the *stakes*—whereas in the present, having someone appear angry may indicate relatively safe emotional expression. The *need* in the past may have been to avoid injury; the need in the present may be to tolerate distress. Given these differences, it is likely that the strategy best suited to address the current stakes and the current needs will be different. Help the child problem-solve to identify what the stakes, needs, and goals are in the current situation, how they differ from those needed in the past, and potential strategies to get those current stakes, needs, and goals met.

  CLINICIAN: Okay, so I'm wondering if we can take a step back here and look at what was actually happening in that car, and not just what it felt like in the moment. When you got in, what was it that you wanted?

  EMMA: I wanted to tell my aunt about my test.

  CLINICIAN: Okay, and what got in the way of that?

  EMMA: She wasn't listening to me.

CLINICIAN: So the problem was that she wasn't listening to you, and you had something you really wanted to tell her. And something that made the problem worse, I think, from what you said before, was that it hurt your feelings that she wasn't listening, right?

EMMA: Yeah, I guess.

CLINICIAN: Okay, so once it started to feel like your aunt wasn't listening, what do you think your goal was then? Was it still to have her listen, or was it for her to know she was hurting your feelings?

EMMA: I don't know. To listen, I guess.

CLINICIAN: Okay, so then let's look at the behavior you used. We talked about the reason this behavior made sense, right? You started yelling and shouting, partly because you felt so upset and partly because that was the way you needed to act to get your mom to listen to you. How did that work with your aunt?

EMMA: *(Laughs.)* Not super well—she started flipping out.

CLINICIAN: *(Laughs.)* Okay, so not the best choice with your aunt, even if that same behavior used to make sense before. So let's think, if your goal was to get her to listen, what kinds of behaviors might work better now?

- *Step 8:* **Build in-the-moment awareness of thematic/fragmented responses.**

→ AFFECT IDENTIFICATION

- ◆ *Overarching point.* Build children's capacity to tune in to and recognize shifts in self-states that signal thematic/fragmented responses in the moment.

- ◆ *The main idea.* Much of the foundational work on the integration of thematic/fragmented self-states happens in the aftermath of these responses, through reflection, observation, and curiosity about patterns of reaction and experience. Ultimately, however, it is important to work toward a goal in which the child is able to recognize and "catch" the response, in the moment, so that he or she can purposely *act*, rather than simply *react*. The capacity to do so is at the heart of the child's ability to engage purposefully with his or her life in the present context.

   Building toward this stage involves helping the child notice and identify internal and/ or external "clues" that previous experiences are driving a current response. These clues will be different for all children. For some, they may be sensory or physiological (e.g., "a funny feeling in my stomach"). For some, they may be cognitive (e.g., "I start thinking I'm really stupid"). Some children can identify specific emotions (e.g., "I just get really enraged, like as mad as I ever get") or lack of emotion (e.g., "I start feeling really shut down, like I can't feel anything at all"). Some children may be able to identify patterns of action or inaction (e.g., "I feel like I need to be moving, like I can't sit still and I have to get out," or "I kind of want to disappear, to not be seen or even exist"). Finally, some children may notice changes in how they interact (e.g., "Well, I usually really like being with my friends, but I suddenly start feeling like I hate them all, and like they don't really care about me anyway").

   Over time, as you work with children to observe and reflect on patterns of behavior, try to identify the clues that signal that they have shifted from one self-state to another. Set as a goal recognizing, as early as possible, the clues, as they appear, in the moment. Keep in mind that this skill is among the hardest to apply. When appropriate, elicit the support of caregivers, who may be able to observe and reflect to the child the presence of these clues.

> Emma was able to identify "this ice-cold but kind of burning feeling—it's hard to describe—that shoots through me, like from the pit of my stomach straight up to my brain, when it feels like she [aunt] isn't paying attention to me. When it happens, it feels like my energy just shoots up too, like crazy-quick."

- *Step 9:* **Build in-the-moment modulation strategies.**

→ MODULATION

- ♦ *Overarching point.* Increase the child's capacity to use modulation strategies to manage in-the-moment distress.

- ♦ *The main idea.* The goal of this step is for children to be able to pair specific modulation strategies with observations of clues of state shifts (i.e., patterns of response generated by previous experience), in the moment, so that they are able to remain engaged in the present, rather than be driven by past experiences. This step should be paired specifically with the previous one (i.e., identification of clues), and specific strategies should be designed to target the affective, cognitive, physiological, and relational patterns identified by each child. The strategies that will work for a child who shuts down and withdraws, for instance, are not likely to be effective for a child who escalates into a rage.

  With older children, it may be important to identify strategies that can be independently used. With younger children (and children who are younger developmentally), it will be crucial to integrate caregivers into this stage, as it is unrealistic to expect a young child to independently observe and identify patterns and engage in modulation strategies. Rather, the "observer" and "modulator" will be external, and the strategies will be engaged within the context of the attachment system.

CLINICIAN: *(Responding to Emma's self-identified clue)* So you get this "ice-cold but kind of burning feeling" that shoots through you, and it kicks up your energy really quickly. That's a tough one, because it sounds like your energy shifts so fast it's hard to control. Do you think you notice that feeling when it happens?

EMMA: I mean, yeah, I guess, but by the time I notice it, I'm like already pissed off and shouting.

CLINICIAN: Okay, so it's going to take a lot of practice, probably, for you to be able to catch it before it gets to that point—which makes sense because this is a new skill, and new things always take time to get good at.

EMMA: *(Nods.)*

CLINICIAN: So we've talked about some different things that bring your energy up and bring it down. It seems like we're looking for something to bring it down, is that right?

EMMA: Yeah, but it's got to be able to like, bag the energy really quickly, and then bring it down, because nothing's going to work that fast.

CLINICIAN: I'm not sure I know what you mean by "bag the energy."

EMMA: Like, if something was trying to run away from you, and you threw a bag over it to capture it, and it's still squirming inside, but you're keeping it from escaping, and then you can calm it down afterward.

CLINICIAN: Oh, okay—you mean like something to help you just get a hold of it first, without bringing it down, and then being able to take the time to bring it down?

EMMA: Yeah, exactly. It's almost like I just kind of have to take a breath and hold it, as soon as I feel that feeling in my stomach, and almost like—(demonstrates throwing her arms around herself and holding herself tightly)—like that, or something.

CLINICIAN: Do you think that would help you bag the energy, or grab hold of it, as a first step?

EMMA: Maybe.

CLINICIAN: It seems like when you do that, your aunt's going to need to know what's happening, so she doesn't say or do something to make it feel worse. Would it make sense for us to talk to her about this?

EMMA: Yeah, I guess so, otherwise she'll just think I'm nuts when I stop talking and start hugging myself.

CLINICIAN: Okay, so once you've stopped talking and start hugging yourself, what do you think you can do next to bring the energy down?

EMMA: I don't know. I liked that breathing thing we did, with that chant over and over, that kind of calmed me down. But if I do that, I'm really gonna have to tell Aunt S____ what I'm doing.

CLINICIAN: I think that'd be a good idea anyway. Because she might even know some clues that she sees from the outside when this kind of thing happens, and since it happens so fast, it might help to have an outside eye, also, so that she can help remind you to get your energy down.

- *Step 10:* **Act in the present moment.**

→ EXECUTIVE FUNCTIONS, SELF-DEVELOPMENT

 ♦ *Overarching point.* Actively and realistically assess the present moment, identify current goals, and make an active choice.

 ♦ *The main idea.* As a child begins to be able to recognize and modulate distress in the moment (and/or the child's caregiving system begins to support these skills), the next step is for the child to harness the capacity to observe and remain in the present moment in the service of identifying and working toward child-identified goals. This involves the use of problem-solving skills, as described in the Executive Functions chapter, and also taps into many other domains, including Self-Development, Affect Identification, and Affect Expression.

   Work with children to apply problem-solving skills to identify the problem (e.g., "What is it that's really bothering me?"), the goals (e.g., "What is it that I really want? What's getting in the way of that?"), and the range of possible solutions (e.g., "What is it that I can/want to do, and what will happen if I make choice A or choice B?"). Work to access and acknowledge the range of states, both past (e.g., "I know that part of me is feeling really sad right now because I'm remembering sad things") and present (e.g., "Right now my feelings are just kind of hurt"). Help children identify areas of strength and resources they can harness to solve problems (e.g., "I don't like it when my friends are mean, but I know when I speak to my grandma about it, I feel better"). Ultimately, support the child in applying solutions, observing and reinforcing the *act* of making active choices, rather than the outcomes. In other words, any instance in which the child makes an active choice, in the present moment, in the service of meeting a goal is a success—regardless of the outcome of the choice.

It is likely not necessary to state this, but this step is the most challenging, and generally occurs only after a great deal of exploration, practice, and after-the-fact reflection. Successes may accrue slowly and will likely be reached in small, age-appropriate steps. It is important to recognize and acknowledge these successes as they occur, both with the child and with the child's caregivers.

> Emma comes to therapy about 2 months after her flareup with her aunt, and after several more escalations, outbursts, and explorations of these outbursts in therapy. She enters the therapy room, flops in the chair, and says, "So you'll never guess what I did." When the clinician asks what she did, Emma says, "I totally did the hold-my-breath-hug thing and didn't freak out!"

CLINICIAN: You mean, like you had that icy, burning feeling and you caught it?

EMMA: Yeah, I totally did.

CLINICIAN: So, what happened?

EMMA: I was with Leslie and Aisha—I told you about them, right? Anyhow, I was trying to talk, and they kept interrupting me and talking to each other, and then I said something, and Leslie did this thing with her hand, like, shut up, right? And I just got super-mad, really quick—I could feel it just shooting through me. Normally I would have just exploded, which would have stunk, because Leslie and I just got back to being friends after we got mad last month. But then, before I said something, I just took a big breath and held it, and I didn't totally do the hug thing, but I like grabbed my shirt in my fists, and just kept thinking, "Bag it, bag it"—like the energy, you know? And I couldn't chant, because we were in the mall, but I did some deep breaths, and got my energy to go down, and then I was still irritated, but you know, not like crazy mad.

CLINICIAN: So then what happened?

EMMA: Not much of anything. It was fine, it really wasn't a big deal, you know? It just felt like it, for a minute. It was like that not-listening thing that we talked about—it just pushed my buttons.

CLINICIAN: I'm so, so impressed, I can't even tell you! I know you've been working on this, and it's really, really hard to catch it when it's happening. And not only did you catch it, but you did it all on your own, and without Leslie and Aisha even knowing what was happening. I'm so proud of you!

EMMA: Yeah, me too! Can we play on the computer today?

SUMMARY. Taken together, the above steps offer a guide toward supporting clients in (1) recognizing and understanding thematic/fragmented self-states that arise from chronic and complex early traumatic experiences; (2) shifting automatic patterns of response; and (3) ultimately integrating multiple aspects of self into a more coherent response that is contextualized in the present moment. As stated earlier, much of this work is a process that builds over time; the integration of historical experience for clients with complex adaptations often involves repeated engagement around present experiences and associated response sets that have their origins in the past. It is important to note the manner in which all steps are embedded within the caregiving system and simultaneously to address the child's own felt mastery: We believe that clients with complex adaptations need to have both the external support and internal resources to safely explore and integrate traumatic experiences that dominate critical periods of development and that occur within the context of early caregiving.

Target #2: Processing Specific Memories and Experiences

THE RATIONALE FOR PROCESSING OF SPECIFIC MEMORIES

- The processing or integration of specific memories and experiences into a broader narrative of self is often what is classically thought of as "trauma processing."

- The processing of specific memories and experiences involves reflecting on the past from the perspective and, ideally, safety of the present. For children and adolescents who have experienced trauma, elements of the past frequently continue to intrude in the form of fragmented memories and their intertwined elements, which may include language, visual images, intense affect, physiological sensation, sensory input, and systems of meaning. These elements often include not just the details of the experience but the aspects of self and other that are embedded in the experience and that now define the self in the present. For instance, as a memory emerges that involves a moment of intense vulnerability, the power of the memory lies only partly in the memory of that helplessness; it also encompasses the extreme helplessness experienced in the present. In that moment, the child is not simply *remembering* vulnerability; he or she is currently *experiencing* the self as vulnerable. There is a dual assault from traumatic memory: the reliving of the overwhelming elements of the experience itself, and the felt helplessness in the face of this intrusion in the present moment.

- Particularly for older children and adolescents, the response in the present may parallel the past experience but may also expand upon and compound it. In the past, for instance, the child may have felt terror, loss, or confusion; in the present, as the past intrudes, the adolescent may feel all of those, and additionally be filled with rage or shame.

- Because of the intensity of traumatic memory and the fear of the present response, many trauma survivors learn to avoid, disconnect from, and shut down memory intrusions. This disconnection prevents mastery over the memory: So long as the response and experience are fully feared in the present, the power of the experience is sustained.

- The processing of traumatic experiences involves careful exploration of aspects of memory and the intertwined/associated affect, physiological sensation, and cognition, both in the past and in the present. Through supporting the child in sitting with, tolerating, moving through, and observing his or her own experiences, the child is able to integrate these experiences into a larger and more coherent story of self; to decrease the intensity and power of these experiences, and therefore of their intrusive nature; and to gain mastery over them.

CONSIDERATIONS IN THE PROCESSING OF MEMORIES

- In working with children who have experienced complex trauma, there are two types of more specific processing that are likely to be relevant:

  1. *Life narrative*—the development of a broader narrative that encompasses the many experiences of the child's life, across time and place, and includes traumatic exposures as well as more positive life experiences.
  2. *Specific memories*—the processing and integration of specific memories, fragments of memory, or composite memories that are particularly distressing for the child and/or intrude into his or her life.

- The development of a life narrative is clearly a process that takes place over time and includes, but is not specific to, trauma exposures. We refer the reader to the chapter on Self-Development and Identity, and particularly to the section, The Coherent Self, on the construction of life books, as an example of the process of constructing a life narrative.

- The following three factors are among those to be considered when addressing specific memories with children.

  TIMING. When is it appropriate to target specific memories?

- Historical experiences are incorporated into the language of skills development throughout this framework, and when treating a child who has experienced complex developmental trauma, these experiences are present in the room and named from early in the therapeutic process. This acknowledgment is often simple, for instance: "When kids have really hard things happen, like what happened with your dad, it can be really tough to manage feelings."

- This broader frame is distinct from the more detailed exploration encompassed in the processing of specific memories. The exploration of traumatic memory has the potential to elicit intense, potentially overwhelming affect, physiological sensation, and cognitive and behavioral dysregulation. It is crucial to consider the child's current functioning as well as current context when discerning whether to open, versus contain, traumatic memories. To safely explore memory, a child must have some capacity to modulate affect and physiology; must have developed some sense of safety in the therapeutic relationship; and must have a sufficiently stable context outside of the clinical space. In the absence of these factors, extensive exploration of the details of memory may lead to further harm and destabilization, rather than healing.

- Having acknowledged the caution, the reality is that specific memories and experiences are likely to emerge in various ways and at many different times, regardless of whether we judge a child to be "stable" or not. Although some trauma processing work will be planned, a great deal will occur in the moment, in response to material the child presents. The professional's capacity to attune to the child and to be ready to respond to this material is crucial. The decision about whether to expand or contain material will depend on clinician judgment regarding the factors delineated above. Regardless of the decision, it is important to observe, acknowledge, and reflect the child's experience. Consider the following example:

> Delia is an 8-year-old girl who is in a short-term foster placement, having recently transitioned out of a longer placement that was disrupted. She has experienced a sharp increase in distressed functioning over the past several weeks, including statements about wanting to hurt herself. When meeting with her therapist, whom she has seen for several years, Delia positions two dolls in a sexual position and states, "That's how my dad liked to do it." The therapist responds, "It seems like you're thinking about your dad." Delia nods, then grabs the dolls and puts them in separate rooms in the dollhouse. The therapist states, "I know those can be scary thoughts, when they come up. Have you been thinking about him a lot?" Delia shrugs and then nods. The therapist responds, "I'm sorry to hear that. It looks like you're feeling kind of sad and mad, just thinking about it now." Delia takes the male doll out of the dollhouse and throws it. "I don't like it!" The therapist validates Delia's current experience by stating, "Those are such big feelings you're having. What happened with your dad was really scary, and even though we've talked about the fact that you're never going to have to live with your dad again, I'm wondering if part of you might be scared about that." Delia shrugs but doesn't answer. The therapist says, "It seems like these are really important thoughts and feelings. Would you like to draw or write about some of the feelings and then find somewhere to put them so that you don't have to take them home with you?" Delia nods. The therapist works with Delia to do an energy and feelings self-check, and then to practice a modulation strategy, before drawing a picture of her feelings. When they have finished, the therapist lets Delia choose where to put the drawing; Delia selects a drawer in the therapist's desk she has used before for this purpose. The therapist and Delia then take several deep breaths, with the therapist guiding Delia in breathing in "calm" and breathing out any scary feelings or distress. The therapist makes sure there is sufficient time for less intense material (e.g., a game) before the session comes to a close.

In this example, the clinician is confronted with emerging intrusive material in a child who has experienced recent instability of living arrangements (placement disruption), along with destabilized presentation. Given these factors and the tenuous nature of the child's current relationship with her caregivers, the clinician chose not to explore in detail the child's intrusive memories; however, the clinician must still acknowledge and, in some way, explore the child's experience. By acknowledging the important nature of the memory, gently exploring the child's current experience, allowing the child to express a key component of the memory (i.e., the affect), and carefully containing the material, the clinician allows the child to achieve some mastery over her distress, without increasing the intensity of it beyond her capacity to manage. At another time, and in another context, the clinician might have further explored the details or nature of the child's memory or experiences.

WHAT TO TARGET. For children who have had many overwhelming experiences, it may be difficult to identify the focus of a trauma narrative. Consider the following.

- *Specific emerging memories*. Some children will identify specific memories that are intruding into daily life. These memories, or memory fragments, are typically an important target for processing.

- *Composite experiences.* When children have had multiple experiences of similar acts (e.g., repeated sexual or physical violence), memories may merge and overlay each other. In creating a narrative, it is likely that memory will encompass details of multiple experiences. It is possible to explore experiences in more thematic, rather than specific, ways. For instance, when working with a child who has a history of exposure to ongoing domestic violence, details explored may include memories of the father's voice, memories of noises, places in which the child hid, feelings in the child's body when hiding, thoughts and fears while listening to parents fight, etc. These details may encompass multiple experiences rather than a single one.

- *High-impact experiences.* For many children who have experienced repeated and multiple early trauma exposures, the experiences that stand out may not be the ones we would anticipate. When asked about worst experiences, an adolescent may identify abruptly leaving a favorite foster mother and leaving a school without a chance to say goodbye to peers, as more distressing than early experiences of violence. Many of these experiences will emerge over the course of the therapy process, particularly in the context of constructing a larger life narrative (e.g., while identifying "significant events" or creating a timeline). These high-impact experiences are important to explore both in the details of the memory and in their influence on present systems of meaning.

FORMAT. The mechanism for processing memories in childhood will vary depending on the child's age, developmental stage, and specific tolerance and preference. In the "Tools" section we discuss various techniques for exploring memory.

STEPS TOWARD PROCESSING SPECIFIC MEMORIES

In the following material we highlight five steps involved in the processing of specific memories. As with the examination of thematic/fragmented self-states, this work often proceeds over a period of time, with layers of detail and understanding added to narratives as the work progresses. Although each of these steps may happen in some way within a single session, it is likely that the creation and exploration of a narrative around an experience, and the integration of that experience into a larger narrative of self, will unfold over an extended time.

- *Step 1:* **Support the child in self-assessment and modulation strategies.**

  ♦ To truly process and explore traumatic memory, a child must be able to sustain connection to the experience of exploring it. When entering into this work, invite the child to do a self-check regarding affect and physiological state (or reflect observed affect/state). Number scales, such as those discussed in the "Degrees of Feeling" section of modulation (e.g., "How do you feel on a −1 to +10 scale?") are often helpful. Many therapies that focus on the processing of memory recommend the use of a "SUDS" (subjective units of distress) scale (e.g., 0–10 or 0–100) to assess a child's level of distress in relation to a memory, and to ensure that he or she is not shutting down or disconnecting. It is helpful to assess level of distress and arousal at the start of the work and in an ongoing way, as the work progresses. Use modulation strategies to achieve a state that is tolerable for the child and effective for the work. Consider the range of coping skills developed with the child while building a "feelings toolbox" (see Modulation section). Also consider specific strategies that may be useful in safely building a narrative, such as (1) helping the child achieve distance from the memory (e.g., "When you tell me this memory, tell me as if you are watching it from outside, like on a TV screen, instead of being in it"); (2) helping the child increase his or her sense of safety by introducing protective mechanisms (e.g., "While we talk about this, imagine that the little girl you're talking about has a safety bubble around her, so that no one can hurt her") or protective people/figures (e.g., "Imagine that your favorite superhero is standing right next to you"); and (3) increasing ties to the present (e.g., "While we're talking about this, I'm going to remind you every little bit to wiggle your toes against the floor, so you can remember that you're sitting here in the room with me, okay?").

- *Step 2:* Guide the telling of the story in a careful, paced way.

  ♦ This step involves the telling of the story, whether through narrative, play, drawing, or other techniques. Support the child in the creation of a narrative: At what point does the child's memory start? What happened next? Work to create a narrative with a beginning, a middle, and an end. Move slowly in this work; allow the child choice in pacing and depth. Often, narratives are created over time. If returning to a previous narrative, review the work and add detail. In the "Tools" section of this chapter, we discuss examples of ways to facilitate the creation of narratives. Use SUDS or other concrete markers to explore the level of distress a memory evokes over time; an important goal of trauma processing is to diminish distress around specific memories as the child's exploration of them unfolds.

  ♦ It is very important to be aware of indications that a child's processing or narrative is "stuck," or that the child is reexperiencing, rather than mastering, traumatic memory. In young children look for indicators of posttraumatic play, such as play with repetitive themes that may include literal or symbolic aspects of traumatic experience, and that appear rigid and difficult to redirect, and in which the child's affect appears constricted or driven rather than enjoyable (Gil, 1991; Terr, 1990). With older children and adolescents be on the lookout for demonstrations of intense affect or sudden constriction, shifts in presentation (e.g., an adolescent who suddenly switches into a baby voice, or who speaks about him- or herself in the third person), and evidence that the child is reliving, rather than remembering, the experience (e.g., an adolescent who is shaking, crying, and pushing outward with his or her arms, as if to push someone away, and who appears unable to respond to clinician statements). If any of these occurs, the child is no longer "processing," and it will be important to focus on modulation, reestablishment of safety, and reengagement with the present.

- *Step 3:* Facilitate self-appraisal and expand and explore the memory in context.

  ♦ Establishing the details of a memory is only the first step in creating a narrative. Over time, work with the child to go beyond the "facts" of the memory and facilitate the child's appraisal of his or her experience, including thoughts and beliefs, feelings, physiological sensations, and actions. Support the child in creating connections across elements, for example: "When they started to yell, I got really scared. My body just went all tense and my stomach got tight, like I was going to be sick. I wished I could stop them, but I was so scared I just couldn't move." For very young children (or for children who are younger developmentally), this connection may occur through the reflected lens of the clinician or caregiver: (with dollhouse play) "I can see that that little girl is hiding in the corner. So much scary stuff is happening, and she looks very scared. I wonder if her whole body is feeling scared, like her tummy hurting or her muscles feeling all tight." Over time, go beyond the specific memory and expand, at age-appropriate levels, on the larger context in which the experience took place. This may include incorporating (1) other experiences (e.g., was this experience representative of other times or distinct from them?); (2) nuances of relationship (e.g., acknowledging and exploring the range of feelings, including positive ones, a child may have about someone who hurt him or her; exploring role and feelings about other individuals who may, or may not, have been involved); and (3) other relevant and contributing factors (e.g., a parent's substance abuse or mental health issues).

- *Step 4:* **Engage in modulation to sustain connection to affect.**

  ♦ As the work progresses, it is important to repeatedly revisit the child's level of arousal and affective state. Check in frequently and support the child in using modulation skills, as needed, to remain "present" and connected to the process.

- *Step 5:* **Explore and develop systems of meaning.**

  ♦ In the final stage of processing, we work with the child to take perspective on the past from the context of the present. This step involves observing past experience and its influence on the child's life, his or her sense of self, relationships with others, and systems of meaning. It is in this stage that we work with the child to explore, for instance, not just past affect but also the thoughts and feelings that occur in the present moment when reflecting on that experience (e.g., "I just feel so mad at myself for not doing anything"). Psychoeducation and reality testing are often an important component of this stage and may involve acknowledgment and exploration of the thought/feeling/wish in the moment (e.g., "It's my job to protect my mom"), as well as the building of more realistic appraisals from the present perspective (e.g., "Even though part of me still wishes I could have, he was just so much bigger than me, there's no way I could have stopped him").

  Move beyond past and present to consider the future: In the past, for instance, no one may have helped; in the present and future, who might the child be able to trust? What skills, strengths, and resources does the child now have with which to protect him- or herself? In what ways has the child developed parts of self that go beyond this single (or multiple) experience(s)? Take note of ways to build coherent links from past to present to future. Over time, we may link this memory to other behaviors and experiences (as in the example of Emma, above) and explore relevant themes. Ultimately, an important goal is to contextualize intense and fragmented memories into the larger narrative of the child's life, so that various aspects of self and experience can be examined as part of a larger whole.

☐ *Teach to Caregivers*

- *Reminder:* Teach caregivers the Key Concepts.

- *Reminder:* Teach caregivers relevant Developmental Considerations.

- As with all aspects of treatment, caregivers play a crucial role in trauma experience integration. Caregivers may be the partial bearers of children's memory; they may be witnesses as well as participants in historical experiences, and/or may have access to details, contextual information, and concrete reminders (e.g., photographs, letters) that represent aspects of that experience. In the present, caregivers may play a role both as participants in the creation of a narrative with their children and as witnesses to it. For caregivers who played a role in historical experiences, even inadvertent, an important component of trauma experience integration is often some reparative experience between caregivers and child, including an acknowledgment of the child's suffering.

- In "Behind the Scenes," above, we discuss the important role of Caregiver Affect Management. Given the intensity of this work and the potential for eliciting strong emotions, it is crucial that caregivers receive support in exploring and addressing their own emotional responses, and that they set aside space for individual processing of traumatic memories and experiences, prior to engaging in this work with their children.

- Consider the following when integrating caregivers, whether professional or primary, into this work:

  ♦ Education about the nature and goals of treatment is vital. It is a common (mis)perception among caregivers that "trauma work" is almost exclusively focused on the exploration and detailing of memory. This misperception may lead caregivers (and clinicians) to dismiss the many other important components of treatment, as detailed throughout this framework, either as superfluous to, or as a simple foundation for, the "real" work, which in turn may create pressure to explore memory before a child is ready. Education about the impact of trauma, the role of developmental competency in its treatment, the pacing of memory exploration, and the importance of modulation and mastery of overwhelming affect should begin at the start of treatment and be revisited as necessary.

  ♦ Because emotional and behavioral dysregulation may occur in the aftermath of exploring traumatic material, it is important that caregivers be prepared and informed.

    ○ When exploration of memories occurs in a planned way (as in the construction of a life book during a particular phase of treatment), it is helpful to discuss with caregivers in advance the goals and format of the work, the child's potential responses, and ways to support the child using skills described in the Attunement and Modulation chapters of this text. When possible, integrate children into this preparation, and integrate caregivers into the work itself.

    ○ When memories emerge and processing occurs in the moment, as with intrusive traumatic material, it is crucial to share information with caregivers, in a manner that is appropriate, about the material and/or ways to support the child.

    ○ The child's age, developmental stage, and nature of relationship with caregivers may impact the type and extent of information that is shared:

      ◊ With a young child living with primary caregivers, for instance, it is important that caregivers understand both the nature of the work and the child's actual and potential responses, as young children rely strongly on their caregivers to provide modulation and support. Consider integrating caregivers into the session, sharing/discussing the material, inviting the child to share with caregivers his or her current feelings, and talking together about what to do if "big feelings" should arise.

      ◊ In other circumstances, more general/broad integration of caregivers may be indicated. For instance, with an older child/adolescent or a child in a milieu, concerns about privacy and confidentiality should be considered along with safety. It may be enough, for example, to share with a caregiver or staff member that a child "talked about some hard experiences today" and might need some extra support in the days to follow.

◊ The more the child/adolescent is integrated into this decision, the better. This may involve letting the child know that the professional would like to talk to the caregivers about what was discussed and asking the child's preference about format (e.g., "Do you want me to tell Mom what we talked about, or do you want to tell her?"); it may involve getting permission to share details (e.g., "I think it's important for staff to know you did some hard work today. What types of things is it okay for me to tell people about, and what would you like me to keep private?"); and it may involve getting the child's input about type of support needed (e.g., "When kids talk about the kind of memories we talked about today, feelings can sometimes come up afterward. What kinds of things do you think would help if you start to feel sad, like you did while we were speaking today? Who should we talk to about helping with those feelings?").

♦ As particular themes and patterns relevant to historical experience and a child's current functioning are identified within the context of treatment, it is important to discuss and explore these with caregivers as well. In the example of Emma, above, for instance, consider the importance of discussing with Emma's aunt the ways in which Emma's behavior and responses may relate to, and be representative of, historical experiences of rejection and danger. By engaging the caregiver's own reflective process, the likelihood of an attuned, purposeful, and empathic response is increased. Pay attention to the ways that the child's patterns may intertwine with those of the caregiver, recognizing that in many families, relevant themes repeat across generations. It is crucial to pair this discussion with empathy and support for the caregiver, and an empowerment of and belief in the caregiver's capacity to take positive action.

♦ Caregivers may play an important role as modulation resources for a child engaging in trauma experience integration. A caregiver's presence may help a child to tolerate distressing affect, to organize disorganized thought, and to regulate physiological arousal. Particularly for children whose caregivers are relatively attuned and responsive, consider inviting those caregivers into sessions to support children in doing this work.

♦ Ideally, whenever appropriate, caregivers will play a role in trauma experience integration not simply as their children's supporters and resources (within and between sessions), but as participants in the process. When safe, indicated, and permissible to the child, invite caregivers to take part in aspects of this work. Consider, for instance, inviting caregivers to be an audience as a child reads his or her story; to observe and take part in play; to support a child in construction of a narrative; and to "co-create" depictions of experience (e.g., individually generated pictures or stories in which each family member depicts a piece of the shared story, based on individual perspective and experience).

✐ Tools: Trauma Experience Integration

In the above sections we describe in detail the steps, or stages, involved in the exploration of both specific memories and fragmented self-states, as relevant to children who have experienced multiple and/or chronic stressors. Below, we briefly describe various techniques that may be useful in working with children to create narratives. In addition, a number of intervention frameworks have been developed that specifically focus on the processing and integration of traumatic experiences in childhood. These include trauma-focused cognitive-behavioral therapy (TF-CBT; Cohen, Mannarino, & Deblinger, 2006) and eye movement desensitization and reprocessing (EMDR; Greenwald, 1999; Lovett, 1999; Shapiro, 1995; Tinker & Wilson, 1999); other treatments, such as *Real Life Heroes* (Kagan, 2007a, 2007b), create a structure that guides storytelling, through the use of workbooks, to support children in the creation of their own narrative. We encourage professionals to familiarize themselves with the available range of strategies for processing and integrating traumatic experience.

Techniques for the Creation of Narrative

- The experience of trauma and overwhelming stress is laid down across physiological, sensory, affective, cognitive, and relational levels. Particularly when experienced in early childhood, a great deal of the impact and memory of trauma is held on a nonverbal level.

- Although much of our work with children and adolescents involves exploration of, and mastery over, physiological sensation, arousal, and action, it is ultimately through language that human beings make meaning of and filter their experience. By taking the *experienced* and making it conscious, we are able to engage higher-order cognitive processes, reflect on our experiences, integrate them into an understanding of self, monitor and understand our own responses, and engage purposefully in our lives by *acting*, rather than merely reacting.

- The creation of a narrative involves activation and integration across cortical structures: engaging in felt experience while reflecting upon it, and eliciting and tuning in to internal experiences across "channels." Because true integration requires this multilevel engagement with material, it is crucial that narrative creation occur at a pace and in a manner in which the child or adolescent can sustain connection to it.

- *The role of "containers."* An important ingredient to safety in trauma experience integration is the role of the container for the child's memories and experiences. Containers can be symbolic (e.g., a visualization that what is discussed in session is being held in a clinician's file cabinet) or concrete (e.g., folders, envelopes, and boxes). When exploring and integrating experience through play, the process of cleaning and putting away toys and figures is often a powerful metaphor for the containing of traumatic material. Regardless of the technique being used, pay attention to the role of containers in supporting children in managing traumatic material.

- When building a narrative, consider the following techniques.

WRITING OR STORYTELLING

Storytelling in written format is perhaps the most straightforward way to create a narrative. Narratives can be created in an open-ended manner (i.e., through exploration of memory as detailed above) or by using specific prompts or worksheets. Children may choose to write the narrative themselves or to dictate their stories to the clinician. In most cases, the clinician will guide the telling of the story through paced and careful questions or prompts. When used to create coherent narrative across experiences, specific memories can be examined separately and then pieced together in chronological (or other meaningful) order to create a larger story.

DYADIC STORYTELLING. For very young children, an alternative to individually generated narrative is the creation of a narrative in a "storybook" format by a primary caregiver. This narrative can be created by the caregiver, typically with the support of a professional, and then read to the child in the context of treatment. The child can be invited to contribute to or enhance the narrative through drawing or verbal statements. It is important that this type of narrative include not just the "trauma story" but also the reassurance of current safety and the protection of trusted adults.

SYMBOLIC NARRATIVE

Aspects of experience can be represented in more symbolic written form, such as in poetry, short stories, and plays. When using symbolic narrative to explore and process a child's experience, it remains important to pay attention to the steps outlined in Behind the Scenes, above, for creating connection, contextualization, and meaning making.

DRAWING

Drawing may be a preferred way to symbolize aspects of experience across developmental stages. As memories are explored, drawings can be used to represent all aspects of experience, including "the story" or experience itself, feelings associated with the experience, perceptions of self and other, body sensations, etc. As with narrative, drawings can be revisited over time, placed in varying order, and reexamined from varying perspectives, including development of future-oriented wishes, solutions, and goals.

PLAY

The young child's natural means of expression is play, and a great deal of processing for young children may occur in the context of symbolic play. Children will represent key themes, important relationships, fantasy outcomes, and frightening experiences in their play. Through the vehicle of play, clinicians can support children in the following:

- Identifying emotion
- Building modulation strategies
- Naming and responding to appropriate and inappropriate boundaries in relationships
- Acknowledging and developing mastery over frightening experiences, losses, and other traumatic exposures
- Acknowledging and working with less-than-ideal outcomes
- Working toward the creation of more positive solutions and future outcomes

A full treatise on play therapy is beyond the scope of the current text; we refer the reader to the many excellent resources that describe the important role of play in the treatment of childhood trauma (e.g., Gil, 1991, 2006; Webb, 2007).

"OUTSIDE-THE-BOX" TECHNIQUES

Strategies for creating narrative are limited, in many ways, only by the imagination of the clinician and the child. Consider the interests and most comfortable medium for the child, as well as cultural influences on storytelling. As examples, in recent years, we have worked with clinicians who have employed strategies such as the following:

COMPUTER PRESENTATION. Creation of an electronic slide presentation symbolizing child experiences and memories (as a substitute for the classic "All about Me" book with a child who hated talking but loved computers).

BOARD GAME. Creation of a board game, with phases of life represented by different sections of the board; difficult experiences represented by "Pitfall" cards; and resources and positive experiences available through special dice rolls to buffer and counteract the Pitfall cards (created by a child who loved collecting and playing with action figures and their associated "action" cards).

LYRICS COLLAGE. Creation of an extensive "story" of self, using individual lines cut from the printed-out lyrics of hundreds of songs (created by an adolescent who loved to listen to, and write, songs).

LIFE RAP. A colleague who works with inner-city youth helps them to create raps and songs about their lives, and records these songs with them using a laptop computer. These children, ranging from young children to adolescents, love the process of creating, recording, and sharing their life through this medium (Toombs, personal communication).

♦♦♦ DEVELOPMENTAL CONSIDERATIONS

Developmental stage	Trauma experience integration considerations
Early childhood	Trauma experience integration with young children is strongly embedded within the attachment system. Young children rely on caregivers to observe and reflect experience, to make links across time and space, to support and provide modulation, and to facilitate engagement in present life. As such, the reflective process necessary for trauma experience integration during this developmental stage will largely be held by the adult caregiver, whether primary or professional. Particularly when approaching fragmented self-states, it is perhaps more important during this stage to work with caregivers to follow the described steps (i.e., to observe and understand these thematic patterns, validate current experience, support and provide modulation, make simple links, and facilitate children's engagement in the present), than it is to work with children directly to do these things.
	Identification of patterns at this stage relies strongly on the observations of caregivers. Communication about these patterns to young children should generally be kept simple (e.g., "I know that it always feels so bad when people aren't paying attention").
	The memories of young children appear to be more fluid than those of older children and adolescents, in that experiences may intrude suddenly, in a manner that seems "omnipresent" (e.g., the child sitting at the dinner table, who suddenly speaks of an event from several months ago as if it occurred yesterday). These memories may seem to recede just as suddenly, as the child shifts quickly from "Daddy is gone" to "I want to color." This disjointed presentation may lead caregivers to both under- and overestimate the current impact of past experiences. It is important, with young children, to "catch" these moments as they intrude and validate and respond to the child's statements and affect (e.g., "Yes, Daddy is gone," as well as, "You're looking a little bit sad"), rather than simply dismissing them or distracting the child from them. It is equally important, however, to *not* press the child to expand upon or

Developmental stage	Trauma experience integration considerations
	remain in the experience longer than he or she can tolerate. Use attunement skills to assess when a child has "had enough" and is ready to move on. Processing experience with young children is likely to occur in many small moments over time.
	Very young children have more limited ability to engage in verbal discussion and exploration of experience than older children and adolescents. Because of this, although some processing will necessarily be verbal, a great deal of work with young children may be displaced and/or symbolic. Processing can be done through symbolic play as well as through the reading of storybooks, the story lines of which parallel the child's experiences in some way. Often, young children will make direct links between these displaced vehicles and their own life. When these more direct links do not occur, a great deal of work may still be done in displacement, as the clinician or other caregiver can explore and name thoughts, feelings, actions, and sensations in the projected-upon characters.
	Modulation is referenced throughout this section as a crucial ingredient for effective trauma experience integration. For young children, modulation relies largely upon caregiver support and cuing. It is therefore important for both professionals and primary caregivers to pay attention to the child's energy and arousal level when engaging in this work, and to provide appropriate supports.
Middle childhood	Children in this developmental stage are increasingly able to reflect upon their experiences. The extent of tolerance for this reflection will vary widely, and it is crucial to meet the child where he or she is at; some children work best initially in displacement, whereas others will be ready and able to talk about and explore personal experiences.
	Many children may be resistant to talking about difficult experiences, including memories as well as current behaviors and experiences that may link to previous ones. As with all work in this framework, it is important to provide psychoeducation, in age-appropriate language, about the rationale and goals for this work. This may be particularly true for this age group, who may be less drawn by play but not yet drawn to the insight-oriented discussion of the older adolescent.
	Children at this stage are frequently drawn to structure, and the establishment of a structure within which to create narrative is generally useful. Children during this stage may respond to worksheets and/or prompt questions better than to open-ended exploration.
	As children enter the late elementary school years, cognitive skill is increasingly sophisticated, and their more nuanced observations of "self," their growing identification of values, and the awareness of "right and wrong" may lead to an incorporation of complex emotions and cognitions, such as shame and self-blame in the perception of self and historical experiences. In working with children to reflect upon their historical experiences, the role of psychoeducation, an exploration of systems of meaning, and the development of realistic appraisal become increasingly important.
Adolescence	Adolescents have many of the same capacities as adults to reflect on their experiences, including the potential for abstract thought and an understanding of links across time and space. However, particularly early in adolescence, there is often an incapacity to take a larger perspective (i.e., what adolescents think and feel *now* may be all-consuming); an intense and often uncomfortable focus on the self and on self in comparison to other; and a wrestling with the more extreme emotional states that accompany the many physiological and cognitive changes of this developmental period. As a result, trauma experience integration—particularly an examination of experiences in the context of self and identity—is both essential and challenging at this stage.
	Because of its prominent nature as a developmental stage task, exploration of identity is often a starting point for work with adolescents. Reflection upon traumatic experiences and their impact on the self is a balancing act at this stage: Some adolescents may be anxious to dive in, at times before they have sufficient skills and resources to manage the experience, whereas other adolescents may be protective and guarded, as the need to be "normal" overrides any rationale for exploring such experience. Clinicians must be able to validate and observe both sides of this dichotomy, while offering containment, pacing, and expansion, as appropriate.

Developmental stage	Trauma experience integration considerations
	It is particularly important with adolescents to link the work done in the clinical setting with their experiences in the "real world": In other words, why is this work relevant to his or her life? More than with any other age group, adolescents must feel that they have a stake and an investment in the treatment process. In creating links with adolescents, consider not just the links between present and past, but also the links with the future; work with adolescents to consider goals and hopes for the future, and the ways in which their current actions have the capacity to shape that future.
	When working with adolescents, it is important to have realistic expectations. For all clients, it is normative to regress in the face of distressing content and experience and/or to operate from a fragmented aspect of self. Keep in mind that the adolescent's chronological age may not be the best predictor of his or her tolerance, cognitive level, or skill set when engaging in trauma experience integration. Pay attention to the adolescent's response to material and pace the work in the same manner as with younger children.

APPLICATIONS

Individual/Dyadic

The foundations for trauma experience integration begin to be laid at the start of treatment. As described above, trauma experience integration encompasses all other skills in this framework. Perhaps more than with any other target described in this framework, trauma experience integration will largely be facilitated within the context of individual or dyadic/familial work. As noted throughout this section, however, the eventual goal is for this work to move beyond the therapy room and into the child's or adolescent's current life, in a way that allows him or her to engage more fully in the present. Supports are often crucial for that application to take place, and integration of caregivers and other collaterals, as appropriate, is a key component of this work. It is also important for clinicians to support the child in making connections between what is discussed in the office and what is experienced in the world.

The acknowledgment of historical experiences and the role of the child's adaptation to those experiences are key overarching frames for this text. As the child gains skill in negotiating current life, and the child's caregiving system is increasingly equipped to support this negotiation, there is increasing capacity to deepen and explore the details of those historical experiences. For children with more chronic/complex trauma histories, it is important to consider trauma experience integration as a process that extends over time: Early in the work, the past will be named in the service of examining the present; increasingly, however, there may be enough safety to sit with, connect to, and reflect upon the past.

Because trauma experience integration is a process, consider the steps described in this chapter to be something the clinician, child, and potentially other caregivers will revisit over time. Begin to assess and explore patterns early in treatment and engage children and caregivers in this process as well. As the work proceeds over a period of time, help children and their caregivers examine the links between and among experiences (e.g., the way that the current reaction, for instance, is similar to the time the child got in trouble at school, and the ways that both may link to systems of meaning related to historical experience). A shared language is often essential in effectively exploring and integrating experience; over time work to build an understanding of key concepts in terms that "fit" for the child and caregiving system (e.g., in the case of Emma, above, an understanding of "push buttons," of "danger brain," and of "energy").

Trauma experience integration requires the capacity to observe and reflect upon behavior and experience. We strongly believe that, for children (and possibly across the lifespan), trauma experience integration is embedded within relationship. As with all new skills in childhood, the attachment system first provides, then supports, then ultimately transfers autonomous "owner-ship" of competencies to the developing child. Particularly for young children, the provider and the caregiver are the primary initial holders of the reflective lens that facilitates trauma experience integration. Increasingly, however, it is important for children to become the owners of the lens: Work to support children in developing an age-appropriate awareness of, and curiosity about, experience. Consider this to be a process that unfolds over time, and that will have wide variation by developmental level, by life experience, by current context, and by child individual differences.

🏠 Group

Trauma experience integration should be approached cautiously in a group setting. Group treat-ment may focus less on sharing and exploring specific details of individual children's experi-ences than on the foundations, skills, concepts, and psychoeducation that facilitate this process. Having said that, for children who are ready, group settings may provide powerful felt aware-ness that a child is not alone (e.g., in having experienced sexual abuse, in having been adopted, in having lived in a shelter).

Consider the role of broad psychoeducation and integrative activities that limit details of individual experience in thematic groups. For instance, a group for female survivors of sexual abuse might (1) provide education about the ways that sexual abuse impacts ideas about relation-ships, (2) invite group members to discuss why abuse might affect relationships, and (3) conduct a group activity defining "positive relationships." It is often helpful for groups that focus on trauma experience integration to make links, in some way, with individual therapy, whether through individual goals (e.g., "This week try to talk with your therapist about your own beliefs about relationships"), prompts (e.g., "This week write in your journal about a good and a not-so-good relationship you've had, and share that with your therapist"), and/or broader communica-tion between the group leader, the individual therapist, and the group participant.

Groups can also effectively address concepts relevant to integration of thematic/fragmented self-states. Consider, for instance, ways to integrate into group curricula the various components of the 10 steps highlighted earlier in this chapter. Educational activities can be built around trauma, the trauma response, the role of adaptation, and why these adaptations continue. Exer-cises, worksheets, and discussion can be used to facilitate group members' self-awareness of triggers, themes, and functional responses, as well as the ways in which these responses appear in current life. Fictional characters (e.g., in film clips) can be a useful way to explore these concepts in displacement, before linking them back to group members' own lives. In order to build links between "real-world" experiences and the group, as well as to build in-the-moment reflective processes, it may be helpful to challenge group members to observe and document key concepts during the intervening time between group meetings (e.g., if a group member has described a particular theme as relevant, such as rejection: "This week, pay attention to any time that you feel rejected. Write about what was going on; what you thought, felt, and did; and what was happening in your body. What was your first clue that it was happening?"). Discuss these assignments either in the group or in individual therapy.

🏠 Milieu

Systemic applications of trauma experience integration are, in many ways, challenging; it is obviously important to be careful about exploring historical experiences in more "open" environments (i.e., outside the protection of a therapy space); however, historical experiences will, without doubt, intrude into these settings. Therefore, it is important that staff in settings such as residential programs, schools, and hospitals gains comfort in understanding, recognizing, and reflecting current youth behaviors and actions as they relate to historical experiences.

In regard to the integration of fragmented self-states, components of the 10 steps described in this chapter can be integrated into staff understanding of, and approach to, students/residents. A clear formulation, including an understanding of a child's prominent historical experiences, potential triggers, and functional responses, is an important shared lens for staff across levels within a program. Consider ways to integrate, in an ongoing and concrete manner, staff observations of child patterns into routine clinical discussions, treatment plans, parent meetings, and other forums in which children are discussed. Build staff capacity to reflect (simply) observed behaviors and responses (e.g., "You seem like you're starting to get charged up"), to cue and support modulation strategies (e.g., "Would you like to take some space or to use something from the sensory cart to get your energy under control?"), and to support youth, as appropriate, in using problem-solving skills in the service of remaining engaged in the present moment (e.g., "What is it that you think you're wanting to accomplish here? Let's think about what options you have."). Beyond observing when these behaviors *do* happen, it is as crucial to begin to observe when they *don't:* For instance, when the adolescent who typically becomes angry and shuts down when confronted is able to engage in conversation about a behavior, or when a child who struggles with boundaries is able to engage appropriately with another. Work as a team to observe and reflect any active choice a child is making that speaks to present, rather than historical, engagement.

Because children and adolescents in more intensive levels of care such as residential programs are, by definition, frequently struggling with severer levels of symptoms, it is likely that staff members will, by necessity, negotiate their responses as children shift among and across self-states. This presentation can be confusing, and the intensity of the embedded emotion and behavior can, at times, be overwhelming for caregivers. It is crucial that staff, across levels, gains an understanding of the fragmented nature of child functioning and gains some facility in responding to children/adolescents in the moment, in their current state, and with an understanding that the particular state is filling some need for the child. The support of a coherent team and a process for exploring staff members' own reactions are often important ingredients in this process.

In regard to specific processing, it is very common for students/residents in milieu settings to disclose specific, intrusive memories and associated elements at unpredictable and uncontained times during the day. It is important for staff in milieu settings to have a well-established response to this type of disclosure. For example, when disclosures occur in the milieu, counselors can be instructed to validate relevant aspects of the experience, complete a brief check-in focused on modulation strategies, and remind the student that communication will occur between the counselor and the therapist.

🌐 REAL-WORLD THERAPY

🌐 **Are we there yet?** One of the most commonly recurring refrains we have heard (from parents, new clinicians, and other providers alike) goes something like this: "I know that he [she] needs to learn to manage his [her] feelings and do better in school and with friends, but I think what he [she] really needs is trauma work." In working with children who have lived their lives surrounded by layer upon layer of stress, and who have organized their lives around survival, don't lose sight of what trauma work really is. It's not just a race to get to the memories. All of the targets embedded in this framework are trauma work; it is the foundation of these skills, resources, and competencies that will support a child in building, over time, a coherent understanding of self and life experience. Don't downplay the importance of all that other work.

🌐 **Everyone's story is different.** The integration of traumatic experiences is a process that occurs over time. Every child metabolizes experience in different ways and at a different pace. Some children may be ready to do this work right away; others won't want to touch it with a 10-foot pole. Although it is important to acknowledge, name, and incorporate historical experiences as a frame for approaching the work, not every child will be ready, at every stage, to examine these experiences in detail. The creation of a narrative about the self is built in layers and can be explored and constructed over time in many different ways. Provide the foundation and the support, but allow children the freedom to develop their story in the way that works for them.

🌐 **Pay attention to your own story.** We enter into this work with our own experiences, beliefs, and responses, and our systems of meaning may both influence and be impacted by the work that we do. As we work with children to integrate and understand their life experiences, it is crucial that we do the same with our own.

A Postscript

Over the years that we have been in clinical practice, we have had occasion to bear witness to the ultimate strength—as well as the immense suffering—of children and families who must live with and negotiate layers of overwhelming stress.

During the year we worked on this text, within our own small clinical team, we watched three families successfully negotiate the sometimes perilous route of "preadoption"; having held our collective breath the many times crises and stress threatened to lead to disruption, we have witnessed with great joy the growing confidence and attunement of the parents, the increasing comfort and competence of the children, and ultimately, were immensely moved as we celebrated the finalized adoptions of all six children.

We watched two other children languish in foster care, their futures and goals still bound in uncertainty, and while also advocating within the larger system for their needs, have worked to support our clinicians in the painful process of sitting with and providing protected space for children who remain in a state of constant crisis. For some children, we acknowledge that our successes come sometimes not in what we build and achieve in the present and for the future, but in what we are able to hold and protect during the time we are involved.

This year we have watched one young adult, whom we knew throughout her adolescence, transform her childhood and begin to build a new future, and we have watched another young adult struggle to transition from the known—chaotic as it has been—into the confusing and somewhat frightening world of adulthood. We acknowledge the joy in watching seeds planted and watered begin to take hold and flower, and we acknowledge the awareness that this work often continues long past childhood, as the hurt children of yesterday negotiate new developmental stages, often without the protective resources of family and community.

Over the past year we have watched residential programs challenge themselves to build an understanding of trauma into their clinical and milieu teams, bring change to their systems in both small and large ways, and negotiate the very real-world constraints with which programs must struggle, while still trying to offer ethical, empathic, and comprehensive services. We have heard about the impact that a growing understanding of trauma has had on the attuned responses of foster parents, through programs that manage therapeutic foster homes, and we have seen the impact of this understanding in Head Start programs, preschools, and classroom settings.

We have learned at every step, and we continue to learn. We are struck, over and over, by the inventiveness and creativity, the positive intentions, and the impressive instincts of caregivers—both professional and familial—and the capacity of caregivers to thrive and to support the growth of children, once they are sufficiently supported themselves. We are struck, over and over, by the resilience of children, by their capacity to emerge from (and sometimes continue to negotiate) layers of stress, and still bring joy, curiosity, connection, and enthusiasm to their worlds, when given the foundation, resources, and permission to do so.

The successes we witness are sometimes small and sometimes large, and often come after long periods of plugging away, hanging in, and sitting with. Despite the setbacks, despite the crises and the pain, we leave this year with a great deal of hope. This is fitting, because in our own discussions of the ingredients of success, hope is among the strongest. Success is built on a faith in the potential of every child, every caregiver, and every system with whom we work. It is built on an acknowledgment of the many strengths that already exist, on the belief that most people are doing their best with the resources that they have, and on the hope that our work will expand upon and foster new resources. Success is built on a foundation of support across levels: the child supported by the caregiver, the caregiver and child supported by the provider, the provider supported by a team. It is built on a respectful underpinning of partnership; an acknowledgment that empowerment lies in allowing the child, the caregiver, and/or the system to be the true agent of change; and an understanding that our role is as collaborator and team member, rather than sole orchestrator.

We are grateful for the opportunities we have had to enter into the lives of children and families, across settings and contexts, and we are immensely appreciative of the education we have received from the many clinicians, educators, program directors, milieu staff, nurses, child welfare workers, and foster, adoptive, and biological parents who have shared their wisdom with us, and with the children whose lives they touch, as well as for the immense wisdom from the children themselves, who have been perhaps our most important teachers.

It is our hope that this text offers some small portion of that wisdom back, to support others in this journey. We look forward, with pleasure, to continuing our own.

Provider Materials

Session Checklist/Tracking Sheet

Session Date: _____   Client ID: _____

Session Number: _____

Therapist: _____

Individual _____   Group _____   Dyad/Family _____   Caregiver(s) _____

Session Component	Yes	No	Comments
Completed Check-In			
Completed Modulation Exercise			
Completed Child-Specific Treatment Goal Activity			
Worked on Self-Development Project			
Provided Child-Directed Free Time			
Completed Check Out			
ATTACHMENT DOMAINS			
A1: Caregiver Affect Management			
A2: Attunement			
A3: Consistent Response			
A4: Routines and Rituals			
SELF-REGULATION DOMAINS			
R1: Affect Identification			
Identifying Own Emotions			
Understanding Trauma Response/Triggers/Body's Alarm System			
Connection (Body/Thought/Behavior)			
Contextualization (Internal/External Factors)			
Identifying Other's Emotions			
R2: Modulation			
Understanding Degrees of Feeling			
Understanding Comfort Zone/Effective Modulation			
Building a Feelings Toolbox			
R3: Affect Expression			
Identifying/Accessing Safe Resources			
Appropriate Physical/Emotional Boundaries			
Nonverbal Communication Skills			
Verbal Communication Skills			
Self-Expression			

(cont.)

Session Component	Yes	No	Comments
COMPETENCY DOMAINS			
C1: Executive Functions			
Impulse Control			
Problem-Solving			
C2: Self-Development and Identity			
Unique Self (Cultural Identity, Values, Likes)			
Positive Self (Efficacy/Competency)			
Coherent Self			
Future Self			
TRAUMA EXPERIENCE INTEGRATION			
Trauma Experience Integration			
Thematic/Fragmented Self-States			
Specific/Narrative			
Other (describe):			

Treatment Planning and Priority Checklist

Domain:	Priority Level		
	Low: Support for continued use of skills	Moderate: Support and coaching in use of skills	High: Vulnerable domain, need for priority focus
Attachment			
Caregiver Management of Affect	1	2	3
Attunement	1	2	3
Consistent Caregiver Response	1	2	3
Routines and Rituals	1	2	3
Self-Regulation			
Affect Identification	1	2	3
Modulation	1	2	3
Affect Expression	1	2	3
Competency			
Executive Function	1	2	3
Self-Development	1	2	3
Developmental Tasks	1	2	3

Please list *concretely* priority treatment goal(s) and potential tools for above domains:

Goal	Potential Tool(s)
Example: Caregiver Affect Management: Increase mother's ability to tolerate child anger	*Psychoeducation; practice monitoring strategies; engage in parent support group*
1.	1.
2.	2.
3.	3.
4.	4.
5.	5.
6.	6.
7.	7.
8.	8.
9.	9.
10.	10.

Caregiver Educational Materials and Worksheets

CAREGIVER EDUCATIONAL MATERIALS

CAREGIVER WORKSHEETS

Introduction: Children and Trauma

WHAT IS TRAUMA?

Many different things may be called "traumatic." *Trauma* refers to experiences that are overwhelming and may leave a person feeling helpless, vulnerable, or very frightened.

Trauma may include specific types of events, such as being in an accident or experiencing a natural disaster like a hurricane or an earthquake. Trauma may also include *ongoing stressors*, such as physical or sexual abuse.

For children, trauma is often about more than physical harm. For instance, separation from a caregiver, emotional neglect, and lack of a stable home (such as living in many different foster homes) are often very traumatic.

HOW DOES TRAUMA IMPACT CHILDREN?

Children who have experienced ongoing trauma may have many different reactions. Children may:

- Develop an expectation that bad things will happen to them.

    When children have many bad things happen, they may come to expect them. They may over-estimate times when they are in danger, or be fearful or withdrawn even in situations that feel safe to other people.

- Have a hard time forming relationships with other people.

    Trauma often involves children being hurt by others and/or not being protected by others. When early relationships are not consistently safe, children may develop a sense of mistrust in relationships.

- Have difficulty managing or regulating feelings and behavior.

    Traumatic stress is overwhelming, and children are flooded by strong emotions and high levels of arousal. Children may feel like they are unable to rely on others to help them with these feelings—for instance, they may believe no one is safe; they may worry that other people will think they are bad; and so on.

    Without tools, children may try to overcontrol or shut down their emotional experience; may try to manage feelings and arousal through behaviors (such as being silly or getting in fights); or may rely on more dangerous overt methods (such as substance abuse or self-injury).

- Have difficulty developing a positive sense of themselves.

    Children who experience trauma may feel damaged, powerless, ashamed, and/or unlovable. It is often easier for children to blame themselves for bad things happening, than to blame others. Over time, children may develop a belief that there is something wrong with them.

Understanding Triggers

THE BODY'S ALARM SYSTEM

We all have a built-in alarm system that signals when we might be in danger. Evolution has helped human beings to survive by creating efficient systems in our brain that recognize danger signals and prepare us to respond. We become particularly efficient at recognizing signals that have been associated with past danger experiences. In the human brain, this system is known as the *limbic* system.

NORMATIVE DANGER RESPONSE

When our brain recognizes danger, it prepares our body to deal with it. There are three primary ways that we can respond to something dangerous: We can FIGHT it, we can get away from it (FLIGHT), or we can FREEZE.

What we choose to do often depends on the type of danger. So, for example:

- A large dog begins attacking your dog. You are bigger than the threat and motivated to help your dog. Response? FIGHT
- You are standing in the street and hear the squeal of brakes. You realize a car is speeding toward you. Response? FLIGHT
- You are a small child being hit by your father. You are not big enough to fight him, and not fast enough to run away. Response? FREEZE

Note: The "freeze" response is often the least understood and/or talked about, but may be the response most accessible to young children. It is a survival response that is used when someone cannot fight the danger and cannot physically escape it (and, in fact, doing either one might increase the danger). The only option, then, is to become very still, try not to be seen, and at times, to mentally escape.

THE DANGER RESPONSE AND AROUSAL

When the brain labels something in the environment as dangerous, it must rapidly mobilize the body. The brain initiates the release of chemicals that provide our body with the energy needed to cope with danger (for example, to run from the car, or to fight the attacking dog). The brain is remarkably efficient—within milliseconds of perceiving danger, the body's arousal level goes up, sensory perception shifts, and "nonessential functions" (such as digestion) shut down. Interestingly, higher cognitive processes—such as logic, planning, and impulse control—are considered *nonessential* in the face of danger. (Think about it—if a car is speeding toward you, do you want to be *thinking*, or do you want to be *running*?)

It is important to understand that this sequence will be initiated, whether the danger is *real* or simply *perceived*.

(cont.)

THE OVERACTIVE ALARM

Typically, when the danger signal first goes off, the "thinking" part of our brain evaluates the immediate environment. If there is no apparent danger (for example, it's a "false alarm"), the alarm system is shut off, and we continue with previous activities. For example: You are walking up a busy street and hear a car backfire. Within moments of your initial startle response, your brain will activate the sensory systems that scan your environment, assess the cause of the noise, and label it as nonthreatening. Almost immediately, you are able to continue on your way.

For some people, however, the brain's danger signal goes off too often. This generally occurs when there has been repeated danger in the past (remember, the more our brain engages in any activity, the more efficient it becomes at that particular activity). Children who have experienced repeated or chronic trauma often have *overactive alarms*—they may perceive danger more quickly and/or may label many nonthreatening things as potentially dangerous.

Consider again the example used above—you are walking down the street and a car backfires. Now imagine, however, that you have been in combat or have lived in an area that has frequent gunfire. As soon as the noise occurs, your body immediately prepares for danger. In this scenario, your "thinking brain" is less likely to get involved—or to take the time to assess whether the danger is real or not. This is because in the past, waiting would have put you at risk for being shot. In order to keep you safe, then, the "thinking brain" stays out of the way and lets the action brain take over. This overactive alarm is therefore adaptive—in times of actual danger, it kept you alive, but in the present, it may cause you to react too strongly to things that may really be safe.

WHAT TRIGGERS THE ALARM?

False alarms can happen when we hear, see, or feel something that reminds us of dangerous or frightening things that happened in the past. Those reminders are called "TRIGGERS." Our brain has learned to recognize those reminders because in the past when they were around, dangerous things happened, and we had to respond quickly.

Different children have different reminders. For instance, for a child who has witnessed domestic violence, hearing people yell or watching adults argue might activate the alarm. For children who have not received enough attention, feeling alone or scared might turn on the alarm.

Often, these reminders, or triggers, are subtle. For example, trauma is often associated with unpredictability, chaos, or sudden change. As a result, even subtle changes in expected routine may activate a child's danger response.

Common triggers for traumatized children include:

- Unpredictability or sudden change
- Transition from one setting/activity to another
- Loss of control
- Feelings of vulnerability or rejection

(cont.)

- Confrontation, authority, or limit setting
- Loneliness
- Sensory overload (too much stimulation from the environment)

Triggers may not always seem to make sense. For instance, some children may be triggered by positive experiences, such as praise, intimacy, or feelings of peace. There are many possible reasons for this. For example:

- A child who has experienced previous losses, rejection, or abandonment may be frightened or mistrustful of positive relationships.
- A child who has received praise or bribery while being sexually abused may fear ulterior motives.
- A child who has experienced consistent chaos may find calmness or routine unsettling.

It is important that children learn to tolerate these positive experiences, but it is also important for caregivers to be aware of the potential for distress.

HOW DO YOU KNOW YOUR CHILD HAS BEEN TRIGGERED?

The primary function of the triggered response is to help the child achieve safety in the face of perceived danger. Remember, there are three primary danger responses available to human beings:

FIGHT   FLIGHT   FREEZE

What do these look like in children?

FIGHT may look like:
- Hyperactivity, verbal aggression, oppositional behavior, limit testing, physical aggression, "bouncing off the walls"

FLIGHT may look like:
- Withdrawal, escaping, running away, self-isolation, avoidance

FREEZE may look like:
- Stilling, watchfulness, looking dazed, daydreaming, forgetfulness, shutting down emotionally

Emotionally, children may appear fearful, angry, or shut down. Their *bodies* may show evidence of increased arousal: trembling, shaking, or curling up.

Look for moments when the intensity of the child's response does not match the intensity of the stressor, or when a child's behaviors seem inexplicable or confusing. Consider—might your child's alarm system have gone off?

Learning Your Child's Language

IT'S NOT WHAT I SAY . . .

Trauma can impact children's ability to understand, tolerate, and manage feelings. Even minor stressors can act as **triggers** that flood children with emotion. Often, children do not even know what it is that is upsetting them—only that there is a strong, bad feeling inside of them, and that *something* needs to happen to make it go away. In the face of these overwhelming feelings, and without strategies to cope with them, children will simply *react*: They work out the distress with their bodies and their actions.

Often, the only thing harder than dealing with feelings is talking to other people about them—especially for children who don't know themselves what they are feeling, or why they are feeling it. Furthermore, for children who have been hurt in the past by other people, or who did not have their needs met early in life, reaching out for help may feel dangerous or frightening.

WHAT I'M TRYING TO SAY IS . . .

Most children communicate to some degree through behavior; the ability to use words to share feelings and experience grows naturally over the course of development, particularly as caregivers use their own words to reflect back experience. Consider these examples:

A 4-year-old returns home from preschool. She is quieter than usual, and when her mother asks if she wants to play, she shakes her head and curls up in a chair. Her mother sits next to her and says, "You're so quiet today. Do you feel sick?" The child shakes her head.

A 10-year-old comes home from school and slams the door. He throws his bag onto the kitchen table and says, "I'm never riding that stupid bus again!"

A 15-year-old has been nervous about her first date. She spends an hour in her room, trying on clothes, then finally comes downstairs, tearful. "Everything looks so stupid on me—I'm not going!"

Most caregivers are familiar with situations such as these, and—even if the precipitating event isn't yet known—will quickly recognize that feelings are driving these behaviors. Through their own words or actions, caregivers help children name and work through the emotion-inducing life events that they experience day to day.

The experiences driving traumatized children's behaviors may be less obvious, and the feelings may be bigger, stronger, or more sudden, but at core, the emotions are the same: fear, sadness, anger, anxiety, and even joy.

(cont.)

TUNING IN

Attunement is the ability to "read" (understand) your children's cues and respond in a way that helps them manage their emotions, cope with distressing situations, and/or make good choices. When a caregiver is attuned, he or she can respond to the emotion underlying a child's actions, rather than simply reacting to the most distressing behavior.

Consider two different scenarios for one of the above examples:

A 10-year-old comes home from school and slams the door. He throws his bag onto the kitchen table and says, "I'm never riding that stupid bus again!"

Scenario 1: His mother is going through mail in the kitchen and looks up as he enters the house.

MOTHER: How many times have I told you not to slam that door!?

CHILD: (*Kicks his bag.*) What's the big deal—it's just a stupid door!

MOTHER: That's it—if you can't be polite, you can just go to your room!

Scenario 2: His mother is going through mail in the kitchen and looks up as he enters the house.

MOTHER: Whoa—you seem pretty mad. Did something happen on the bus?

CHILD: (*Looks down, kicking his bag gently.*) Stupid bus driver hates me—he won't let me sit with my friends. I'm not riding it anymore!

MOTHER: (*Pulls out a chair.*) C'mere—why don't you tell me what happened, and we'll see if we can figure it out?

In the first scenario the child's mother responds to the behavior—slamming the door—and the emotion escalates, leaving both mother and child frustrated. In the second example the mother responds to the emotion—anger? frustration?—and provides the child with support, calming the situation.

Most situations aren't quite this straightforward, and no caregiver can be attuned at all times. The goal is not to be the "perfect parent," but to try—more times than not—to understand the feelings driving children's behavior.

PUTTING ON YOUR DETECTIVE HAT

Attunement requires caregivers to be "feelings detectives." Every child gives cues that help signal what might be going on.

Learn your child's individual communication strategies. Pay attention to the following areas and consider: How does your child look when he/she is angry? Sad? Excited? Worried? For each of these emotions, ask yourself the following questions:

(cont.)

Facial expression	What does your child show on his face? This may include intense expressions, but may also include a lack of expressiveness.
Tone of voice	Does your child's voice become louder? Softer? Higher-pitched?
Extent of speech	Does your child suddenly have more to say than usual? Does she become quiet? How pressured (in a rush) is her speech?
Quality of speech	Do your child's words become disorganized? Is he rambling or having a hard time getting words out? Do his words seem more babyish or regressed than usual?
Posturing/muscular expression	What does your child's body look like? Is she curled up? Are her fists clenched? Are her muscles tense or loose? Is her posture closed or open?
Approach versus avoidance	Does your child become withdrawn and retreat? Does he become overly clingy? Does he seem to want to do both at the same time?
Affect modulation capacity	Does your child seem to have a harder time than usual being soothed, and/or self-soothing? Does she start to need more comforting from you or someone else? How receptive is she to comfort—does this change in the face of stress?
Mood	Does your child's mood overtly change? For instance, is he normally even-tempered, but becomes more reactive in the face of intense emotion? If so, pay attention to signs of moodiness—it can serve as a warning sign that something is going on.

(cont.)

NOW WHAT?

When your detective skills tell you that something is going on with your child, it's time for action. But what kind of action? Often, we rush to solve children's problems for them or try to help them "solve" things themselves. Sometimes, though, the most important action is simply to be there, to provide support, and to help children name, understand, and regulate their feelings. Only after doing that can children move toward solving problems.

Consider a possible example from your own life: You've had a hard day, your boss is irritating you, people are making demands, and you come home ready for a little sympathy. Your spouse notices that you are upset and asks what is going on. You begin to unload: "My boss is so unreasonable! Can you believe he asked me to . . . " Your spouse listens to your story, then shrugs, and says, "Well, you could have . . . " (or "Why don't you just . . . ?").

Do you feel more frustrated, or less?

Most of us want someone to *listen to* us before they solve our problems or tell us what we could have, should have, or what *they* would have done. When people listen to us, understand us, and give us empathy, it validates our experience, shares the burden, and often, helps us begin to feel better.

The following five rules/steps for reflective listening can help caregivers (or partners in any type of listening situation) become better listeners.

Reflecting Listening Skills for Caregivers

Step	Description
1. Accept and respect all of a child's feelings.	There should never be a hidden agenda to "change" the child's feelings. A child feels what he/she feels. We may not like the child's *behaviors*, or we may not completely understand the reaction, but it should always be okay to be mad, or sad, or excited.
2. Show your child that you are listening.	Use active listening skills: Use eye contact, nod your head, respond verbally, etc. Don't interrupt too much or take over the conversation. Use all the techniques that you like someone to use when they are paying attention to *you*.
3. Tell your child what you hear him/her saying.	Reflect back what you hear. Validate the importance of the situation to the child (even if you, yourself, do not think it was that big of a deal): *"So, you didn't think your teacher was listening to you? Wow, that must have been really hard."* Ask questions if you're not sure what part affected the child.
4. Name the feelings.	Reflect back the child's feelings. If your child doesn't state a feeling, offer a guess (name at least two possibilities), but be prepared to be wrong: *"You seem kind of worried or maybe angry. Is that right?"*

(cont.)

	Name the cues—*why* do you think the child seems worried or angry. Always allow the child to correct you. If your child denies any feelings at all, let that be okay, but then either

1. Name the behaviors:

"Okay, maybe you're not mad, but you're throwing your things around and yelling. What do you think might be going on?"

Or

2. Normalize feelings in general:

"Okay, maybe you're not mad, but I can understand how someone might feel really mad or upset if someone wasn't listening to them." |
| 5. Offer advice/ suggestions/ reassurance/ alternative perceptions *only* after helping the child to express how he/she feels. | Don't jump to problem solving until you've taken the time to listen to what your child has to say. Validate the feelings and the situation *first*, then collaborate with your child to come up with a solution, if appropriate. Keep in mind that solutions may simply be about how to express and cope with the feeling. If a child rejects your attempts at help, let him or her know that the offer stands:

"It's okay if you don't want to talk about it right now, but if you start to feel like it, you can come find me." |

Understanding the Trauma Cycle

	Youth	Parent/Caregiver
Cognitions	"I'm bad, unlovable, damaged." "I can't trust anyone."	"I'm ineffective." "My child is rejecting me."
Emotions	Shame, anger, fear, hopelessness	Frustration, shame, anger, fear, worry, sadness, hopelessness/helplessness
Behavior/Coping Strategies	Avoidance, aggression, preemptive rejection	Overreacting, controlling, shutting down, being overly permissive
The Cycle	"I'm being controlled; I have to fight harder."	"He keeps fighting me; I better dig in my heels."

Praise and Reinforcement

Teaching Points	Trauma creates significant distress that impacts individuals and their families. Over time, it is not uncommon for a negative pattern to develop, in which family members focus almost exclusively on difficulties, stressors, and symptoms.	
	When overwhelmed by distress, there may be a loss of awareness of the positives. Children (and their caregivers) may begin to identify primarily with the "bad": "I'm a bad kid." "I'm a bad parent."	
	This pattern may lead to feelings of helplessness and/or hopelessness: *"This will never change!"*	
	The use of positive praise and reinforcement can . . . • Increase positive interactions with your child • Increase desired behaviors • Increase attunement • Increase felt safety • Build self-esteem and self-efficacy for both child and caregiver • Increase feelings of child and caregiver mastery	
	Praise and reinforcement must be a conscious choice. Surprisingly, the good things are often *much* more difficult to notice than the hard ones! Noticing the positives often requires effortful focus and selection of behaviors to target.	
Selecting Targets	**Don't praise everything.**	Be selective. If you praise everything you see, it will feel false to you and to your child. Pick things that are tangible, that are important, that are goals, etc., and focus on those.
	Start small.	Start by picking one behavior to notice. Try to tune in to it and praise it whenever it appears. Track your use of praise.
	Choose behaviors that are desired, and that (at least occasionally) occur.	Specifically select targets based on those behaviors that you are trying to increase. For instance, if tolerating frustration without tantrumming is an important goal, then any sign that your child is doing this should be noticed and reinforced. Try to specifically link the praise to the behavior or effort. For example, don't just say "Good job." Instead say something like this: "Wow, I'm so proud of you. I just told you that you had to wait a few minutes before we went outside, and you said okay. I know that can be hard, and I'm really proud of how you handled it."
		Remember: Choose your targets wisely. If the initial target is the one thing the child never does, neither you nor your child will experience success.
	Redefine "success."	Think step by step rather than hoping for overnight success. If the ultimate goal is for the child not to punch a wall when angry, for instance, then reinforce the first time the child yells and screams but doesn't punch.
	Go beyond "being good."	Praise should not always be linked to actions. Praise is not just about shaping behavior, but about fostering a positive sense of self. Try to reinforce your child's qualities and efforts.

(cont.)

Examples of Praise Statements	Behavior related:	"You did a really good job finishing your homework."
		"I like how well you're sharing with your sister."
		"I feel so proud when you find safe ways to tell me what you're feeling."
	Effort related:	"I can see how hard you're working at that."
		"Thank you for trying to compromise, even though it's hard."
		"I can see how frustrated you are, and I'm really proud of you for not yelling."
	Child qualities:	"I'm so proud of how kind you are."
		"You're so adventurous—I think it's great!"
		"What a great sense of humor you have."
	Open-ended:	"You're such a great kid, I have such fun being with you."
		"I love it when we play games together."
		"It made me so happy to see you smile yesterday."

Responding When Children Are Triggered by Praise

Don't take it personally.	Be aware that praise may be a trigger. If your child responds negatively to being praised, try not to take it as a personal rejection.
Hang in there.	For many children, part of making meaning about trauma includes self-blame. Praise and reinforcement won't lead to immediate change in this. Try to build tolerance for the emotions (for example, shame, guilt, frustration) that go along with witnessing negative self-statements by your child.
Don't argue it.	It is okay to stand by your praise *without* arguing. Keep your response simple. For instance, if you tell your child that you are proud of him/her, and your child rejects it, your response might be: "Well, *I'm* feeling proud of you, but it's okay for you to feel however you want."
Stay tuned in to child emotions.	If a child begins to escalate, use your attunement skills to name and respond to the underlying affect. For instance, "I can see that was kind of scary for you to hear. Would a hug help you feel better?"
Keep it concrete.	If your child seems to reject global praise (for example, "You're such a great kid"), then keep your praise concrete. Link it to specific behaviors or actions. For instance, "I really like the way you used green in that picture." It may be easier for some children to accept specific praise than global praise.

Trauma Considerations with Limit Setting

Reduce the need for limits.	Children who have experienced trauma often feel the need to be in control. Power struggles can be avoided by providing **limited choice** (for example, "You can do your homework in your room or at the table. Which would you like to do?"). This kind of choice provides the child with the *illusion of control*, while allowing the caregiver to maintain limits around the behavior.
	Use your attunement skills to determine the reason behind your child's noncompliance. Learn to tell the difference between when your child feels overwhelmed by a task and times he or she is just refusing to do it. Try the following: • Ask the child what he/she is feeling, and/or name what you are seeing. For example: "You seem really upset by having to clean your room. What do you think is making you so upset?" • Break large tasks into smaller ones. • Offer to help.
	Compromise. Define for yourself which rules are essential, and on which you are willing to compromise.
Choose your moments.	When traumatized children are in a high state of arousal, they are unable to tap into higher cognitive functions such as logical thinking, problem solving, planning, anticipating, delaying response, etc.
	When children are very emotional or overly energetic, try to do the following: 1. Name the unsafe behavior, if any. 2. Help the child to use coping skills for managing energy and/or emotions (including caregiver support), as necessary. 3. Apply limits only after the child has calmed down.
Be aware of triggers.	All types of limit setting can act as triggers. Time-out and ignoring can trigger fears of abandonment and rejection; setting limits and consequences can trigger fears of punishment, authority, and vulnerability. Although caregivers should not avoid the use of limits for these children, it is important that caregivers are aware of the possible impact. This impact can be minimized by: • *Always naming the rationale for a limit* and linking it to the behavior (rather than to the child). • *Always naming the boundaries around the limit* (e.g., length of time in time-out, amount of time privilege is lost). • *Moving on.* Caregivers should not continue to scold, bring up the behavior, or express a lot of emotion after setting the limit and carrying it through. Caregivers should let the child know, explicitly, if necessary, that they still love them. • *Making adaptations to limits for specific triggers* (e.g., a child who has been previously punished by being enclosed in a small space might have time-out sitting in a nearby chair, rather than in another room).

Building Daily Routines

Morning	The morning transition is often difficult for everyone, but particularly when families are coping with stress. Think about whether you and your family have a consistent morning routine. If not, are there ways to make the morning process more consistent?
Mealtimes	Meals are often a great opportunity for communication and a place for family together time. For children (and their caregivers) family meals can build social skills, turn taking, manners, and interest in each other's activities. Consider building family meals into your daily routine, as often as possible. • *Note*: Food choice is a common place for children to exert their need for control. Try to avoid power struggles. Find a middle ground between too much flexibility and too much control. For instance, provide a predictable alternative (e.g., child can eat family meal or eat a peanut butter and jelly sandwich).
Play	Play is a child's natural means of expression. Try to find time to play with your children. Consider building time into the week for "family play" as well as solitary and peer-to-peer play. *Although often mistakenly considered less important than chores, homework, etc., play is a crucial part of healthy development.* In addition, play also provides a forum for socialization and skill building. • Together time should *not* be tied to rewards or consequences (e.g., "If you don't clean your room, you don't get to spend time with Mom"). For children with histories of neglect and abandonment, in particular, this can be triggering. • Try to build one-on-one time with each child in the family, as well as full family time.
Chores	Chores help to build a sense of responsibility and self-efficacy. Of course, chores should be age-appropriate, but it is okay for even very young children to expect to be responsible for certain (however small) chores. This distribution of chores builds in the idea that all family members are integral to the successful functioning of the family, and that the child makes an important contribution. Try to develop child-appropriate and realistic daily expectations.
Homework	School achievement and success are important areas of competency building for children. Caregivers can contribute here by emphasizing the importance of homework, providing an appropriate environment to support homework completion, being available to offer help or encouragement, and emphasizing effort over success.
Family Together Time	It is important to build into family daily routines a formal or informal time for caregivers and children to come together to share experience. For instance, some families may consider holding a weekly "family meeting" in which to share significant events; it could be incorporated into mealtime, bedtime, etc. Regardless of the forum, it is important that family members have opportunities to share experience on a routine basis.

(cont.)

EXPANDED EXAMPLE: BEDTIME ROUTINES

Teaching Points	Bedtime is often a difficult time for children and adolescents who have experienced trauma, particularly those whose abuse occurred at a similar time or in the place where they are now expected to sleep.
	For children whose arousal is high during the day, it may be hard for them to calm their bodies in preparation for sleep.
	Bedtime routines help children decrease their arousal and learn to transition into sleep.

Things to Consider	<ul><li>*Develop a consistent bedtime routine.* Have your child put on pajamas, brush teeth, have quiet time, etc. Pay attention to the location where your child is sleeping; try to help your child sleep in the same place each night.</li><li>*Trouble-shoot.* How can you keep bedtimes and their routines as consistent as possible? What might (or sometimes does) interfere with a regular routine? Think about how you will handle this.</li><li>*Identify nighttime boundaries and ways to cope with nighttime fears.* For example, what will you do if your child awakens during the night? Try to be consistent in follow-through.</li><li>*Minimize your child's engagement in highly arousing activities near bedtime.* Decrease your child's involvement in activities such as video games, overstimulating television shows, loud music, active play, etc.</li></ul>

General Activities	Nurturing	Read a story, cuddle, or listen to soft music together.
	Bathing	Have your child take a bath or shower about an hour before bed; this may help bring down arousal. Pay attention to issues of privacy, boundaries, and the possibility of this area being a trigger.
	Safety check	Help children feel safe. Leave on a night-light, hang a dream catcher, check under beds or in closets, rub on "no-monster" lotion, etc.
	Relaxation/ quiet time	Allow child to read, listen to quiet music, etc.

Bedtime Routines: Developmental Considerations	Early Childhood	Routines at this age should include the caregivers. Nurturing activities (e.g., reading a bedtime story) are a good way to build attunement and relax the child.
		Night is a time when generalized fears often emerge. Predictable nighttime routines are particularly important during this developmental stage.

(cont.)

	Middle Childhood	Although children at this age will desire greater independence, bedtime is a natural place for nurturance, and traumatized children may show some developmental regression around bedtime.
		Developmental changes may shift the mechanics of bedtime: for example, caregivers may now read *with* their child instead of *to* him/her; may include independent activities (child brushes teeth, showers, gets into pajamas) as well as together time (caregiver enters room to say "good night").
	Adolescence	Balance is very important at this developmental stage. The important areas to balance include: • *Independence versus nurturance*: Adolescents need privacy. However, like younger children, they may also experience developmental regression around bedtime. Check in with your teen before bed—does he/she want a hug good night? Etc. • *Flexibility versus limits*: Although adolescents are independent, don't lose sight of the need for limits. Maintain expectations around bedtime (e.g., must be in room by 10:00 P.M.), but allow flexibility (e.g., can have quiet time—read, listen to music—and turn off lights when ready).

Supporting Modulation

Consider a scenario in which your child's emotion escalates.

Steps toward supporting modulation:

1. **Be attuned:** Notice the feeling (tune into the energy).
2. **Keep yourself centered**: Check in with yourself.
3. **Ask yourself:** Where is your child's energy? Where does it need to go (up or down)?
4. **Reflect (simply) what you're seeing** (e.g., "I can see you just got really mad. Let's see if we can calm it down a bit so we can talk.").
5. **Cue child in use of skills** (e.g., breathing, sitting quietly, calming down space, stress ball).
6. **Reinforce use of modulation skills** (e.g., "I'm really proud of you for trying to calm down your energy").
7. **Invite expression**/communication when child is calm.

Tuning In to Yourself

Situation: _____

Using the following questions as a guide, write down observations about yourself during difficult interactions or situations. Fill in any additional observations at bottom.

Domain	Prompt Questions	Caregiver Observations
Body	What are you experiencing in your *body*? Pay attention to cues such as heart rate, breathing, muscle tension, temperature, and feelings of numbness or disconnection.	
	What warning signs does your body provide of "losing control" or hitting a danger point?	
Thoughts	What do you *think* in this situation? Consider both thoughts about yourself (e.g., "I can't handle this," or "I should have _____") and thoughts about your child (e.g., "He's doing this on purpose," or "She'll always be this way").	Thoughts about self:
		Thoughts about child/adolescent:
Emotions	What do you *feel* in this situation? Consider anger, guilt, shame, sadness, and helplessness.	
Behavior	What do you *do* in this situation? Do you freeze? Withdraw? Dig in your heels? Scream?	
Other	What else do you notice about yourself? Consider your ability to cope with emotion, ability to use supports, unhealthy (or healthy) coping responses, etc.	

Taking Care of Yourself

Situation: _____

Use the following techniques for ideas and consider possible self-care strategies you might apply in difficult or challenging situations. Fill in any additional ideas at bottom.

Self-Care Strategies		
Technique	**Tips**	**Might this technique work in this situation? Describe when and how you might use this:**
Deep Breathing	**When?** • Well, hopefully always! • Particularly when faced with surging or intense emotions **How?** • In through the nose, out through the mouth • Through the diaphragm, not your chest or shoulders • Pair with a calming visual image, verbal mantra, or saying	
Muscle Relaxation	**When?** • When the tension is building up . . . • As an alternative focus for energy (instead of exploding) **How?** • As big or small as you want it to be • Under-the-table methods (tense and release) • Progressive muscle relaxation	
Distraction	**When?** • Dealing with a problem you can't solve immediately. • Caught in a negative mental thought cycle. **How?** • *Self-soothe*: Consider your five senses. • *Find alternatives*: Switch activities.	

(cont.)

Technique	Tips	Might this technique work in this situation? Describe when and how you might use this:
Self-Soothing	**When?** • As an ongoing tool, to prevent stress build-up • When you want to pamper or reward yourself • When you are upset or stressed and need to calm down • When you are feeling disconnected and need to reconnect **How?** • *In-the-pocket techniques*: Carry small objects that feel soothing or pleasurable; consider all five senses (e.g., a pleasant lotion, a small stone or piece of velvet, a picture of a favorite place). • Identify and incorporate pleasurable activities into daily routine (e.g., a long, hot bath; going for a walk; listening to music).	
Time-Outs	**When?** • In the moment, to delay a negative response • Preventive, as an ongoing measure to "charge the batteries" **How?** • In the moment: For example, go for a walk, go to your room, go to the bathroom. • Preventive: Build in self-care time daily/weekly/ monthly.	
	Ask yourself: Is this a safe situation in which to take a time-out?	
Other techniques?	What other techniques can you think of? Describe **when** and **how** you might use these techniques:	

Learning Your Child's Emotional Language

Emotion: _____

Using the following questions as a guide, write down "clues" that tell you that your child is experiencing the selected emotion. Fill in any additional clues at bottom.

Domain	Prompt Questions	Caregiver Observations
Facial expression	What does your child show on his/her face?	
Tone of voice	Does your child's voice become louder? Softer? Higher-pitched?	
Extent of speech	Does your child suddenly have more to say than usual? Does he/she become quiet? How pressured (in a rush) is his/her speech?	
Quality of speech	Do your child's words become disorganized? Rambling? Stilted? Regressed?	
Posturing/muscular expression	What does your child's body look like?	
Approach versus avoidance	Does your child become withdrawn? Clingy? Both?	
Affect modulation capacity	Does your child seem to have a harder time than usual being soothed, and/or self-soothing?	
Mood	Does your child's mood overtly change?	
Other?	What other "clues" are there that your child is experiencing a given emotion?	

What Does Your Child Look Like When Triggered?

It may be hard to identify a specific trigger, but you can learn to read signs that your child is showing the danger response

Fight Response:

Description: Signs of high arousal levels, which often appear sudden: for example, irritability, swearing, sudden anger, hyperactivity

Your child's behaviors that may indicate "fight":

_____

_____

_____

_____

_____

Flight Response:

Description: Physical withdrawal or escape: for example, avoiding contact with others, isolating self from friends or family, refusal to do homework

Your child's behaviors that may indicate "flight":

_____

_____

_____

_____

_____

Freeze Response:

Description: Shutting down or disconnecting from experience: for example, child looks numb; blank stare; child appears dazed

Your child's behaviors that may indicate "freeze":

_____

_____

_____

_____

_____

Identifying Your Child's Triggers

Name: _____ Date: _____

Example of Trigger	**May Remind Child of . . .**
1. Hearing people yell in loud tone of voice	Times when child was yelled at a lot
2. Feeling alone or being ignored	Times when child did not get enough attention when he/she was little
3. Smell of smoke	A bad fire
4. _____	_____
5. _____	_____
6. _____	_____
7. _____	_____
8. _____	_____

Group Activities

Sample Group Activities

ACTIVITY: GUESS WHO?

- **ARC Target(s): Affect Expression, Identity; Icebreaker activity**
- **Purpose:** Increase group members' awareness of/attunement to other members and awareness of ways in which they already know each other. Have fun.
- **Materials:** Preprinted slips of paper with questions (see examples).
- **Directions:** Each group member receives five slips with prompts on them (e.g., favorite movie, song). Each member writes answers to each prompt and puts folded slips in a hat. Members take turns picking a slip out of the hat and guessing whose answer it is. If they guess right, they get a point. If short on time, you can leave slips out of hat after all guesses, right and wrong, so the hat goes around five times, and then those that were guessed wrong can be claimed by those who wrote them. If you have more time, you can put wrong guesses back in hat and keep going around until all have been guessed.
- **Sample Prompts:** favorite type of pet, favorite food, favorite movie, favorite song, favorite actor or actress, favorite TV show, favorite color, favorite band or musical artist, place you'd like to travel to, favorite book

ACTIVITY: BODY DRAWING

- **ARC Target(s): Affect Identification**
- **Purpose:** To increase participant ability to tune in to ways that feelings are expressed in the body.
- **Materials:** Silhouette drawing of body (such as *"Where Do I Feel . . .,"* Appendix D), crayons or colored pencils (preferable to markers)
- **Directions:**
  - ♦ Provide participants with body drawing and six colored pencils or crayons.
  - ♦ Ask participants to create a key, selecting colors to represent the following feelings: happy, angry, sad, scared, excited, worried.
  - ♦ For each identified feeling, participants should use crayons/pencils to color . . . *Where in their body they feel _____.*
  - ♦ *Discussion:* Following completion of this activity, discuss with participants:
    - ○ How easy/hard was this?
    - ○ Were some feelings easier than others to locate in the body? Which feelings were the easiest? Which were the hardest?
    - ○ Did any feelings overlap in location? Which ones?
    - ○ Which feeling was the most distinct (i.e., the only one held in a particular part of the body)?

DISCUSSION: THE FUNCTION OF FEELINGS AND "MASKING" FEELINGS

- **ARC Target(s): Affect Identification, Modulation, Affect Expression**
- ***Ask:*** What function do feelings serve? Elicit ideas from the group.
  - ♦ If group members are not able to think of reasons, provide examples: Fear may tell us we need to run, and it helps us survive; anger may help us feel powerful in a difficult situation; and so on.
  - ♦ *General idea:* Feelings provide us with information (about external world and internal experience) and pull us toward specific actions or responses.

(cont.)

- **Ask:** "Are feelings always accurate? In other words, is what we're *AWARE* that we're feeling always the true feeling we are having?"
  - *Teaching points:*
    - One feeling sometimes acts as a "mask" for another.
    - This can happen for many reasons:
      - ◊ To decrease feelings of vulnerability (e.g., anger substituting for sadness or fear).
      - ◊ Because past experience made it dangerous to exhibit or acknowledge a particular emotion (e.g., showing fear might increase vulnerability, *or* showing anger might increase abuse).
      - ◊ Cultural or family norms: How acceptable it is to show particular feelings, as well as different ways feelings are expressed.
- **Ask:** "Are there feelings that you don't like to show? Do you know why?"
- **Ask:** "How do you know when feelings are 'true feelings' versus 'mask feelings'?"
- **Ask:** "Is there any risk that comes with consistently masking feelings?"
  - *Teaching point:* Feelings that don't come out in one way will often come out in other ways (e.g., held in the body, interfering with sleep or eating, irritability, etc.)
- **Ask:** "Why might you want to shift your feelings?"
  - *Teaching point:* Feelings may be too intense, interfere with current activities, be inappropriate to the situation, lead to impulsive behavior, etc.
- **Ask:** "How do you shift to a different feeling?"
  - Review or discuss skills associated with managing feelings (e.g., relaxation, breathing, music).
- **Ask:** "What skills do you use?"

ACTIVITY: FIGHT, FLIGHT, FREEZE GAME, PART 1: IDENTIFICATION OF DANGER RESPONSE

- **ARC Target(s): Affect Identification (Advanced), Trauma Experience Integration**
- **Purpose:** To facilitate application of the learned concept of the body's alarm system and the human danger response.
- **Materials:** Scenarios
- **Directions:**
  - The group facilitator reviews the body's alarm system and the trauma response. See teaching points below:
    - **The Body's Alarm System:** *"Everyone has a built-in alarm system that signals when we might be in danger. One reason why human beings have been able to survive over time is because our brain recognizes signals around us that tell us that danger might be coming. This helps our bodies prepare to deal with danger when it comes."*
    - **The Human Danger Response:** *"When our brain recognizes danger, it prepares our body to deal with it. We can deal with something dangerous in three major ways: We can fight it, we can get away from it (flight), or we can freeze."*
    - **Our Response May Be Different in Different Situations:** *"What we pick to do sometimes depends on the kind of danger. So, for example, if a really small squirrel is attacking you, you might fight it, because you're bigger and stronger than it is. If a car comes speeding at you, and you're standing in the street, you'd probably run, because you can't really fight it, and if you stand still, you'll get hit. If you saw a big bear or some other animal nearby, you might freeze, because you can't really fight it, and you're probably not fast enough to run away."*

(cont.)

    ○ ***Our Body Gives Us the Fuel/Energy that We Need to Survive:*** *"When it's time for our body to fight, or run, or freeze, we need a lot of energy to do those things. So, once the brain recognizes danger, the "action" or "doing" part of our brain sends a signal to our body to release a bunch of chemicals, like fuel for a car. That gives us the energy we need to cope with the danger."*

♦ Following review of the concepts, the group leader facilitates the "Fight, Flight, Freeze Game." Each member takes a turn listening to one of the scenarios below. The task is to identify whether the person in the scenario is actively engaged in the *fight*, *flight*, or *freeze* response. Group members can earn points for guessing the correct response (goal should be cooperative, rather than competitive).

FIGHT, FLIGHT, FREEZE GAME, PART 1—SAMPLE SCENARIOS

1. Joey is crossing the street and all of a sudden a car comes racing toward him. Without thinking he runs to the other side of the road as fast as he can. *(flight)*
2. Bobby is taking a nature walk and all of a sudden he sees a bear standing 10 feet away looking at him. He has learned that bears react to sudden movement and noise. He stays as still as he possibly can until the bear finally moves away. *(freeze)*
3. Jennifer is in school and one of her peers calls her a name and starts to threaten her. She starts screaming and yelling as loud as she can "NO, NO, NO . . . you don't threaten me." *(fight)*
4. Holly just started a new program. One of her roommates is having a difficult time and starts slamming things around the room. Holly bolts out of her room and out of the front door of the building. *(flight)*
5. Gage is at the hospital waiting for news about a family member who is in surgery. He sees the doctor walking toward him and then everything feels as if it were in slow motion: He can't move, he can't talk, and time stands still. *(freeze)*
6. Nate is walking down the street and a small dog begins to attack his leg. Nate starts screaming at the dog and kicks his leg back and forth, over and over again, until the dog finally lets go of him. *(fight)*
7. Betty is walking down the street and a large, large dog starts to walk toward her. Without thinking she starts running toward the nearest building and is able to narrowly escape the dog. *(flight)*
8. Bobby just left the movie theater after watching a scary movie. Walking down a dark road, he hears a weird noise nearby. His heart starts beating, his body feels jumpy, his arms go up, and his fists are ready to strike. *(fight)*
9. A deer is crossing the road and a car starts coming toward it. The deer just stands there—"a deer caught in the headlights." *(freeze)*
10. Joey's dad comes home in a really angry mood and starts calling for him. Joey runs into his room and hides under the bed. *(flight)*
11. Lilly is sitting in class and one of her classmates starts to throw things at the teacher. Lilly gets up from her desk, grabs her classmate's arm to stop her, and puts a book in front of the object that is being thrown. *(fight)*
12. Johnny is tiptoeing out of his room, trying to sneak down the hallway to get some water even though he does not have permission. All of a sudden he hears a staff member calling his name. Johnny tries to stay as still and as quiet as possible because he is very scared of getting in trouble. *(freeze)*

(cont.)

ACTIVITY: FIGHT, FLIGHT, FREEZE GAME, PART 2: RECOGNIZING TRIGGERS

- **ARC Target(s): Affect Identification (Advanced), Trauma Experience Integration**
- **Purpose:** To facilitate application of the learned concept of triggers, or "false alarms."
- **Materials:** Scenarios
- **Directions:**
  - ♦ The group facilitator reviews the concept of triggers, or "false alarms," using the teaching points outlined below:
  - ♦ *False Alarms:* "*False alarms can happen when we hear or see or feel something that reminds us of bad things that used to happen. Those reminders are called Triggers. Our brain has learned to recognize those reminders, because in the past when they were around, dangerous things happened, and we had to react pretty quickly. Different people have different reminders. So, if someone got yelled at a lot, hearing people yell might activate the alarm and make the 'doing' part of the brain turn on. If someone didn't have enough attention paid to them when they were little, feeling all alone or scared might turn on the alarm.*"
  - ♦ *What Happens When the Alarm Goes Off?:* "*Once our alarm turns on, our brain preps our body for action. When that happens, our body fills with 'fuel' to prepare us for dealing with danger. This is really important if it's real danger (like a bear, or a speeding car, or a really mean squirrel), but not so helpful if it's a false alarm, and there isn't really any danger around. Imagine if you were in math class, and something felt dangerous—suddenly, your body is filled with fuel.*"
  - ♦ **How Our "Danger Energy" Affects Us:** "*Remember that the fuel gives us the energy to fight, or get away, or freeze. When our body has all that energy, we have to do something. So—some kids suddenly feel really angry, or want to argue or fight with someone. Some kids just feel antsy or jumpy. Some kids want to hide in a corner or get as far away as they can—and sometimes they don't even know why. Other kids suddenly feel really shut down, like someone flipped a switch and turned them off. All of these are ways your body is trying to deal with something it thinks is dangerous.*"
  - ♦ **The Problem with the False Alarm:** "*Sometimes, though, what sets off the alarm isn't really dangerous—it's just something that feels bad or reminds us of something bad that happens. When kids have a false alarm like that, it can be hard for other people to understand what just happened, and to help. Sometimes, kids even get into trouble.*"
  - ♦ *Recognizing Triggers:* "*It's important to learn about what kinds of reminders might feel dangerous to you, and how your body reacts when those reminders are around. Everyone has different triggers and different ways to respond when the alarm goes off. If we know what sets off your alarm, and how you respond, we can get your thinking brain on board to help figure out when danger is real and when it's a false alarm.* **Triggers can be people, places, sounds, smells, touch, change, etc.**"
  - ♦ Following review of these concepts, the group leader facilitates the "Recognizing Triggers Game." Each member takes a turn listening to one of the scenarios written below. The task is to identify the current trigger that reminds the person in the scenario of past experiences. Group members can earn points for guessing the correct response (goal should be cooperative, rather than competitive).

(cont.)

278

RECOGNIZING TRIGGERS GAME—SAMPLE SCENARIOS

1. Lavert grew up in a neighborhood where there was a lot of violence. He often heard scary sounds outside of his window at night, including the sound of gunshots. One day Lavert was in school and someone dropped a book on the floor. He reacted quickly by yelling and then crying. *(sound of book dropping)*

2. Francisco's dad was really strict and often became very, very angry at home when Francisco broke a rule or made a mistake. Francisco learned to be very good at following rules, and he worked very very hard to *never* make mistakes. He couldn't even have fun because he always had to think and plan to make everything in his life perfect. He would not do things that felt good if they broke one of his rules. *(mistakes)*

3. Tammy's mother used to hit her a lot when Tammy lived with her. Her mother's perfume smelled like oranges. At snack time Tammy started to peel an orange. All of a sudden she appeared frozen. She didn't say or do anything and couldn't answer staff's questions about whether or not she was okay. *(orange scent)*

4. When Debbie did something wrong at home, like broke the rules or didn't do her chores, she would get into trouble and her dad would hit her. One day at her school Debbie was told that she was in trouble for breaking a rule and was going to earn a consequence. Debbie stopped talking, did not move, and appeared frozen. *(being in trouble)*

5. When Jimmy was a little boy his mother always promised to do something special with him on Saturday afternoons. But, every Saturday afternoon Jimmy's mother would drink too much and break her promise. Jimmy would feel so disappointed and scared when his mom would drink. Yesterday, Jimmy's mom cancelled a visit. Jimmy started yelling at a female staff person, saying, "You are the worst staff person! You don't want me to see my mother! It's all your fault!" *(being let down/cancelled visit)*

6. Vivian had three younger sisters in her home growing up. Her mom wasn't around to take care of the younger kids, and they often took Vivian's things without asking. When Vivian complained, her mom always took her sisters' side. One day at the program, Vivian's roommate picked up one of Vivian's CDs and put it in the radio to play. Vivian ran over to her and punched her as hard as she could, screaming, "That's not yours!!!!!!!!!!" *(taking CD)*

7. When Evan was 8 years old, he was taken suddenly from his parents home by DCF because his home was not a safe place for him. He didn't get any warning and was so, so scared, not knowing what was going to happen next. One day at the program he was living in, Evan learned that one of his favorite staff members had to leave the job suddenly for personal reasons. Evan found this out and went immediately to his room. He crawled under his bed and refused to come out. *(sudden departure/change)*

8. Gerald's dad used to hit him in the head with an open hand all the time. Gerald can't really remember why this happened—just that it did. One day one of his friends came walking up to him and started to move his arm and hand to give Gerald a side hug. Seeing the hand moving toward him, Gerald flinched and ducked his head. *(raised hand)*

(cont.)

9. Briana loved making things for her grandmother, with whom she lived as a little girl. She would spend all day working on cards, drawings, and other nice things to give to her grandmother when she returned home from work. Most of the time her grandmother, returning from work, would glance at the art work that Briana gave her and say "What's this? I can't even tell what it is. Do you call this a drawing?" She would often throw it away. Briana usually won't even try to make things now that she is living with a foster family, but one day she did participate in an art project at school. She handed it to her foster mom when she got home, who started to ask a question about it. As soon as Briana heard the word *what*, she grabbed the paper back, ripped it up, and said "I suck at doing art." *(the word* what*)*

10. Benjamin's mother had a boyfriend who often hit his mother when angry. Benjamin was scared and angry watching his mother get hurt by someone so much bigger and stronger than she, and he would often try to help her/protect her. Now, in his program, Benjamin always makes sure that he pays attention to helping smaller animals or kids when they need it. Like at home, Benjamin feels that his job is to be the protector. One day one of the other kids was having a hard time and started threatening to hurt the program dog. Benjamin, without thinking, jumped in between the dog and the other student and started fighting back. *(threatened dog)*

ACTIVITY: TUNING INTO YOUR BODY/CHANGES IN PHYSIOLOGICAL AROUSAL

- **ARC Target(s): Modulation**
- **Purpose:** To increase participants' awareness of their own level of physiological arousal, and ways that various activities might increase or decrease arousal level.
- **Materials:** Worksheet for measuring pulse rate. *(See worksheet, "Checking My Pulse," Appendix D)*
- **Teaching Points:**
  - ◆ "In order to regulate your body, you need to be able to tune in and know where you're at."
  - ◆ "Although your body responds automatically to different cues in the environment, and to internal and external experiences, there are things you can do to change your own arousal level."
  - ◆ "What kind of cues does your body give that you're in a comfortable or uncomfortable state of arousal?"
- **Measure Your Heartbeat:**
  - ◆ **Baseline pulse:** Teach participants how to take their own pulse by placing their index and middle fingers on the wrist or neck; be sure participants are not using their thumb. Have each participant measure his or her pulse for 20 seconds and multiply by 3 to get the baseline pulse rate. Write down the baseline pulse on the worksheet.
  - ◆ **Exercise pulse:** Have participants do 10–15 jumping jacks (and/or other brief strenuous activity—e.g., jogging in place for at least 20–30 seconds). Immediately after stopping, have participants remeasure their pulse and write down the results on the worksheet.
  - ◆ **Resting pulse:** Have each participant take five deep breaths while seated. Show participants how to breathe slowly in through the nose, out through the mouth. Immediately after completing the deep breaths, remeasure the participant's pulse and write down the result on the worksheet.
- **Discussion:** Ask participants: "How did your heart rate change across the three measurements? What other changes did you notice in your body? How effective was breathing in slowing down your heart rate? If not, why do you think this is? When else do you notice that your heart rate speeds up? Slows down?"
- **Note:** Other activities or exercises can be substituted or added at the discretion of the group leader; it is helpful to teach multiple exercises for each component (up-regulation, down-regulation).

(cont.)

ACTIVITY: BALL TOSS/GROUP JUGGLE

- **ARC Target(s): Affect Expression, Attunement**
- **Purpose:** To build awareness of key skills involved in effective communication.
- **Materials:** For every six participants, four to six small balls (ideally, round Nerf balls, beanbag balls, or similar)
- **Directions:**
  - ◆ Participants should stand in a circle. The group leader explains: "We are going to make a pattern using this ball. I will throw to someone, saying the name first. That person should then throw the ball to someone else. Make sure that you throw the ball to someone who has not yet received it. The rules are simple: We are going to make a pattern with our throws. Everyone should get the ball once, and no one should get it more than once. The last person to get the ball should throw it back to me, completing the pattern. Every time you throw the ball, say the name of the person you are throwing to first. There are no winners or losers in this game. If you drop the ball, just pick it up and keep going."
  - ◆ The group leader should then start the pattern, making sure that all participants receive the ball once. When the group leader receives the ball back, practice the pattern several times to make sure all members remember from whom they receive the ball and to whom they throw the ball.
  - ◆ Once the group has become comfortable with the pattern, the group leader explains: "We are going to introduce more balls into our pattern, one by one. Our goal is to see how many balls we can throw at the same time, and keep the pattern going."
  - ◆ Make sure the group is comfortable with adding more balls, and then slowly add additional balls into the pattern. The group should be comfortable with two balls before a third is added, with three before a fourth is added, etc.
- **Postactivity Discussion:** Start open-ended: Ask group members what they noticed about the activity, whether they liked it or not, etc.
  - ◆ Specific questions:
    - ○ "What did you notice about what made it easier or harder to be effective in this game? What helped keep the pattern moving smoothly?"
    - ○ If not mentioned, tune in to the following ideas:
      - ◊ Making eye contact with the person who is throwing to you, and with the one who is receiving from you.
      - ◊ Saying the person's name [offering a cue that you are about to throw the ball].
      - ◊ Not throwing too hard or too soft.
      - ◊ Indicating with body language, eye contact, etc., that you are ready to throw/receive.
      - ◊ Tuning out distractions, concentrating only on the person who is throwing to you, and the person to whom you throw.
      - ◊ Lack of pressure: If you drop the ball, you can pick it up and continue the pattern.
    - ○ Discuss with the group: "All of these skills were important in being successful at this activity. These skills are also all important in being effective at communicating." Ask: "How does each of these skills play into good communication?"

(cont.)

ACTIVITY: CIRCLES OF TRUST

- **ARC Target(s): Affect Expression, Identity**
- **Purpose:** To build awareness of relationship resources; to build awareness of variations in intimacy across relationships.
- **Materials:** "Circles of Trust" worksheet (see Appendix D); pencils/pens
- **Directions:** Participants are given worksheets (concentric circles) and asked to consider the various relationships in their life. The center circle represents them; each participant is then asked to place names/initials of significant people in their life in the remaining circles, with distance from the center circle indicating strength/closeness of the relationship.
- **Postactivity Discussion:** Questions/discussion points may include: "Notice how many/few people are in your circles; notice where people tend to cluster. What does this tell you about your pattern of relationships? Do you tend to keep many people close? Most people at arm's length? Are you comfortable with the number of people in your life? Are there resources that you had forgotten about?"
- **Examine Specific Relationship Types**
  - ♦ **Have participants circle or mark in different colors, who in their circle are . . .**
    - ○ People with whom they have fun?
    - ○ People to whom they speak about important decisions?
    - ○ People to whom they go to for emotional support?
    - ○ People whom they consider family?
    - ○ People who really know them?
  - ♦ **Using arrows, have participants indicate people to whom they would want to be closer, or from whom they would want more distance.**
  - ♦ *Discuss:* "Notice who in your life fills which functions. Are there any functions that are missing?"

DISCUSSION: "I" STATEMENTS

- **ARC Target(s): Affect Expression**
- **Purpose:** To teach participants about "I" statements and how these are linked to effective communication.
- **Materials:** None
- **Directions:**
  - ♦ Provide participants with an example of two statements, such as:
    - ○ "I can't believe you did that! You're such a jerk!"
      versus
    - ○ "I'm really angry about what you did. I need some space from you right now."
  - ♦ **Ask:** "What is different about these two statements? What kind of reaction might there be to the first one? To the second one?"
  - ♦ **Teach:** "I" statements are an effective way to communicate:
    - ○ Rather than blaming, insulting, being aggressive, or putting someone on the defense, "I" statements focus on our own feelings and reactions.
    - ○ Someone can challenge a "you" statement (the obvious answer to "You're such a jerk" is "No, I'm not, you are!"), but it's harder for someone to challenge an "I" statement (if I say I'm angry, it's hard for you to tell me I'm not!).
    - ○ "I" statements express to someone how we feel and why we feel that way. They allow us to work on solutions and resolve conflicts. "You" statements often increase conflicts or negative situations.

(cont.)

ACTIVITY: CRAZY "I" STATEMENT TRANSLATION

- **ARC Target(s): Affect Expression**
- **Purpose:** To provide practice in using "I" statements rather than "you statements."
- **Materials:** Prompts for "I" statement translation; large Post-its and markers for Part 2 application/discussion.
- **Directions:**
  - ◆ *Part 1:* Demonstration: Crazy "I" Statements
  - ◆ Ask participants if they have ever seen movies in which words are translated from one language to another. Tell them: "In this activity you will act as the translators for people speaking in the foreign 'You language'; your job is to translate each statement from *you* into *I*."
  - ◆ Group leaders demonstrate:
    - ○ One leader reads a crazy "you" statement. For example: "You yellow-bellied, no-good rotten horse's pimple! You're a sniveling good-for-nothing who couldn't get something right if your life depended on it!"
    - ○ The second leader offers a translation: "I'm very frustrated with how you did that."
    - ○ *Note: Leaders should play up the humor/contrast between the two statements.*
  - ◆ Participants are then asked to translate further statements. Activity may consist of dialogue between the two group leaders or individual statements, with translations offered by two participants. **(See below for sample statements.)**
  - ◆ *Part 2:* Application: "You" versus "I" Statements
  - ◆ Ask participants to generate a list of "you" statements. These can be statements they've heard or ones they find themselves making. If participants have difficulty, offer examples (e.g., "You're such a jerk," "You make me so mad," "You ruin everything"). The goal is to generate a list of *realistic* "you" statements that are commonly experienced.
  - ◆ For each "you" statement generated, ask the group to offer translations: What kind of "I" statements might go with these? Write these next to the "you" statements.
- **Postactivity Discussion:** How did the statements change when they were *you* versus *I*? Which statements seemed more respectful? Which ones were likely to make the situation worse versus lead to solution? How would you rather be talked to?

"I" STATEMENTS TRANSLATION GAME—SAMPLE PROMPTS
"You" Statement:
"You yellow-bellied, no-good, rotten horse's pimple! You're a sniveling good for nothing who couldn't get something right if your life depended on it!"
> ***Sample "I" statement:***
> "I'm very frustrated with how you did that."

"You" Statement:
"This school assignment is lame! It's only for stupid pea-brain donkeys! Your directions stink! And I already did this last year!"
Sample "I" Statements:
> "I don't know how to do this assignment."/"I don't like doing this type of work."

(cont.)

"You" Statement:
"You must be a complete and utter moron, if you think I am so stupid/insensitive/dumb/worthless/inconsiderate/hopeless that I wouldn't know already that I shouldn't have done that!"
> *Sample "I" Statements:*
> "I already feel really bad about what happened."/"I'm sorry."

"You" Statement:
"You're getting on my last, worn-out, overstretched nerve! You annoying, pestering, aggravating, irritating, bothersome turnip head! Cut it out!!!"
> *Sample "I" Statement:*
> "I want you to stop that."

"You" Statement:
"You brainless, dim-witted, moronic nincompoop! You make me absolutely, certifiably, completely insane! You big baboon! How does someone get to your age without a brain!?"
> *Sample "I" Statements:*
> "I'm really angry with you."/"I'm feeling frustrated."

"You" statement:
"You're so pushy and annoying. Why are you always shoving into my business? You don't know what you're doing. You can't help me. You're always getting involved in stuff you don't know anything about."
> *Sample "I" Statements:*
> "I need some time alone."/ "I'd like some space."/ "I don't want to talk about that."

"You" Statement:
"Like your life is so big and important—you're just sooooo busy, and then you don't want to do anything, and here I am just twiddling my thumbs having nothing to do because you're just a stupid jerk!"
> *Sample "I" Statement:*
> "I want you to spend more time with me."

ACTIVITY: OWN YOUR ZONE

- **ARC Target(s): Affect Expression**
- **Purpose:** To recognize personal "comfort zones" with physical boundaries and to practice asserting personal preferences around boundaries.
- **Materials:** Strips of paper or masking tape, marker
- **Directions:** Participants can either be paired up, or paired one at a time with a group leader.
  - ◆ Participants should face their partner at a 10-foot difference (distance should be great enough that it is larger than most individuals' spatial needs).
  - ◆ One partner should begin to walk slowly toward the other. The person who is not moving should say "Stop" when the partner reaches a distance that feels comfortable.

(cont.)

- ♦ Once stopped, the partner should be directed to "check in" with the other person, asking whether the distance is comfortable or whether he or she should move in/out. Once a comfortable distance is reached, the group leader should measure the distance with a strip of paper or piece of tape, and mark it with the participant's name. This is his or her "physical comfort zone."
- ♦ For each participant, introduce at least one novel variable (e.g., pretend that your partner is your . . . best friend, mother, therapist, school principal, kid you hate, etc., *or* you are in a . . . great mood, terrible mood, feeling sick, feeling jumpy, etc.). Redo the distance—how does this change the comfort zone?
- ♦ Each participant's comfort zones (primary plus added variables) should be hung on the wall.
- **Postactivity Discussion:**
  - ♦ What are "physical spatial needs"? How do participants understand these?
  - ♦ What influences our spatial needs (if not named, introduce concepts such as relationship to other person, current mood state, family norms about space, cultural names about space, current situation, etc.)?
  - ♦ How do you know if your spatial need is different from other people's? Group leaders can demonstrate physical cues: What does it look like if you step into someone's personal space? Pay attention to cues such as the other person stepping or leaning back, avoiding eye contact, looking pained.
  - ♦ How do you/should you handle different spatial needs? *Teaching point:* In interpersonal interactions, boundaries are generally determined by the person with the furthest/greatest boundary need.
  - ♦ Are you ever in situations where people inadvertently violate your boundaries—for example, in a crowded train? How can you deal with this?

ACTIVITY: EMOTIONAL BOUNDARIES

- **ARC Target(s): Affect Expression**
- **Purpose:** To explore personal "comfort zone" with emotional boundaries, and to illustrate differing boundary needs across interaction partners.
- **Materials:** List of interview questions (see sample questions, below) with increasingly intimate questions
- **Directions:** Participants are paired up and given the following instructions:
  - ♦ "Each of you is being given a list of interview questions to ask your partner. The questions start out as broad but become increasingly personal. Each of you gets to choose which of these questions you answer. The person being interviewed may answer whichever questions he or she is comfortable with; once you reach a question you do not feel comfortable answering, let your partner know you are ready to stop."
  - ♦ Once the first partner has had an opportunity to act as interviewer, the roles should switch, and the second person should be interviewed.
- **Postactivity Discussion:**
  - ♦ How many questions were you willing to answer?
  - ♦ Were your boundaries the same as your partner's, or different—that is, did you stop on the same question?
    - ○ *Teaching Point:* Often, we reciprocate social intimacy—we go only as deep as our social partner.

(cont.)

♦ What factors influenced how many questions you were willing to answer? Consider who your partner was, the setting, the mood you were in, etc. Is there anyone you can think of for whom you would have answered all of the questions? Any situations where you might answer none?

♦ General boundary discussion point: How do you know when something has intruded upon your boundaries? What internal cues do you have that your boundaries are being pushed?

SET YOUR BOUNDARIES: SAMPLE INTERVIEW QUESTIONS

1. What is your favorite color?
2. Who is your favorite musical artist?
3. How many people are in your immediate family, or what you consider immediate family?
4. What book or books have influenced you?
5. Who is the person that you admire the most?
6. Who is the person that you feel closest to in your family?
7. What is the best experience you ever had in school?
8. What is a dream you have for your future?
9. If you could have three wishes, what would they be?
10. What is one of your earliest memories?
11. What is the worst experience you ever had in school?
12. What is something you don't like people to know about you?
13. Who is the person in your family you feel most disappointed by?
14. What is the scariest thing that ever happened to you?
15. What is something that you're ashamed of?

DISCUSSION: HEALTHY RELATIONSHIPS

- **ARC Target(s): Identity, Affect Expression, Trauma Experience Integration**
- **Purpose:** To distinguish healthy from unhealthy relationships.
- **Materials:** Large Post-its, markers
- **Discussion Points:**
  - ♦ What does it mean to have a "healthy" relationship? What qualities do you think are seen in healthy relationships? Write participant responses on Post-it sheets.
    - ○ If not listed, include qualities such as *respect, not exploitive, appropriate to role*.
  - ♦ How do you know you are safe in a relationship? What does it mean to be "safe" in a relationship?

ACTIVITY: RELATIONSHIP CONTINUUM

- **ARC Target(s): Identity, Affect Expression, Trauma Experience Integration**
- **Purpose:** To distinguish healthy from unhealthy relationships.
- **Materials:** Sheets of paper or preprinted handouts with horizontal lines anchored at each end by "Healthy/Unhealthy" to create a continuum; relationship description prompts (see below); pencils; large Post-it with continuum line; marker

(cont.)

286

- **Directions:** Read participants the following Relationship Description Sample Prompts one at a time (select four to six, depending on the group, or generate appropriate scenarios based on group composition). After reading each one, have participants mark whether they think the relationship is healthy or unhealthy by placing a vertical line on the continuum and marking it with the description number (i.e., 1–5).
- **Postactivity Discussion:**
  - ◆ After all prompts have been read, go back to each description and survey the group. Mark on a large sheet of paper how the group rated each scenario. Note differences in group ratings, and elicit why group members made the ratings they did.
  - ◆ Possible follow-up questions:
    - ○ "How can you tell if a relationship is healthy or unhealthy? What struck you about these descriptions?"
    - ○ "What do you think influences your perception of whether a relationship is healthy?" (Help participants to consider family norms, cultural norms, past experience in relationships, etc.)
    - ○ "How can you make a relationship healthier? Do you always have control over this?"
    - ○ "Is there ever a reason to stay in an unhealthy relationship? If yes, why? Are there things you can do to protect yourself in less healthy relationships?"

RELATIONSHIP DESCRIPTION SAMPLE PROMPTS FOR RELATIONSHIP CONTINUUM

1. Joshua and Tanya have been going out for 6 months; they are both 16. They started spending all their free time together right away. Josh gets really jealous if Tanya spends time away from him, whether with her girlfriends or even with her family. He wants her to prove that she loves him, and he suspects that she is cheating on him. Sometimes he accuses her of cheating and calls her names. Recently, he got so angry that he pushed her into the wall. Later, he apologized and said that he really loved her and didn't want to hurt her.

2. Kenny has always looked up to his father. His dad spends time with him, and has taught him how to do many things, like drive a car (when he was 13 years old) and fix things around the house. A lot of times, Kenny's dad is funny and fun to be around. However, at other times, Kenny's dad will get angry with him for little things. When Kenny doesn't understand how to do things right away, his father calls him "stupid" and an "idiot." Kenny tries really hard to do things the right way so that he will stay on his father's good side.

3. Jamie and Maria have been friends since they were small; they grew up next door to each other. They like to do things together, such as go to the mall or just hang out. Sometimes they argue and get angry with each other, but usually they work it out pretty quickly. When Jamie is upset about things at home, she sometimes talks to Maria about it. Maria doesn't say much, but she knows Jamie very well, so she understands.

4. Larry is 15 and lives with his mother and younger sister, Amelia, who is 13. He works after school until 10 o'clock every night at the supermarket, bagging groceries. Half of this paycheck goes to his mother to help pay the rent, and he brings food home every night when he gets off work. Amelia has been getting into trouble at school and was suspended today for getting into a fight with another girl. When Larry came home and found out about Amelia's suspension, he became upset and began to yell at her and took away her cell phone as punishment.

(cont.)

5. Joe and Mark have been friends forever. They both graduated high school and Mark went off to college 100 miles away. Joe works a steady job, owns a car, and lives at home with his mother and father. Every weekend, Joe drives over to Mark's school and hangs out with Mark and his friends, often staying over in Mark's dorm on Saturday nights. Sometimes Mark has schoolwork to do but is unable to get it done because Joe wants to hang out and party.

6. Jennifer and Tommy have been going out for a few months. Jennifer is 17 and graduating this year. Tommy is 18 and going to GED classes along with working. Jennifer loves sports and has joined a team each season and spends all her extra time studying or seeing Tommy. Tommy expects her to be home in the evenings when he calls to talk. Jennifer has had the opportunity to go out with the girls on her team after practice but doesn't do this because she doesn't want to miss Tommy's calls.

7. Johnny and Lindsey have been dating for about a month. It is the first time that Lindsey has had a boyfriend. She is excited that Johnny calls her a dozen times a day, both at home and at her after-school job. He says that he really loves her and is concerned about her, so he just wants to check to make sure she's okay. Recently he has wanted to spend a lot of time with her and asks her to cancel any plans that she has made with her friends. Lindsey's parents are concerned because she doesn't help out with her younger sister anymore.

8. Ryan lives with his mother, stepfather, and younger brother Joey. Ryan gets along with his family okay, but would rather spend time with his friends. He usually does the chores he is supposed to do at home. He has a curfew of 11 on weekdays and 12 on weekends, and he usually follows it, but sometimes he doesn't. When he comes home late, his mother and stepfather are angry and they ground him or take away his Game Boy or something else that he likes to do. He thinks he should have more freedom, since he is 16, so sometimes he gets angry at his parents, especially his stepfather, who, after all, isn't his "real" father. But he also knows that his parents are usually there for him when he needs them, and last year when he got in trouble in school for something he really didn't do, they went to bat for him.

9. Jordan is 13 years old; his next-door neighbor, Ray, is 17. Jordan has always looked up to Ray, but Ray has barely paid any attention to him. Lately, Ray has allowed Jordan to hang out with him and his friends, as long as Jordan does them favors, like go and get them cigarettes or beer out of Jordan's house when his parents aren't looking. Sometimes Ray pushes Jordan around and laughs with his friends about it, but Jordan knows it is all in fun. Recently, Ray suggested that Jordan might help him and his friends out with some other things; for example, Ray and his friends are planning to break in to a house where they know there is a lot of money, and Ray says Jordan might be able to help.

10. José and Marie have been hanging out together for about 9 months. José is 18 and Marie is 17. They spend a lot of time together, but also have other friends, too, so sometimes they might go several days or even a week without seeing each other. They each get along with each other's families as well, which is nice. They are having sex together but do use condoms, even though they trust each other, because they don't want Marie to get pregnant.

11. Jim is having trouble understanding his math homework. He has sat in the study hall for almost an hour without getting more than two problems done. Other people can see him getting more upset over not knowing how to do the math. Finally, Armand walks in and notices what is

(cont.)

happening. Armand walks over to find out how Jim is doing. After seeing what Jim is working on, Armand shows Jim how to come up with the answer to the next problem, and later, Jim gives Armand a good idea for a story he has to write for English class.

12. Rihanna practiced for many months to get ready for volleyball tryouts. When the tryouts were over, she found out that she did not make the freshman team. Rihanna went home feeling very angry with the coaches and was disappointed in herself. When she walked in the house, her older sister Juleesa asked Rihanna if she made the team. When Rihanna said no, Juleesa laughed at her and said, "What can you expect from a klutz?"

ACTIVITY: GIVING COMPLIMENTS TO OTHERS

- **ARC Target(s): Affect Expression, Identity**
- *Note:* See worksheet, "Giving Others Compliments," Appendix D
- **Purpose:** To build group members' ability to tune in to and name positive qualities in others; to build understanding of how other people see them.
- **Materials:** "Giving Others Compliments" worksheet, crayons or markers
- **Directions:** *(Group leaders say:)* "Most of us like the feeling that we get when people say nice things to us or recognize what we do. Today we are really going to practice giving compliments to each other in order to celebrate things about each one of us that we really like or see as positive." Group participants should be invited to list one positive quality about each group member on their worksheet. Participants then share these compliments with other members. *Note:* Participants may need to have adults write their answers or may choose to verbalize answers without writing.

ACTIVITY: ALTERNATE VERSION—GIVING COMPLIMENTS TO OTHERS

- **ARC Target(s): Affect Expression, Identity**
- **Purpose:** To highlight competencies and positive aspects of self; to build group members' ability to tune in to and name positive qualities in others; to build understanding of how other people see them.
- **Materials:** Giant Post-it notes (one per group member, with member's name written on top); smaller Post-its on which members write comments; pens/markers
- **Directions:**
  - ◆ Group members are handed a stack of smaller Post-its and a pen/marker.
  - ◆ Members are asked to write at least one positive comment about each member of the group. Comments *must* illustrate something positive about the other person. Comments can be anonymous, or group members may sign their names to the Post-it.
  - ◆ When all group members have written their comments, they should attach their Post-its to the giant Post-it sheets; all comments should be attached. Group leaders should ensure that all comments are appropriate/positive.
  - ◆ Group leaders then read aloud each member's list.
    (*Alternative directions:* Group members may write directly on other members' giant Post-its, with a rule that no two comments should be the same.)
- **Postactivity Discussion:** Possible questions include: "Did anything surprise you in what other people wrote about you? What is it like to hear all of these positive things about yourself?"

(cont.)

ACTIVITY: POSITIVE SELF-RECOGNITION

- **ARC Target(s): Identity (Positive Self), Affect Expression**
- ***Note:*** Complete this activity in association with the worksheet, "Giving Myself Compliments", in Appendix D.
- **Purpose:** To highlight competencies/positive aspects of self.
- **Materials:** "Giving Myself Compliments" worksheet, crayons or markers
- **Directions:**
  - ◆ Group leaders: "Sometimes it's hard to focus on what we like about ourselves, or what we're proud of. Today we want to practice giving ourselves compliments. This is important to do because it helps us to feel good about ourselves. We are going to hand out a worksheet for you to complete. The worksheet focuses on things that you think you do well in different areas of your life, such as school, activities, relationships, the residence, etc. After you complete the worksheet, you can choose whether or not to share your self-compliments with the group."
  - ◆ Distribute worksheets and writing materials to all group members. When all participants have completed their worksheets, invite members to share.
  - ◆ *Note:* Participants may need to have adults write their answers, or they may choose to verbalize answers without writing.
- **Postactivity Discussion:** Possible questions include: "What was it like to give yourself compliments? Were there some areas where it was easier to compliment yourself than others? Were there areas where it was harder? Is it comfortable to compliment yourself? Why, or why not?"

ACTIVITY: DESERT ISLAND

- **ARC Target(s): Executive Functions, Affect Expression**
- **Purpose:** To apply skills, including problem solving, negotiation, "I statements," conflict resolution, etc., to a group problem-solving task.
- **Materials:** Forty index cards listing array of objects, including essentials (e.g., food, matches, bedding), personal items (e.g., shampoo, toothpaste), and "luxury" items (i.e., iPod, radio, deck of cards).
- **Directions:**
  - ◆ Participants are told that they are members of a group that has been stranded on a desert island. As a group, they are able to select 10 objects out of the provided index cards; these will be the objects that have also been stranded with them. The group must negotiate which 10 objects to select, and must negotiate a process for making the selection.
  - ◆ After the initial selection, group leaders should generate a "challenge" scenario. For example: A big storm is coming that will last two days (meaning, participants can't leave shelter to gather food), and the temperature will drop (meaning, participants need to find a way to stay warm). Ask: "Based on the objects you have selected, how will you survive?" The group is given a 5-minute period to consider their items, to re-negotiate selected objects, and to exchange them for other items in the stack.
  - ◆ At the discretion of the group leaders, further challenge scenarios may be provided. After the first selection, group members are no longer allowed to exchange cards and must use problem-solving skills to describe how they will address the challenge using only the selected items.

(cont.)

○ Sample challenge scenarios:
◊ "You are being attacked by a group of natives from another island."
◊ "Wild monkeys steal all the food you have gathered."
◊ "Half of your group develops a nonfatal but uncomfortable illness (e.g., serious poison ivy)."

- **Postactivity Discussion:** "How was the negotiation process? Did everyone feel able to express their opinion? Did it feel like someone 'won' and someone 'lost'? How well do you think, as a group, you did with selecting objects? What factors did you consider? Do you think you considered different alternatives, or did you impulsively select certain objects? Which of the skills we have learned in the group do you think you applied to this challenge?" (Group leaders should note any skills not mentioned by the group.)
- **Sample Items for Desert Island Game:** iPod, flashlight, Game Boy, batteries that are halfway rundown, six-pack of bottled water, sunflower seeds, vegetable seeds, 20 yards of rope, Swiss army knife, tarp, toothpaste, bar of chocolate, toilet paper, matches, bubble gum, balloon, machete, duct tape, potatoes, camera, five large pizzas, big bag of assorted Chinese food, dictionary, encyclopedia, compass, *Harry Potter* series (books), Boy Scout manual, binoculars, hammer and nails, magnifying glass, sunscreen, one set of extra clothes per person, deck of cards, waterproof blanket, one pillow, metal bucket, soap

ACTIVITY: INFLUENCES ON SELF

- **ARC Target(s): Identity**
- *Note:* Complete this activity in association with the worksheet "What Has Influenced My Identitiy?" in Appendix D.
- **Purpose:** To individually examine relative importance of influences on identity, and to concretely represent those influences.
- **Materials:** Small plastic bottles with cork stoppers; sand in different colors (at least six colors); small funnels; measuring cups/spoons in various sizes; paper and pencil
- *Alternative Version:* Modeling clay such as Sculpey can be used instead of sand. In this case, color of clay and relative amount will correspond to values. Prompt may be to make a specific item (e.g., an "identity stone") or leave the sculpture choice open-ended.
- **Directions:** Group members are asked to select up to six key factors that have influenced them; group leaders should give examples (e.g., family, religion, neighborhood, life experiences). Members should pick a color of sand to represent each of these values or beliefs. Using the measuring spoons, members should select amounts of sand to represent how strong/important these values are to them (e.g., the most important belief or value would correspond to the largest measuring cup). Members then use the funnels to fill their bottles with the different colored sand.
- **Postactivity Discussion:** "How well do these influences represent you? What's missing? Was it hard to select what to include? Do you see any commonalities across group members? Any differences?"

ACTIVITY: IDENTITY SHIELD

- **ARC Target(s): Identity**
- *Note:* Complete this activity in association with the worksheet "Identity Shields" in Appendix D.
- **Purpose:** To examine multiple aspects of self; to acknowledge that all people have facets of identity that change in different contexts.

(cont.)

- **Materials:** Paper, colored pencils/markers/crayons
- **Directions:** Group members are provided with an outline drawing of a shield divided into four sections. Instruction is to complete sections of the shield using prompts such as the following (select four):
  - ♦ "Something that symbolizes you as you are with your friends"
  - ♦ "Something that symbolizes you as you are with kids you don't know"
  - ♦ "Something that symbolizes you as you are with your family"
  - ♦ "Something that symbolizes you as you are when you are alone"
  - ♦ "Something that symbolizes you as you are in school"
  - ♦ "Something that symbolizes you as you are in this program"
  - ♦ "Something that symbolizes your hopes for yourself"
  - ♦ "Something that symbolizes an important part of you"
  - ♦ "Something that symbolizes your culture"
- **Postactivity Discussion:** What reactions do group members have to this activity? Were there sections of the shield that were easier to complete? Sections that were harder? What similarities and what differences were there across shield sections? How do each of these sections capture different aspects of group members' identity? Do any sections feel "truer" than others?

ACTIVITY: VALUE LINE (PHYSICAL)

- **ARC Target(s): Identity**
- **Purpose:** To examine one aspect of self that may differ across group members: that is, personal values.
- **Materials:** None
- **Directions:** Group leaders stand in opposite corners. One group leader represents "very important"; the second group leader represents "not at all important." Group leaders provide different prompt values (e.g., importance of education, importance of family, working hard, fairness, being tough, being strong, having friends). Group members are asked to place themselves on the invisible "line" between group leaders to represent how important that value is to them.
- **Postactivity Discussion:** Possible questions include: "Were there any surprises in yourself or in others? Did you find yourself closer to or farther from other group members than you thought? Was it hard/easy to rank values? Were some easier than others? Which ones? What might affect how you rank your values?"

ACTIVITY: VALUE LINE (DRAWN)

- **ARC Target(s): Identity**
- **Purpose:** To individually examine relative importance of personal values.
- **Materials:** Paper, pen or pencil
- **Directions:** Students are asked to draw a line down the middle of a piece of paper. Group leaders provide a list of values (e.g., importance of education, importance of family, working hard, fairness, being tough, being strong, having friends). Members are asked to place the words on the line in order of relative importance.

(cont.)

- **Postactivity Discussion:** Possible questions include: "Were any of these hard to rank? Do any feel like they're equally important? Do any feel completely unimportant? Completely important? Where do you think these came from? What kinds of things affect your values?"

ACTIVITY: QUALITY OF INFLUENCE

Note: Activity is based on a technique taught by Janina Fisher, PhD.
- **ARC Target(s): Identity**
- **Purpose:** To explore past influential relationships and to build awareness of important qualities for future relationships.
- **Materials:** Quality-of-Influence Pyramid worksheets (see Appendix D); pens or pencils
- **Directions:** Participants use the worksheets to identify past influential relationships and to identify qualities they want to develop or avoid in future relationships.
  - ◆ Using the worksheets, identify five people who have most influenced you in your life (either in a positive or a negative way). *Note:* If participants do not want to write actual names, they can use initials or some other "code" to identify the person.
  - ◆ In the space next to that person's box, write one quality that was important within that relationship, either as something you would want to experience in future relationships, or as something you would want to avoid.
- **Postactivity Discussion:** "How hard or easy was it to identify the people who have most influenced you? Did you find yourself purposely leaving out some people who were probably influential? How easy/hard was it to identify the key qualities? How many relationships do you have in your life right now that capture these qualities? What kind of relationships do you think you might want/need to build in the future?"

293

Feelings Toolkit Creation

ACTIVITY: FEELINGS TOOLKIT—INTRODUCTION

- **ARC Target(s): Modulation**
- **Purpose:** Ongoing project; goal is for each participant to build a "toolkit" for use in managing feelings and emotional experience over time.
- **Materials:** Cardboard boxes, markers/paint, other decorative materials
- **Directions:** Ongoing project is introduced. Participants are each given a cardboard box, which they can decorate in any way they like. One thing will be added to the toolkit at each subsequent session.

ONGOING INSTRUCTIONS:

- **Materials:** Toolkit objects
- **Directions:** At end of group sessions, provide a variety of materials within each category (e.g., several scents of lotion, several types of stress balls, several picture postcards). Each participant may choose one object for his or her toolkit.

FEELINGS TOOLKIT: SAMPLE ITEMS

- Biofeedback dots
- Cedar squares/balls
- ChapStick tube (flavored)
- Cloth swatches (fabric, felt, velvet, etc.)
- Feathers
- Hard candy
- Index cards (participants to write positive self-statements on cards)
- Mini bottles of lotion
- Mini bottles of bubbles
- Mini glitter wands
- Mini thought-for-the-day book
- Mini stuffed animal
- Picture postcards
- Plug-in lights (night-lights)
- River stones (or other small polished stones)
- Plastic Slinkys
- Scented sachets
- Stress balls/other textured balls (e.g., Koosh balls, stretch balls)
- Water snakes
- Wikki stix

Progressive Muscle Relaxation Technique

Note: Wording as follows is directed toward participants who are lying on their backs. For participants who are seated, modify language accordingly.

"Get into a comfortable position and relax. Now begin by clenching your right fist, tighter and tighter, studying the tension as you do so. Keep it clenched and notice the tension in your fist, hand, and forearm. Now relax. Feel the looseness in your right hand and notice the contrast with the tension. Repeat this with your right fist again, always noticing, as you relax, that this is the opposite of tension—relax and feel the difference. Repeat this entire procedure with your left fist and then with both fists.

"Now bend your elbows and tense your biceps. Tense them as hard as you can and observe the feeling of tightness. Relax, straighten out your arms. Let the relaxation develop and feel that difference.

"Turning your attention to your head, wrinkle your forehead as tight as you can. Now relax and smooth it out. Let yourself imagine your entire forehead and scalp becoming smooth and at rest. Now frown and notice the strain spreading throughout your forehead. Let go. Allow your brow to become smooth again.

"Close your eyes now, squint them tighter. Look for the tension. Relax your eyes. Let them remain closed gently and comfortably.

"Now clench your jaw, bite hard, notice the tension throughout your jaw. When the jaw is relaxed, your lips will be slightly parted. Let yourself really appreciate the contrast between tension and relaxation.

"Now press your tongue against the roof of your mouth. Feel the ache in the back of your mouth. Relax. Press your lips now, purse them into an o. Relax your lips. Notice that your forehead, scalp, eyes, jaw, tongue and lips are all relaxed.

"Press your head back as far as it can comfortably go and observe the tension in your neck. Roll it to the right and feel the stress; roll it to the left. Straighten your head and bring it forward, pressing your chin against your chest. Feel the tension in your throat and the back of your neck. Relax, allowing your head to return to a comfortable position. Let the relaxation deepen.

"Now shrug your shoulders. Hold the tension as you hunch your head down between your shoulders. Relax your shoulders. Drop them back and feel the relaxation spreading through your neck, throat, and shoulders—pure relaxation, deeper and deeper.

"Give your entire body a chance to relax. Feel the comfort and the heaviness. Now breathe in and fill your lungs completely. Hold your breath. Notice the tension. Now exhale, letting your chest become loose, letting the air hiss out. Continue relaxing, letting your breath come freely and gently. Repeat this breathing pattern several times, noticing the tension draining from your body as you exhale. Next, tighten your stomach and hold. Note the tension, then relax. Now place your hand on your stomach. Breathe deeply into your stomach, and notice how your stomach pushes your hand up. Hold—then relax. Feel the contrast of relaxation as the air rushes out. Now arch your back, without straining. Keep the rest of your body as relaxed as possible. Focus on the tension in your lower back. Now relax, deeper and deeper.

(cont.)

"Tighten your buttocks and thighs. Press down on your heels as hard as you can. Relax and feel the difference. Now curl your toes downward, making your calves tense. Study the tension. Relax. Now bend (flex) your toes toward your knees, creating tension in your shins. Relax again.

"Feel the heaviness throughout your lower body as the relaxation deepens. Relax your feet, ankles, calves, shins, knees, thighs, and buttocks. Now let the relaxation spread to your stomach, lower back, and chest. Let go more and more. Experience the relaxation deepening in your shoulders, arms, and hands. Deeper and deeper. Notice the feeling of looseness and relaxation in your jaw and all of your facial muscles.

"Let the tension dissolve away. . . . "

Icebreaker Prompts

Group Opening Activity

OPENING CIRCLE

- *Purpose:* Build group cohesion and attunement; share information; create a consistent routine/ritual.
- Ask each group member to respond to the icebreaker question of the day (e.g., "If you were any car, what kind would you be?").

CLOSING CIRCLE

- *Purpose:* Build group cohesion and attunement; create a consistent routine/ritual.
- Go around the circle and ask "Who can remember from the check-in what car _____ would be?" for each member.
- Ask: "What is one thing you learned about this person today in group?"

IDENTITY-FOCUSED ICEBREAKER SAMPLE PROMPTS

- "If you were any musical instrument, what kind would you be?"
- "If you were any car, what kind would you be?"
- "If you were any form of weather, what kind would you be?"
- "If you were any magazine/book title, what would you be?"
- "If you were any animal, what would you be?"
- "If you were any celebrity, who would you be?"
- "If you had any type of magical power, what kind would it be and why?"
- "If there was one activity you had to do every day, what would you want it to be?"
- "If you could be any age, what would you be?"
- "If you were guaranteed success at any job in the world, what would you do?"
- "If people could only use one word to describe you, what would you want that word to be?"

RELATIONAL-FOCUSED ICEBREAKER SAMPLE PROMPTS

Name . . .

- "One quality you are proud of that you bring to your friendships."
- "One quality that you would want in a friend."
- "One quality you have improved in yourself that is important to relationships."
- "One quality that you appreciate in authority figures."
- "Something that you like to do for fun with friends."
- "One quality you are proud of that you bring as a son/daughter [or in other family relationships]."
- "One quality that you would want to have as a father/mother."
- "One quality that you would look for in a spouse or intimate partner."
- "One quality that you want to work on in yourself that affects relationships."

(cont.)

- "One quality that you would *not* want to have as a father/mother."
- "The number of friends you feel you need in your life."
- "Something you like to do with your family."
- "Something you would rather *not* do with your family."
- "One quality important to you in parents/program staff/teachers/therapists/adults."

AFFECT-FOCUSED ICEBREAKER SAMPLE PROMPTS

Name . . .

- "Something that you really love to do."
- "Something that relaxes you."
- "Something that you like to do when you're mellow."
- "Something that you like to do when you're really excited."
- "Someone you like to talk to when you're annoyed."
- "Something that makes you really frustrated."
- "Something that you're proud of."
- "Something that you think is scary."
- "Something that puts you in a good mood."
- "Something that puts you in a bad mood."
- "Something that you like to do when you want to think."
- "Something that you like to do when you don't want to think."
- "Something that brings your energy down."
- "Something that brings your energy up."
- "A way that other people could tell if you were really happy."
- "A way that other people could tell if you were really angry or upset."
- "A way that other people might know you wanted to be left alone."
- "A way that other people might know you wanted company."

Sample Group Session

Session 5: Learning about the Connection between Behavior, Feelings, and Energy

GOALS

1. To practice advanced affect identification skills: connecting behavior to affect and energy states
2. To continue practicing self-appraisal and affect modulation
3. To continue to work on self-development skills

MATERIALS

Paper "leaves"

Markers

Lunch bags

Different objects/materials for guessing game (one for each group member)

"Going on a Vacation" script

OVERVIEW

1. Review program rules and group expectations.
2. Opening modulation activity: "Guess what's in the bag using your sense of touch."
3. Process the opening check-in; invite each member to share his or her experience (energy check-in).
4. Group members fill out their identity leaf.
5. The group facilitators lead discussion and worksheet activity that focuses on the connections between affect and behavior and energy, building on previous group activities.
6. Closing mindfulness activity: Conduct relaxation exercise using imagery ("Going on a Vacation" script).
7. Process the closing check-in; invite each member to share his or her experience (energy check-in).

GROUP ACTIVITIES

Opening Circle: The facilitator leads the opening energy check-in by asking each group member to identify the level of arousal that he or she is currently experiencing: *high*, *medium*, or *low*. Group members are also asked to determine whether their energy is *comfortable* or *uncomfortable*.

Opening Modulation Activity: Following the initial energy check-in, the facilitator leads the opening modulation activity, "Guess what's in the bag":

"We are going to practice using our sense of touch today to figure out what the item is that's in each of these bags. You are each going to have your own bag. Reach into the bag, without looking in it, and try to figure out what the object is that is in your bag. When you feel like you have figured it out, give the bag back to _____ [facilitator]. There is going to be a

(cont.)

time limit of 2 minutes. When finished, each of you is going to have a chance to share your guess with the group. The goal is to focus on the shape, texture, and weight of the object to determine what it is. Good luck."

The group facilitator repeats the opening energy check-in and observes and discusses any notable changes in energy following the modulation activity.

Competency Activity: The group facilitator leads this identity activity, Personal Leaves. (Leaves will be hung on the "All about Me Tree" in the group room.) The question for today's group is "Tell us about something that you are good at in school."

Self-Regulation Activity: The group facilitator leads a discussion about the connection between affect, energy, and behavior:

"Last week we talked about how feelings are very important because they help us learn many things about ourselves. We played a game to learn about how feelings are connected to the different kinds of behaviors that we all have. Today we are going to take it one step further. We have been teaching you about your energy since the very beginning of this group. The reason that we have been doing that is because our energy is connected to everything that we think or don't think about, say, feel, and do. Today we are going to go back to the behaviors that we talked about last week and we are going to connect those behaviors not only to feelings but also to the energy that we feel in our bodies."

Each group member is given a worksheet "Connections: Learning about Our Energy, Feelings, and Behavior." *See the worksheet below.*

Closing Circle: The group facilitator leads the closing mindfulness activity: relaxation using imagery (see "Going on a Vacation" script below), ending with a final energy check-in. Group facilitator observes and discusses any notable changes in energy.

The facilitator praises the members for their participation in the group and hands out the practice worksheet for homework.

(cont.)

Connections: Learning about Our Energy, Feelings, and Behavior

1. **Behavior:** Staying alone in my room

   ↑ High   → Medium   ↓ Low

   My energy feels: ☐ Comfortable   ☐ Uncomfortable

2. **Behavior:** Crying

   ↑ High   → Medium   ↓ Low

   My energy feels: ☐ Comfortable   ☐ Uncomfortable

3. **Behavior:** Hurting myself

   ↑ High   → Medium   ↓ Low

   My energy feels: ☐ Comfortable   ☐ Uncomfortable

4. **Behavior:** Yelling at other people

   ↑ High   → Medium   ↓ Low

   My energy feels: ☐ Comfortable   ☐ Uncomfortable

5. **Behavior:** Giving up on doing a good job in school

   ↑ High   → Medium   ↓ Low

   My energy feels: ☐ Comfortable   ☐ Uncomfortable

(cont.)

6. Behavior: Hitting or throwing things

↑ High   → Medium   ↓ Low

My energy feels: ☐ Comfortable   ☐ Uncomfortable

7. Behavior: Not wanting to go to bed because I think something bad might happen

↑ High   → Medium   ↓ Low

My energy feels: ☐ Comfortable   ☐ Uncomfortable

8. Behavior: Sharing with a peer

↑ High   → Medium   ↓ Low

My energy feels: ☐ Comfortable   ☐ Uncomfortable

9. Behavior: Trying to run away

↑ High   → Medium   ↓ Low

My energy feels: ☐ Comfortable   ☐ Uncomfortable

10. Behavior: Provoking other people so they get mad

↑ High   → Medium   ↓ Low

My energy feels: ☐ Comfortable   ☐ Uncomfortable

(cont.)

"Going on a Vacation" Script

Close your eyes and make yourself comfortable. We are going on a vacation, and this will require you to use your imagination and your senses to try and experience the trip.

Imagine yourself at the beach. You are barefoot walking on the sand. Notice the feeling of the soft, hot sand on your feet. Are your soles sensitive? Does the sand tickle? Can you feel the sand between your toes?

Look around to find a perfect spot on which to lay your towel. You spread out your towel and notice the color of the stripes—red, blue, green, and black. Look out at the ocean. Can you see the horizon? What color is the water? Is the surf calm or choppy? Notice the ocean breeze on your skin and the smell of the tide? Do you taste the ocean air?

Take out your sunscreen and begin to rub it on your skin. How does it feel? How does it smell? Does the fragrance remind you of anything?

Lie down and get your body comfortable in the sand. How does the sand feel under your back? Notice your body relaxing. How does the sun feel beating on your skin?

Listen to the surf hitting the shore and the sounds of nature around you.

Enjoy the peacefulness and quiet for a few minutes . . .

(cont.)

ARC Practice Sheet: Tracking Positive Behaviors and Energy

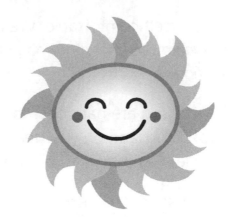

Name: _____ Date: _____

1. I participated in a group activity.

                                               _____
                                               (Staff check-off and initial)

2. I gave someone a compliment.

                                               _____
                                               (Staff check-off and initial)

3. I gave myself a compliment.

                                               _____
                                               (Staff check-off and initial)

4. I encouraged someone to do well.

                                               _____
                                               (Staff check-off and initial)

5. I helped someone out with
   chores or something else.

                                               _____
                                               (Staff check-off and initial)

APPENDIX D

Youth Educational Handouts and Worksheets

Giving Others Compliments

- This worksheet supports positive interactions with others (Affect Expression) by helping a child identify/describe positive attributes of others. This worksheet may be particularly useful in a group context.

Giving Myself Compliments

- This worksheet supports positive esteem/efficacy (Self and Identity) by helping a child identify positive self-attributes.

What Has Influenced My Identity?

- This worksheet should be used in conjunction with the "Influences on Self" group or individual activity described in Appendix C. This worksheet and associated activity support a child in exploring influences on identity (Self and Identity—Unique Self).

Identity Shields

- This worksheet provides templates for completion of identity shields (Self and Identity—Coherent Self).

About My Feelings

Name: _____ Date: _____

Please come up with examples of times when you have felt the following emotions during the week and why. Notice what was happening in your body and what was going on around you.

This week, I felt <u>happy</u> when . . .

_____
_____
_____
_____

This week, I felt <u>mad</u> when . . .

_____
_____
_____
_____

This week, I felt <u>sad</u> when . . .

_____
_____
_____
_____

This week, I felt <u>worried</u> when . . .

_____
_____
_____
_____

This week, I felt <u>scared</u> when . . .

_____
_____
_____
_____

What Are They Feeling?

Name: _____ Date: _____

Please look in magazines and find one picture of a person. Name all the possible emotions that you think this person/character is feeling.

Place your picture here:

Possible emotions that this person/character is feeling:

1. _____

2. _____

3. _____

4. _____

5. _____

Tuning In to Feelings

Name: _____ Date: _____

Name of Emotion: _____

Rate the intensity of this feeling on the following scale:

_____

| -1 | 0 | 1 | 2 | 3 | 4 | 5 | 6 | 7 | 8 | 9 | 10 |

Shut   Low Energy/   Moderate Energy   High Energy/
Down   Calm   Intense Emotion

Did you like the feeling or not?   Why?

_____

_____

_____

_____

_____

What was going on at the time? What do you think led to this feeling?

_____

_____

_____

_____

_____

_____

_____

Where Do I Feel . . . ?

Name: _____ Date: _____

Key:

Happy ☐
Sad ☐
Angry ☐
Worried ☐
Scared ☐
Excited ☐
Frustrated ☐
Proud ☐
_____ ☐

Where Do I Feel . . . ?

Name: _____   Date: _____

Key:

Happy ☐
Sad ☐
Angry ☐
Worried ☐
Scared ☐
Excited ☐
Frustrated ☐
Proud ☐
_____ ☐

Noticing My Feelings

Name: _____ Date: _____

In order to cope with our feelings, we first must be aware of *what* we are feeling. This week, pick one feeling each day and complete the feelings log.

Day 1: Feeling: _____

When I felt it (what was happening?): _____

_____

Rate the intensity: –1----0-------------5--------------10

Where in your body was the feeling held? _____

_____

Day 2: Feeling: _____

When I felt it (what was happening?): _____

_____

Rate the intensity: –1----0-------------5--------------10

Where in your body was the feeling held? _____

_____

Day 3: Feeling: _____

When I felt it (what was happening?): _____

_____

Rate the intensity: –1----0-------------5--------------10

Where in your body was the feeling held? _____

_____

(cont.)

Day 4: Feeling: _____

When I felt it (what was happening?): _____

_____

Rate the intensity: –1----0-------------5-------------10

Where in your body was the feeling held? _____

_____

Day 5: Feeling: _____

When I felt it (what was happening?): _____

_____

Rate the intensity: –1----0-------------5-------------10

Where in your body was the feeling held? _____

_____

Day 6: Feeling: _____

When I felt it (what was happening?): _____

_____

Rate the intensity: –1----0-------------5-------------10

Where in your body was the feeling held? _____

_____

Day 7: Feeling: _____

When I felt it (what was happening?): _____

_____

Rate the intensity: –1----0-------------5-------------10

Where in your body was the feeling held? _____

_____

The Body's Alarm System

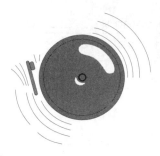

We all have a built-in alarm system that signals us when we might be in danger. One reason why human beings have been able to survive over time is because our brain recognizes signals around us that tell us danger might be coming. This helps our bodies prepare to deal with danger when it comes.

THE HUMAN DANGER RESPONSE

When our brain recognizes danger, it prepares our body to deal with it. We have three major ways to deal with something dangerous: We can **fight** it, we can get away from it (**flight**), or we can **freeze**.

What we pick to do sometimes depends on the kind of danger. So, for example, if a really small squirrel is attacking you, you might fight it, because you're bigger and stronger than it is. If a car comes speeding at you, and you're standing in the street, you'd probably run, because you can't really fight it, and if you stand still, you'll get hit. If you saw a big bear or some other animal nearby, you might freeze, because you can't really fight it, and you're probably not fast enough to run away.

OUR BODY GIVES US THE FUEL/ENERGY THAT WE NEED TO SURVIVE

When it's time for our body to **fight**, or **run**, or **freeze**, we need a lot of energy to do those things. So, when the brain recognizes danger, its "action" or "doing" part sends a signal to our body to release a bunch of chemicals, like fuel for a car. Those chemicals give us the energy that we need to cope with the danger.

THE OVERACTIVE ALARM

When the danger signal goes off, the "thinking" part of our brain checks out what is going on around us. If it is a false alarm, and there is no real danger,

(cont.)

the "thinking brain" shuts off the alarm, and we can keep doing whatever we were doing. If there is danger, the "doing brain" takes over and gives the body fuel to deal with whatever is going on.

Sometimes, though, the danger alarm goes off too much. That usually happens when kids have had lots of dangerous things happen—like their parents hurting them, or someone touching them when they didn't want it, or someone yelling or fighting a lot. For kids who have had to deal with danger a lot, the "thinking brain" has gotten tired of checking things out and just assumes that the signals mean more danger. So now, when the alarm goes off, the "thinking brain" stays out of the way and lets the "doing brain" take over.

FALSE ALARMS

False alarms can happen when we hear, or see, or feel something that reminds us of bad things that used to happen. Those reminders are called "triggers." Our brain has learned to recognize those reminders because in the past when they were around, dangerous things happened, and we had to react pretty quickly.

Different people have different reminders. So, if someone got yelled at a lot, hearing people yell might activate the alarm and make the "doing" part of the brain turn on. If someone didn't have enough attention paid to them when they were little, feeling all alone or scared might turn on the alarm.

WHAT HAPPENS WHEN THE ALARM GOES OFF?

Once our alarm turns on, our brain preps our body for action. When that happens, our body fills with "fuel" to prepare us for dealing with danger. This is really important if it's real danger (like a bear, or a speeding car, or a really mean squirrel), but not so helpful if it's a false alarm, and there isn't really any danger around. Imagine if you were in math class and something felt dangerous—suddenly, your body is filled with fuel.

Remember that the fuel gives us the energy to fight, or get away, or freeze. When our body has all that energy, we have to do something.

(cont.)

So—some kids suddenly feel really angry or want to argue or fight with someone. Some kids just feel antsy or jumpy. Some kids want to hide in a corner or get as far away as they can—and sometimes they don't even know why. Other kids will suddenly feel really shut down, like someone flipped a switch and turned them off. All of these are ways your body is trying to deal with something it thinks is dangerous.

Sometimes, though, what set off the alarm isn't really dangerous—it's just something that feels bad or reminds us of something bad that happens. When kids have a false alarm like that, it can be hard for other people to understand what just happened, and to help. Sometimes, kids even get into trouble.

RECOGNIZING TRIGGERS

It's important to learn about what kinds of reminders might feel dangerous to you and how your body reacts when those reminders are around. Everyone has different triggers and different ways to respond when the alarm goes off. If we know what sets off your alarm, and how you respond, we can get your thinking brain on board to help figure out when the danger is real and when it's a false alarm.

My Body's Alarm System

Name: _____ Date: _____

Please come up with one example of each of the ways that our bodies protect us from danger . . . fight, flight, and freeze.

<u>Fight Response:</u>

Example: A squirrel jumps out of the trash can as you are walking to school. You jump and scream at the squirrel. <u>(high energy—fight)</u>

1. Your Personal Fight Response Example:

_____

_____

_____

_____

_____

<u>Flight Response:</u>

Example: A car speeds toward you as you cross the street. You quickly run back to the sidewalk away from the car. <u>(flight)</u>

1. Your Personal Flight Response Example:

_____

_____

_____

_____

_____

(cont.)

Freeze Response:

Example: A bear suddenly appears while you are out on a walk in the woods. You know that the bear is much bigger, stronger, and faster than you, so you stand perfectly still and quiet so the bear goes away and doesn't chase you. (freeze)

1. Your Personal Freeze Response Example:

_____

_____

_____

_____

_____

My False Alarm Goes Off When . . .

Name: _____ Date: _____

Trigger	Reminds Me of . . .
1. Hearing people yell in loud tone of voice	Times when I was yelled at a lot
2. Feeling alone or being ignored	Times when I did not get enough attention when I was little
3. Smell of smoke	A bad fire

4. _____

_____

_____

5. _____

_____

_____

6. _____

_____

_____

7. _____

_____

_____

8. _____

_____

_____

Identifying Triggers

Name: _____ Date: _____

Trigger: <u>Something that sets off our brain's alarm system and kick-starts our survival strategies: fighting, fleeing, or freezing.</u> Notice your triggers. Pay attention to a time this week (or recently) when you were triggered.

What was the situation? What do you think triggered you?

_____

What was your response? Describe as many as you can:

Body: _____

Thoughts: _____

Feelings: _____

Behavior: _____

Was this a fight, flight, or freeze response? _____

Rate the intensity of your arousal:

-1	0	1	2	3	4	5	6	7	8	9	10
Shut Down		Low Energy/ Calm			Moderate Energy				High Energy/ Intense Emotion		

How did you cope with the situation or the feeling?

_____

_____

_____

_____

My Nonverbal Cues

Name: _____ Date: _____

Please come up with examples of how people would know that you were _____

_____.

(Pick a feeling.)

When I'm _____, my face might look like this . . .

_____

_____

_____

When I'm _____, my body might look like this . . .

_____

_____

_____

When I'm _____, my voice might sound like . . .

_____

_____

_____

When I'm _____, people might notice that I do
this behavior . . .

_____

_____

_____

Emotional Intensity Meter

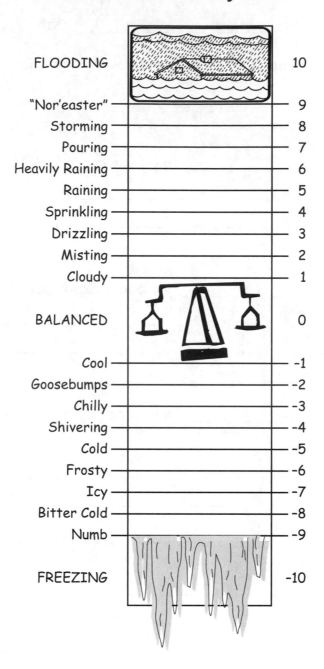

FLOODING	10
"Nor'easter"	9
Storming	8
Pouring	7
Heavily Raining	6
Raining	5
Sprinkling	4
Drizzling	3
Misting	2
Cloudy	1
BALANCED	0
Cool	-1
Goosebumps	-2
Chilly	-3
Shivering	-4
Cold	-5
Frosty	-6
Icy	-7
Bitter Cold	-8
Numb	-9
FREEZING	-10

Checking My Pulse

Name: _____ Date: _____

My resting heart rate is _____ beats per minute.

After exercise my heart rate is _____ beats per minute.

After taking deep breaths my heart rate is _____ beats per minute.

Plot it! On the chart below, color in your heart rate.

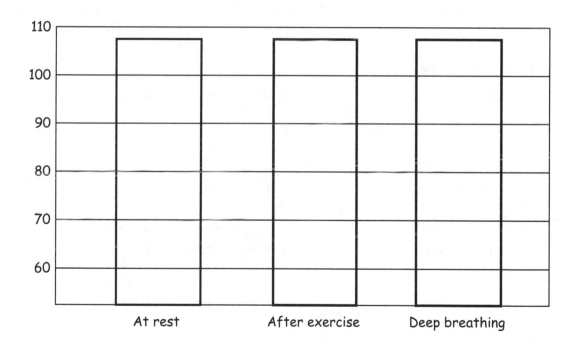

Tracking My Energy

Name: _____ Date: _____

Physical activities can help you cope with emotions and manage energy. Some physical activities <u>increase</u> your body's arousal level, and some <u>decrease</u> it; all of us respond in different ways. We will be exploring different activities and their effect on your arousal—your energy level. Track your response on this sheet.

<u>Start Point:</u> How do you feel right now? What are you noticing in your body? Jot a few notes: _____

_____

_____

Rate your energy level right now on the following scale:

-1	0	1	2	3	4	5	6	7	8	9	10

Shut   Low Energy/   Moderate   High Energy/
Down   Calm   Energy   Intense Emotion

<u>Activity 1:</u> Activity: _____

Starting arousal level: _____ Ending arousal level: _____

Reactions: _____

_____

_____

<u>Activity 2:</u> Activity: _____

Starting arousal level: _____ Ending arousal level: _____

Reactions: _____

_____

_____

(cont.)

Activity 3:   Activity: _____

Starting arousal level: _____ Ending arousal level: _____

Reactions: _____

_____

_____

Activity 4:   Activity: _____

Starting arousal level: _____ Ending arousal level: _____

Reactions: _____

_____

_____

Activity 5:   Activity: _____

Starting arousal level: _____ Ending arousal level: _____

Reactions: _____

_____

_____

Activity 6:   Activity: _____

Starting arousal level: _____ Ending arousal level: _____

Reactions: _____

_____

_____

Bringing Down My Energy

Name: _____   Date: _____

Please practice your coping skills at least one time before our next meeting <u>when you are calm</u> to practice ways to bring down your energy.

You may want to try things like . . .
- Putting a weighted blanket or weights on your shoulders or lap
- Listening to soft, calming music
- Looking at pictures of sand and stones and concentrating on the details
- Squeezing a stress ball or tightening and relaxing your muscles
- Belly breathing

This week I practiced . . .

_____

_____

_____

_____

_____ to bring down my energy.

This is how I knew that my energy changed from higher to lower:

_____

_____

_____

_____

_____

_____

I practiced this skill with . . .

_____   _____
Name   Caregiver (date)

Circles of Trust

Name: _____ Date: _____

Think about all of the different people in your life. Map out how close they
are to you.

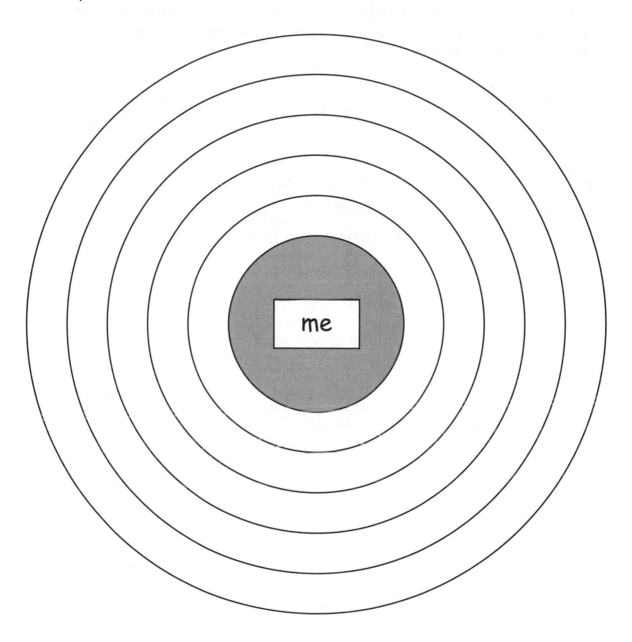

Starting a Conversation

Name: _____ Date: _____

Practice starting a conversation with someone (pick who: _____)
about how you're feeling. Let _____ know ahead of time how you
will let him or her know that you'd like to talk (for example, by using a
hand signal, door sign, words, other?). Practice this at least one time
before our next meeting.

I practiced this with _____ (name of person)
on _____ (date/time).

Remember . . .

Comfortable state (How does your body feel?)

Effective state (Are you in control?)

Good time (What's a good and not-so-good time?)

Right person (Who can meet your needs?)

Communication style (How can you be an effective communicator?)

How did it go?

_____

_____

_____

_____

_____

_____

_____

_____

_____

_____

_____

Giving Others Compliments

Name: _____ Date: _____

One thing that I like about _____ is _____

_____

_____

One thing that I like about _____ is _____

_____

_____

One thing that I like about _____ is _____

_____

_____

One thing that I like about _____ is _____

_____

_____

One thing that I like about _____ is _____

_____

_____

One thing that I like about _____ is _____

_____

_____

One thing that I like about _____ is _____

_____

_____

Giving Myself Compliments

Name: _____ Date: _____

In school I'm really good at _____

_____

_____

_____

I'm really good at playing _____

_____

_____

_____ when I have free time.

I show that I'm a good friend to others by _____

_____

_____

_____

_____

One thing that I really like about myself is _____

_____

_____

_____

_____

_____

What Has Influenced My Identity?

Name: _____ Date: _____

Directions: All of us are influenced by many different things. Below are some examples of things that might influence who you are. Pick six things that you think have had the <u>most</u> influence on you and list them. Assign a different color to each thing on your list (e.g., "family" might be <u>red</u>; "peers," <u>purple</u>). Using those colors, create a sculpture (using colored Play-Doh, modeling clay, or similar) or some other art project (such as a painting, drawing, or tissue-color collage) to represent some of the influences on your identity.

<u>Possible Influences:</u>

- Family
- Neighborhood
- Peers
- Religion
- Cultural background
- Role models

- Music
- Media
- School
- Life experiences
- Other?

Your top six influences:

1.

2.

3.

4.

5.

6.

Color Code:

1.

2.

3.

4.

5.

6.

Negative Quality of Influence

Positive Quality of Influence

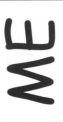

In the box write the name of a person you know who has influenced you in some way.

On the line next to the box, write the quality he/she has that has influenced you.

For instance, one person might write "Grandma" in one of the left-side boxes, and on the line next to it, write "caring," because her caring was a positive influence. Someone else might write "my cousin" on the right side and put "hard to trust" on the line, because it always felt like the cousin couldn't be counted on.

Identity Shields

<u>Directions:</u> All of us have many different qualities—for instance, different parts of our personality, different ways we behave with various people, and things we keep on the inside and things we show on the outside. Use the shield below to create your own personal crest, or identity shield. In each section, draw or write something that symbolizes a different part of who you are.

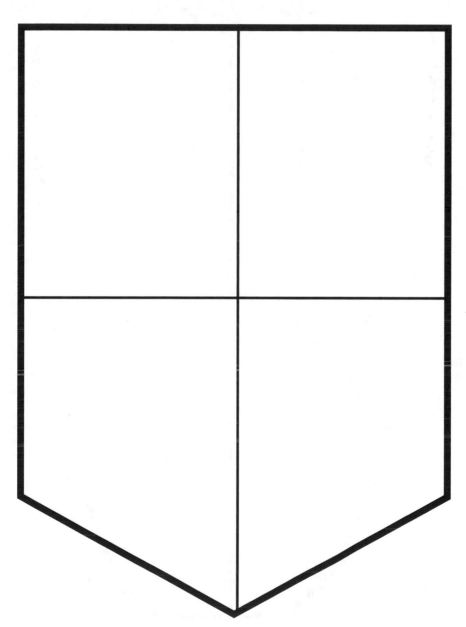

Identity Shields

<u>Directions:</u> All of us have many different qualities—for instance, different parts of our personality, different ways we behave with various people, and things we keep on the inside and things we show on the outside. Use the shield below to create your own personal crest, or identity shield. In each section, draw or write something that symbolizes a different part of who you are.

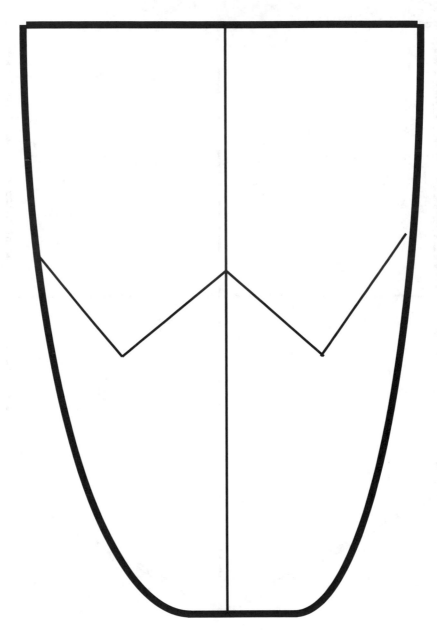

Milieu–Systems Materials

Staff Self-Care Plan

Name: _____ Date: _____

Two **in-the-moment strategies** (e.g., counting to 10, taking three deep breaths, reciting my ABC's) that I will practice when dealing with challenging youth behaviors are:

1. _____

_____

2. _____

_____

Two **long-term strategies** (e.g., getting together with friends, doing something I enjoy) that I will practice upon leaving work are:

1. _____

_____

2. _____

_____

_____   _____
Staff Signature/date of review   Supervisor Signature/date

Sensory Toolbox Guidelines

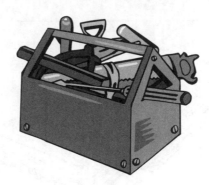

1. Youth should be *supervised* at all times when using tools in the cart/box.

2. Staff person should begin intervention with a *quick energy check-in* prior to selecting a tool: "Where is your energy at right now—high, medium, or low?"

3. Staff person should guide discussion about changing energy: "Do we want your energy to change by getting lower or higher?"

4. Staff person should provide choices and suggestions about tools to try and frame the exercise as an *experiment*.

5. Staff person should engage in each selected activity with the youth for a specified period of time.

6. Following each activity staff person should *repeat the energy check-in*.

7. When staff person and youth agree that "tool time" is finished, youth should *return the sensory tool directly to the staff person* who is leading this intervention.

Note: This process can be used with additional activity-based strategies such as taking walks, playing basketball, doing art, etc.

Taking a Break

Name of Student: _____ Date: _____

Procedure: This form should be completed by staff in discussion with student when a **break or time-out** from the group has been earned due to minor behaviors, such as being disrespectful or failure to follow directions.

I understand that I earned a break because I was:

_____

_____

I think that I was feeling:　　Happy　　Sad　　Mad　　Worried　　Other _____

(circle all that apply) when I earned a break.

Happy　　　　　　　　Sad　　　　　　　　　　Mad　　　　　　Worried

I earned a break from the group because I was not fully in control of my emotions/behavior. I can learn about how much control I have right now by checking the following:
(Use these questions as a guide to help assess student's experience in the moment.)

_____ Where's my energy level?　　Low　　Medium　　High

_____ How does my body feel? Breathing (fast or slow); heartbeat (fast or slow); muscles (tense like uncooked spaghetti or loose like cooked spaghetti) _____

_____ What am I thinking right now? _____

_____ What am I feeling right now? _____

_____ What are my triggers right now? _____

On a scale of 1 to 5, my self-control is:

1--------------------------2--------------------------3--------------------------4--------------------------5
No control　　　　Little control　　　　Not sure　　　　Okay control　　　　Good control

(Give examples of no control and good control: an engine overheating and exploding versus an engine that is running smoothly; a train running off the tracks versus a train running at a comfortable speed for its passengers.)

(cont.)

Staff will know I am in control when I am able to:

_____ Stay in the designated break area until staff gives me permission to leave.

_____ Talk with staff in a safe, respectful way.

_____ Focus on myself, not my peers.

_____ Listen to staff.

_____ Follow staff directions.

_____ Practice a sensory skill of my choice right now *(for at least 1 minute and make note of which skill used)*.

_____ Join routines when staff and I agree I am ready.

_____ Other _____

How will I show staff I am ready to join community routines? _____

_____

_____

_____

I would like staff to help me stay on track by *(try to encourage student input here and note any observations you think are important; consider check-ins, reminders, play a game during quiet time, etc.)*:

_____

_____

_____

When I return to the community, I will do the following in order to help myself stay on track:

_____

_____

_____

Follow up with supervisor/clinician to review student response to this discussion and finalize any decisions regarding repair work, safety agreement, or precaution status.

_____

Staff member/date and time

Processing Form

Name of student: _____

"How Do I Know When I Am in Control
and Ready to Be Part of the Community Again?"

Procedure: This form should be completed by staff in discussion with student when a consequence or time-out has been earned. It should be completed away from the group.

I understand that I earned a consequence/time-out because I was:

_____

_____

_____

This is what happened right before I earned a consequence (*check all that apply*):

_____ Someone said something to me.

_____ I was asked to do something I did not want to do.

_____ Something happened that scared me.

_____ I could not do something that I wanted to do.

_____ I heard bad news.

_____ I was feeling something I did not like.

_____ I was thinking about something I DO LIKE to think about.

_____ My body felt uncomfortable.

_____ I was thinking about something I DO NOT LIKE to think about.

_____ I had an unpleasant memory.

_____ I felt unsafe (because) _____

_____ Other _____

I think that I was feeling: Happy   Sad   Mad   Worried

Other _____ (*circle all that apply*) when I earned a consequence.

| Happy | Sad | Mad | Worried |

(cont.)

I earned a consequence because I was not fully in control of my emotions/behavior. I can learn about how much control I have right now by checking the following:
(Use these questions as a guide to help assess youth's experience in the moment. Responses to all questions are not necessary, but the more information you get, the better able we are to assess readiness for reentry into the program/community.)

_____ Where's my energy level?   Low   Medium   High

_____ How does my body feel? Breathing (fast or slow); heartbeat (fast or slow); muscles (tense like uncooked spaghetti or loose like cooked spaghetti)

_____

_____ What am I thinking right now?   _____

_____ What am I feeling right now?   _____

_____ What are my triggers right now?   _____

On a scale of 1 to 5, my self-control is:

1----------------------------2----------------------------3----------------------------4----------------------------5

No control   Little control   Not sure   Okay control   Good control

Give examples of no control and good control: an engine overheating and exploding versus an engine that is running smoothly; a train running off the tracks versus a train running at a comfortable speed for its passengers.

Staff will know I am in control when I am able to:

_____ Stay in the designated break area until staff gives me permission to leave.

_____ Talk with staff in a safe, respectful way.

_____ Focus on myself, not my peers.

_____ Listen to staff.

_____ Follow staff directions.

_____ Accept my consequence *(if appropriate)*.

_____ Agree to and follow a safety plan *(if I need or have one)*.

_____ Practice a sensory skill or use a sensory tool of my choice right now *(for at least 1 minute and make note of which skill used)*.

_____ Join routines when staff and I agree I am ready.

_____ Other

How will I show staff I am ready to join community routines?

_____

_____

_____

(cont.)

344

I would like staff to help me stay on track by *(try to encourage youth input here and note any observations you think are important; consider check-ins, reminders, play a game during quiet time, etc.)*:

_____

_____

_____

When I return to the community, I will do the following in order to help myself stay on track:

_____

_____

_____

Follow up with supervisor/clinician to review student response to this discussion and finalize any decisions regarding repair work, safety agreement, or precaution status.

_____

Staff member/date and time

Youth Processing Packet

Becoming a "Feelings Detective" by Completing My Processing Packet

Understanding the Link between My Energy, Feelings, Behaviors, and Thoughts

Name _____

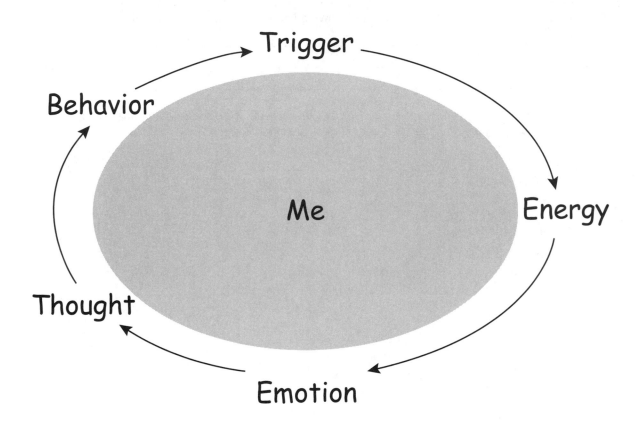

(cont.)

This Happened Right Before I Earned a Consequence/Time-Out

Please check off all of the things that happened right before you earned a consequence:

_____ Someone said something to me.

_____ I was asked to do something I did not want to do.

_____ Something happened that scared me.

_____ I could not do something that I wanted to do.

_____ I heard bad news.

_____ I was feeling something I did not like.

_____ I was thinking about something I DO LIKE to think about.

_____ My body felt uncomfortable.

_____ I was thinking about something I DO NOT LIKE to think about.

_____ I had an unpleasant memory

_____ I felt unsafe (because) _____

_____ Other _____

(cont.)

The Body's Alarm System (for staff to teach or remind students)

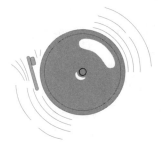

We all have a built-in alarm system that signals us when we might be in danger. One reason why human beings have been able to survive over time is because our brain recognizes signals around us that tell us danger might be coming. This helps our bodies prepare to deal with danger when it comes.

FALSE ALARMS

- False alarms can happen when we hear, or see, or feel something that reminds us of bad things that used to happen. Those reminders are called "triggers."
- Different people have different reminders. Reminders can be people, places, smells, sounds, touch, taste, certain emotions, etc.

WHAT HAPPENS WHEN THE ALARM GOES OFF?

- Once our alarm goes off, our brain preps our body for action. When that happens, our body fills with "fuel" to prepare us for dealing with danger, and this fuel feels like energy in our body.
- The fuel gives us the energy to fight, or **get away**, or freeze. When our body has all that energy, we have to do something.
  - So—some kids will suddenly feel really angry or want to argue or fight with someone. Some kids just feel antsy or jumpy.
  - Some kids want to hide in a corner or get as far away as they can—and sometimes they don't even know why.
  - Other kids will suddenly feel really shut down, like someone flipped a switch and turned them off.
- All of these are ways your body is trying to deal with something that it thinks is dangerous.

(cont.)

My False Alarm Goes Off When . . .

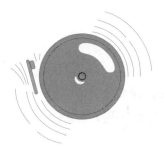

Please think about and have <u>staff</u> write down anything that might have happened before you earned a consequence/time-out that could have reminded you of something bad, sad, or scary that happened to you <u>before</u> you came to this program. It's important to learn about what kinds of reminders might feel dangerous to you and how your body reacts when those reminders are around.

False Alarm or Trigger

Reminds Me of . . .

1. Hearing people yell, loud tone of voice

Times when I was yelled at a lot.

<u>When I think about this now I feel:</u>

Happy   Sad   Scared/Worried   Angry   Other

2. Feeling alone, being ignored

Times when I did not get enough attention when I was little.

<u>When I think about this now I feel:</u>

Happy   Sad   Scared/Worried   Angry   Other

Staff Reminder: When learning about student triggers, please respond by validating what you hear and referring any further detail to therapy. "It makes sense that you feel _____ now or that you react by _____ when _____ happened because you've been through some really hard things. We can't talk a lot about your past now but if it's okay with you, I'd like to let your therapist know that we talked about this today so that you can follow up with her or him."

(cont.)

When my alarm went off, my energy was (please circle):

High   Medium   Low

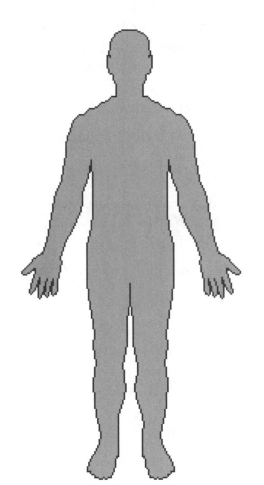

I know that my energy was
_____ **because my body <u>clues</u> were:**

Breathing (please check):

Fast   Medium   Slow

Heartbeat: (please check):
Fast   Medium   Slow

Muscles (please check):

Tense like uncooked spaghetti

Relaxed like cooked spaghetti

Body Temperature: Hot   Warm   Cold

Other Body Clues: _____

(cont.)

When my alarm went off and I was triggered, I felt (please circle all that apply):

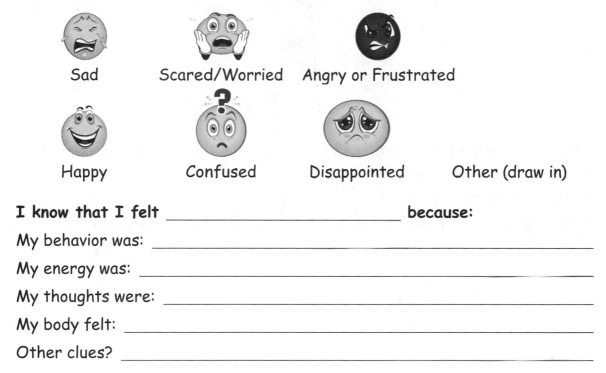

Sad   Scared/Worried   Angry or Frustrated

Happy   Confused   Disappointed   Other (draw in)

I know that I felt _____ **because:**

My behavior was: _____

My energy was: _____

My thoughts were: _____

My body felt: _____

Other clues? _____

(cont.)

Noticing My Behavior Clues

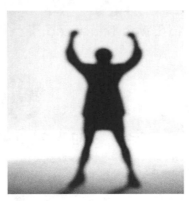

These are the behaviors that show me and others that I was triggered or very upset (circle all that apply):

- Asking to talk to staff
- Asking to go to the nurse because of a stomachache, headache, etc.
- Not following staff directions
- Going to my room to be alone
- Yelling at a staff person
- Yelling at another student
- Trying to break something
- Trying to hurt myself
- Trying to hurt someone else

Other "clue behaviors" that tell me and others that I am triggered or very upset (staff should list):

1. _____

2. _____

(cont.)

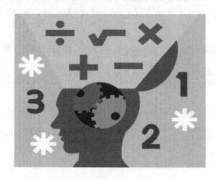

These are the thoughts that show me and others that I am triggered or very upset (circle all that apply):

- Thinking that staff is mean or out to get me
- Thinking that students are mean or out to get me
- Thinking something negative about myself, like that I am bad or stupid
- Thinking that nobody cares about me
- Thinking that things will never get better
- Thinking about hurting myself
- Thinking about hurting someone else
- Thinking about running away

Other "clue thoughts" that tell me and others that I am triggered or very upset (staff should list):

1. _____

2. _____

(cont.)

353

***What Tools Can I Use to Stay in Control and Get What I Need
When I Am Triggered or Very Upset?***

1. The next time that I become triggered or upset, my goal is to _____

_____

_____

   instead of doing something that is hurtful to myself or others or that
   leads to a consequence.

2. When _____ happens the next time, I will try to
   do something to get into my "comfort zone" before I do anything else.

   When _____ happens and my energy is high/low,
   then I will try to practice _____

   _____

   _____ from the list(s) below:

Remember: YOU have the power to change what you feel! When your energy
is HIGH or Medium HIGH and uncomfortable and your feelings are big, start
with one of these TOOLS and then try one from the LOW-energy list.

- Walk around the building one time with staff permission.
- Use the balance board.
- Play catch with someone.
- Play catch by yourself.
- Run in place.
- Do 10 jumping jacks.
- Do 10 push-ups (challenge staff to do more!).
- Dance.
- Sing a song.
- Squeeze a stress ball as hard as you can.
- Hold a weighted ball.
- Try out the body sack.
- Or . . . think of some other ways to MOVE YOUR BODY!

(cont.)

When your energy is LOW or Medium LOW and uncomfortable, and you need to wake up your mind and body, start with one of these TOOLS and then try one other tool from the HIGH-energy list.

- Listen to <u>quiet</u> music.
- Read a book.
- Sit down and play a quick game of cards.
- Blow Bubbles or just BREATHE slowly.
- Draw a picture.
- Write a poem or write in a journal.
- Balance the peacock feather.
- Squeeze a stuffed animal.
- Use the sensory belt.
- Use the weighted lap blanket.
- Play with a Koosh ball or some other sensory tool.
- Manipulate the Rubik's Cube or a puzzle.
- Talk to someone OR think of some other way to WAKE UP YOUR BODY.

3. When I'm triggered or upset, it helps me when staff . . .

_____

_____

_____

4. When I'm calm, I'm going to tell someone that I'm upset and that what I need to reach my goal is one or more of the following resources:

Identifying Resources: Choose the top three people whom you feel comfortable talking to:

1.

2.

3.

Using Your Resources:

a. Picking your moment: Please circle the best time to ask staff member for help:
- When another student is having a hard time.
- When he/she is talking to another student.

(cont.)

355

- ◆ When he/she is talking to another staff person.
- ◆ When he/she is asking you if you need a check-in.
- ◆ When he/she is not busy with something else.
- ◆ Other _____

b. Using My Skills to Get What I need:
- ◆ I will use a _____ tone of voice.
- ◆ The kinds of words that I will use will include:

_____

_____

_____

- ◆ The kinds of behavior that I will show will include: _____

_____

_____

_____

_____

_____

I will know that I have reached my goal when:

_____

_____

_____

_____

I know that I can reach my goal because (identify two positive things about yourself):

1. _____

2. _____

(cont.)

356

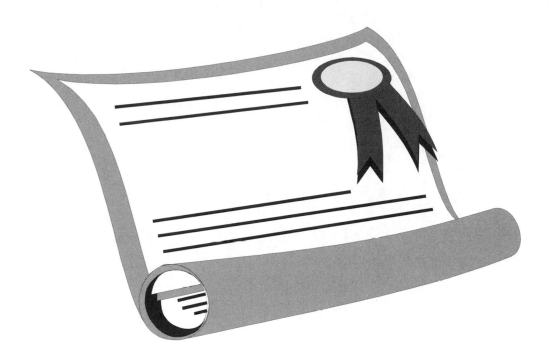

I reviewed my packet with _____ on _____.

_____   _____
Student Name (signature)   Caregiver signature and date

Additional Resources

There are many, many excellent authors, researchers, and practitioners who have made significant contributions to the field of traumatic stress, and who have influenced our own thinking and our practice. Although there are far too many for us to be able to provide a comprehensive list here, we include below some of those who have most influenced us. Some are specifically referenced within this text, while others, though not directly referenced, have impacted our thinking about and approach toward the treatment of children who have experienced trauma. We are lucky enough to consider a number of the authors below to be both our colleagues and our teachers; and we are appreciative of the transmission of knowledge we have received from those we have not yet been fortunate enough to work with directly. We highly recommend these resources to other professionals.

Bloom, S. (1997). *Creating sanctuary: Toward the evolution of sane societies.* New York: Routledge.

Briere, J., & Lanktree, C. (2008). *Integrative treatment of complex trauma for adolescents (ITCT-A): A guide for the treatment of multiply traumatized youth.* Long Beach, CA: MCAVIC-USC, National Child Traumatic Stress Network.

Briere, J., & Scott, C. (2006). *Principles of trauma therapy: A guide to symptoms, evaluation, and treatment.* Thousand Oaks, CA: Sage.

Brom, D., Pat-Horenczyk, R., & Ford, J. (2009). *Treating traumatized children: Risk, resilience and recovery.* New York: Routledge.

Courtois, C. A., & Ford, J. D. (Eds.). (2009). *Treating complex traumatic stress disorders: An evidence-based guide.* New York: Guilford Press.

Damasio, A. (1999). *The feeling of what happens.* San Diego: Harcourt.

DeRosa, R., Habib, M., Pelcovitz, D., Rathus, J., Sonnenklar, J., Ford, J., et al. (2006). *Structured psychotherapy for adolescents responding to chronic stress.* Unpublished manual.

Ford, J. D., & Russo, E. (2006). Trauma-focused, present-centered, emotional self-regulation approach to integrated treatment for posttraumatic stress and addiction: Trauma Adaptive Recovery Group Education and Therapy (TARGET). *American Journal of Psychotherapy, 60,* 335–355.

Gil, E. (1991). *The healing power of play: Working with abused children.* New York: Guilford Press.

Herman, J. L. (1992). *Trauma and recovery.* New York: Basic Books.

Hughes, D. (2006). *Building the bonds of attachment: Awakening love in deeply troubled children.* Lanham, MD: Jason Aronson.

Hughes, D. (2007). *Attachment-focused family therapy.* New York: Norton.

James, B. (1989). *Treating traumatized children*. New York: Free Press.

James, B. (1994). *Handbook for treatment of attachment-trauma problems in children*. New York: Free Press.

Kagan, R. (2007a). *Real life heroes: A life storybook for children* (2nd ed.). Binghamton, NY: Haworth Press.

Kagan, R. (2007b). *Real life heroes: Practitioner's manual*. Binghamton, NY: Haworth Press.

Lieberman, A. F., & Van Horn, P. (2008). *Psychotherapy with infants and young children: Repairing the effects of stress and trauma on early attachment*. New York: Guilford Press.

Monahon, C. (1993). *Children and trauma: A guide for parents and professionals*. San Francisco: Jossey-Bass.

Perry, B., & Szalavitz, M. (2007). *The boy who was raised as a dog, and other stories from a child psychiatrist's notebook: What traumatized children can teach us about loss, love, and healing*. New York: Basic Books.

Putnam, F. W. (1997). *Dissociation in children and adolescents: A developmental perspective*. New York: Guilford Press.

Saxe, G. N., Ellis, B. H., & Kaplow, J. B. (2007). *Collaborative treatment of traumatized children and teens: The Trauma Systems Therapy approach*. New York: Guilford Press.

Schore, A. (1994). *Affect regulation and the origin of the self: The neurobiology of emotional development*. Hillsdale, NJ: Erlbaum.

Sunderland, M. (2006). *The science of parenting: Practical guidelines on sleep, crying, play, and building emotional well-being for life*. New York: Dorling Kindersley.

Terr, L. (1990). *Too scared to cry: Psychic trauma in childhood*. New York: HarperCollins.

van der Kolk, B. (1987). *Psychological trauma*. Washington, DC: American Psychiatric Press.

van der Kolk, B. A., McFarlane, A. C., & Weisaeth, L. (Eds.). (1996). *Traumatic stress: The effects of overwhelming experience on mind, body, and society*. New York: Guilford Press.

Webb, N. B. (Ed.). (2007). *Play therapy with children in crisis: Individual, group, and family treatment* (3rd ed.). New York: Guilford Press.

References

Abitz, M., Nielsen, R. D., Jones, E. G., Laursen, H., Graem, N., & Pakkenberg, B. (2007). Excess of neurons in the human newborn mediodorsal thalamus compared with that of the adult. *Cerebral Cortex, 17*(11), 2573–2578.

Alink, L., Cicchetti, D., Kim, J., & Rogosch, F. (2009). Mediating and moderating processes in the relation between maltreatment and psychopathology: Mother–child relationship quality and emotion regulation. *Journal of Abnormal Child Psychology, 37*(6), 831–843.

American Psychiatric Association. (2000). *Diagnostic and statistical manual of mental disorders* (4th ed., text rev.). Washington, DC: Author.

Anda, R. F., Croft, J. B., Felitti, V. J., Nordenberg, D., Giles, W. H., Williamson, D. F., et al. (1999). Adverse childhood experiences and smoking during adolescence and adulthood. *Journal of the American Medical Association, 282*(17), 1652–1658.

Anda, R. F., Felitti, V. J., Bremner, J. D., Walker, J. D., Whitfield, C., Perry, B. D., et al. (2006). The enduring effects of abuse and related adverse experiences in childhood: A convergence of evidence from neurobiology and epidemiology. *European Archives of Psychiatry and Clinical Neuroscience, 256*(3), 174–186.

Anthonysamy, A., & Zimmer-Gembeck, M. (2007). Peer status and behaviors of maltreated children and their classmates in the early years of school. *Child Abuse and Neglect, 31*(9), 971–991.

Appleyard, K., Egeland, B., van Dulmen, M., & Sroufe, A. (2005). When more is not better: The role of cumulative risk in child behavior outcomes. *Journal of Child Psychology and Psychiatry, 46*(3), 235–245.

Barnes, J., Noll, J., Putnam, F., & Trickett, P. (2009). Sexual and physical revictimization among victims of severe childhood sexual abuse. *Child Abuse and Neglect, 33,* 412–420.

Beers, S., & De Bellis, M. D. (2002). Neuropsychological function in children with maltreatment-related posttraumatic stress disorder. *American Journal of Psychiatry, 159,* 483–486.

Benoit, D., & Parker, K. (1994). Stability and transmission of attachment across three generations. *Child Development, 65*(5), 1444–1456.

Blaustein, M., & Kinniburgh, K. (2007). Intervening beyond the child: The intertwining nature of attachment and trauma. *British Psychological Society, Briefing Paper 26,* 48–53.

Bolger, K. E., Patterson, C. J., & Kupersmidt, J. B. (1998). Peer relationships and self-esteem among children who have been maltreated. *Child Development, 69*(4), 1171–1197.

Bremner, J. (1999). Does stress damage the brain? *Biological Psychiatry, 45,* 797–805.

Bremner, J. D., Randall, P., Scott, T. M., Capelli, S., Delaney, R., McCarthy, G., et al. (1995). Deficits in short-term memory in adult survivors of childhood abuse. *Psychiatry Research, 59,* 97–107.

Breslau, N. (2001). The epidemiology of posttraumatic stress disorder: What is the extent of the problem? *Journal of Clinical Psychiatry, 62*(17, Suppl.), 16–22.

Brock, K., Pearlman, L. A., & Varra, E. (2006). Child maltreatment, self capacities and trauma symptoms: Psychometric properties of the Inner Experience Questionnaire. *Journal of Emotional Abuse, 6*(1), 103–125.

Campbell-Sills, L., Cohan, S., & Stein, M. (2006). Relationship of resilience to personality, coping, and psychiatric symptoms in young adults. *Behaviour Research and Therapy, 44*, 585–599.

Centers for Disease Control and Prevention. (2005). Adverse childhood experience study: Prevalence of individual adverse childhood experiences. Retrieved July 10, 2008, from *www.cdc.gov/nccdphp/ ACE/prevalence.htm.*

Chandy, J. M., Blum, R. W., & Resnick, M. D. (1996). Female adolescents with a history of sexual abuse: Risk outcome and protective factors. *Journal of Interpersonal Violence, 11*(4), 503–518.

Cicchetti, D., & Curtis, W. J. (2007). Multilevel perspectives on pathways to resilient functioning. *Development and Psychopathology, 19*(3), 627–629.

Cicchetti, D., & Rogosch, F. (2009). Adaptive coping under conditions of extreme stress: Multilevel influences on the determinants of resilience in maltreated children. *New Directions in Child and Adolescent Development, 124*, 47–59.

Cicchetti, D., Rogosch, F. A., Lynch, M., & Holt, K. D. (1993). Resilience in maltreated children: Processes leading to adaptive outcome. *Development and Psychopathology, 5*, 629–647.

Cicchetti, D., Rogosch, F. A., & Toth, S. L. (2006). Fostering secure attachment in infants in maltreating families through preventive interventions. *Development and Psychopathology, 18*(3), 623–649.

Cicchetti, D., & Toth, S. (1995). A developmental psychopathology perspective on child abuse and neglect. *Journal of the American Academy of Child and Adolescent Psychiatry, 34*(5), 541–565.

Cicchetti, D., & Toth, S. (2005). Child maltreatment. *Annual Review of Clinical Psychology, 1*(1), 409–438.

Cohen, J. A., & Mannarino, A. P. (2000). Predictors of treatment outcome in sexually abused children. *Child Abuse and Neglect, 24*, 983–994.

Cohen, J. A., Mannarino, A. P., & Deblinger, E. (2006). *Treating trauma and traumatic grief in children and adolescents.* New York: Guilford Press.

Cook, A., Spinazzola, J., Ford, J. D., Lanktree, C., Blaustein, M., Cloitre, M., et al. (2005). Complex trauma in children and adolescents. *Psychiatric Annals, 35*(5), 390–398.

Coster, W., Gersten, M., Beeghly, M., & Cicchetti, D. (1989). Communicative functioning in maltreated toddlers. *Developmental Psychology, 25*(6), 1020–1029.

Crittenden, P. M. (1995). Attachment and psychopathology. In S. Goldberg, R. Muir, & J. Kerr (Eds.), *Attachment theory: Social, developmental, and clinical perspectives* (pp. 367–406). New York: Analytic Press.

Crittenden, P. M., & DiLalla, D. L. (1988). Compulsive compliance: The development of an inhibitory coping strategy in infancy. *Journal of Abnormal Child Psychology, 16*, 585–599.

Cross, T., Bazron, B., Dennis, K., & Isaacs, M. (1989). *Towards a culturally competent system of care* (Vol. I). Washington, DC: Georgetown University Child Development Center, CASSP Technical Assistance Center.

de Bellis, M. D. (2001). Developmental traumatology: The psychobiological development of maltreated children and its implications for research, treatment, and policy. *Development and Psychopathology, 13*, 539–564.

Dexheimer Pharris, M., Resnick, M. D., & Blum, R. W. (1997). Protecting against hopelessness and suicidality in sexually abused American Indian adolescents. *Journal of Adolescent Health, 21*(6), 400–406.

Dinero, R., Conger, R., Shaver, P., Widaman, K., & Larsen-Rife, D. (2008). Influence of family-of-origin and adult romantic partners on adult romantic attachment security. *Journal of Family Psychology, 22*(4), 622–632.

D'Zurilla, T., & Goldfried, M. (1971). Problem solving and behavior modification. *Journal of Abnormal Psychology, 78*, 107–126.

D'Zurilla, T., & Nezu, A. (2007). *Problem-solving therapy: A positive approach to clinical intervention* (3rd ed.). New York: Springer.

Egeland, B., Sroufe, A., & Erickson, M. (1983). The developmental consequences of different patterns of maltreatment. *Child Abuse and Neglect, 7*, 459–469.

Erickson, M. F., Sroufe, L. A., & Egeland, B. (1985). The relationship between quality of attachment and behavior problems in preschool in a high-risk sample. *Monographs of the Society for Research in Child Development, 50*(1–2, Serial No. 209), 147–166.

Felitti, V. J., Anda, R. F., Nordenberg, D. F., Williamson, D. F., Spitz, A. M., Edwards, V., et al. (1998). Relationship of childhood abuse and household dysfunction to many of the leading causes of death in adults: The Adverse Childhood Experiences (ACE) study. *American Journal of Preventative Medicine, 14*(4), 245–258.

Flores, E., Cicchetti, D., & Rogosch, F. (2005). Predictors of resilience in maltreated and nonmaltreated Latino children. *Developmental Psychology, 41*, 338–351.

Ford, J. (2005). Treatment implications of altered affect regulation and information processing following child maltreatment. *Psychiatric Annals, 35*(5), 410–419.

Ford, J., Racusin, R., Daviss, W. B., Ellis, C. G., Thomas, J., Rogers, K., et al. (1999). Trauma exposure among children with oppositional defiant disorder and attention deficit-hyperactivity disorder. *Journal of Consulting and Clinical Psychology, 67*, 786–789.

Ford, J., Stockton, P., Kaltman, S., & Green, B. (2006). Disorders of Extreme Stress (DESNOS) symptoms are associated with type and severity of interpersonal trauma exposure in a sample of healthy young women. *Journal of Interpersonal Violence, 21*(11), 1399–1416.

Fortier, M., DiLillo, D., Messman-Moore, T., Peugh, J., DeNardi, K., & Gaffey, K. (2009). Severity of child sexual abuse and revictimization: The mediating role of coping and trauma symptoms. *Psychology of Women Quarterly, 33*, 308–320.

George, C., & Main, M. (1979). Social interactions of young abused children: Approach, avoidance, and aggression. *Child Development, 50*, 306–318.

Gil, E. (1991). *The healing power of play: Working with abused children.* New York: Guilford Press.

Gil, E. (2006). *Helping abused and traumatized children: Integrating directive and nondirective approaches.* New York: Guilford Press.

Greenwald, R. (1999). *Eye movement desensitization and reprocessing (EMDR) in child and adolescent psychotherapy.* Northvale, NJ: Jason Aronson.

Guber, T., Kalish, L., & Fatus, S. (2005). *Yoga pretzels.* Cambridge, MA: Barefoot Books.

Haggerty, R., Sherrod, L., Garmezy, N., & Rutter, M. (1996). *Stress, risk, and resilience in children and adolescents: Processes, mechanisms, and interventions.* New York: Cambridge University Press.

Haugaard, J. (2004). Recognizing and treating uncommon behavioral and emotional disorders in children and adolescents who have been severely maltreated: Dissociative disorders. *Child Maltreatment, 9*, 146–153.

Hebert, M., Parent, N., Daignault, I., & Tourigny, M. (2006). A typological analysis of behavioral profiles of sexually abused children. *Child Maltreatment, 11*(3), 203–216.

Jaffee, S., Caspi, A., Moffitt, T., Polo-Tomás, M., & Taylor, A. (2007). Individual, family, and neighborhood factors distinguish resilient from non-resilient maltreated children: A cumulative stressors model. *Child Abuse and Neglect, 31*, 231–253.

Kagan, R. (2007a). *Real life heroes: A life storybook for children* (2nd ed.). Binghamton, NY: Haworth Press.

Kagan, R. (2007b). *Real life heroes: Practitioner's manual.* Binghamton, NY: Haworth Press.

Kazdin, A. (1985). *Treatment of antisocial behavior in children and adolescents.* Homewood, IL: Dorsey Press.

Kazdin, A., Esveldt-Dawson, K., French, N., & Unis, A. (1987). Problem-solving skills training and relationship therapy in the treatment of antisocial child behavior. *Journal of Consulting and Clinical Psychology, 55*, 76–85.

Kazdin, A., Siegel, T., & Bass, D. (1992). Cognitive problem-solving skills training and parent management training in the treatment of antisocial behavior in children. *Journal of Consulting and Clinical Psychology, 60*, 733–747.

Kelly, J. F., Morisset, C. E., Barnard, K. E., Hammond, M. A., & Booth, C. L. (1996). The influence of early mother–child interaction on preschool cognitive/linguistic outcomes in a high-social-risk group. *Infant Mental Health Journal, 17*, 310–321.

Kilpatrick, D., Ruggiero, K., Acierno, R., Saunders, B., Resnick, H., & Best, C. (2003). Violence and risk of PTSD, major depression, substance abuse/dependence, and comorbidity: Results from the National Survey of Adolescents. *Journal of Consulting and Clinical Psychology, 71*(4), 692–700.

Kim, J., & Cicchetti, D. (2003). Social self-efficacy and behavior problems in maltreated children. *Journal of Clinical Child and Adolescent Psychology, 32*(1), 106–117.

Kim, J., & Cicchetti, D. (2004). A longitudinal study of child maltreatment, mother–child relationship quality and maladjustment: The role of self-esteem and social competence. *Journal of Abnormal Child Psychology, 32*(4), 341–354.

Kim, J., & Cicchetti, D. (2006). Longitudinal trajectories of self-system processes and depressive symptoms among maltreated and nonmaltreated children. *Child Development, 77*(3), 624–639.

Kinniburgh, K., & Blaustein, M. (2005). *Attachment, self-regulation, and competency: A comprehensive framework for intervention with complexly traumatized youth. A treatment manual.* Unpublished manuscript.

Kinniburgh, K., Blaustein, M., Spinazzola, J., & van der Kolk, B. (2005). Attachment, self-regulation, and competency: A comprehensive intervention framework for children with complex trauma. *Psychiatric Annals, 35*(5), 424–430.

Lansford, J. E., Dodge, K. A., Pettit, G. S., Crozier, J., & Kaplow, J. (2002). A 12-year prospective study of the long-term effects of early child physical maltreatment on psychological, behavioral, and academic problems in adolescence. *Archives of Pediatrics and Adolescent Medicine, 156*, 824–830.

Lieberman, A. F., & van Horn, P. (2008). *Psychotherapy with infants and young children: Repairing the effects of stress and trauma on early attachment.* New York: Guilford Press.

Liem, J., & Boudewyn, A. (1999). Contextualizing the effects of childhood sexual abuse on adult self- and social functioning: An attachment theory perspective. *Child Abuse and Neglect, 23*, 1141–1157.

Linehan, M. M. (1993). *Skills training manual for treating borderline personality disorder.* New York: Guilford Press.

Lipschitz-Elhawi, R., & Itzhaky, H. (2005). Social support, mastery, self-esteem and individual adjustment among at-risk youth. *Child and Youth Care Forum, 34*(5), 329–346.

Lovett, J. (1999). *Small wonders: Healing childhood trauma with EMDR.* New York: Free Press.

Lynch, M., & Cicchetti, D. (1991). Patterns of relatedness in maltreated and nonmaltreated children: Connections among multiple representational models. *Development and Psychopathology, 3*, 207–226.

Lyons-Ruth, K., Dutra, L., Schuder, M., & Bianchi, I. (2006). From infant attachment disorganization to adult dissociation: Relational adaptations or traumatic experiences? *Psychiatric Clinics of North America, 29*, 63–86.

Lyons-Ruth, K., Yellin, C., Melnick, S., & Atwood, G. (2005). Expanding the concept of unresolved mental states: Hostile/Helpless states of mind on the Adult Attachment Interview are associated with disrupted mother–infant communication and infant disorganization. *Development and Psychopathology, 17*(1), 1–23.

Main, M., & Cassidy, J. (1988). Categories of response to reunion with the parent at age 6: Predicted from infant attachment classifications and stable over a 1-month period. *Developmental Psychology, 24*, 415–426.

Main, M., & Goldwyn, R. (1984). Predicting rejection of her infant from mother's representation of her own experience: Implications for the abused–abusing intergenerational cycle. *Child Abuse and Neglect, 8*, 203–217.

Masten, A. S. (2001). Ordinary magic: Resilience processes in development. *American Psychologist, 56*, 227–238.

Masten, A. S., Best, K. M., & Garmezy, N. (1990). Resilience and development: Contributions from the study of children who overcome adversity. *Development and Psychopathology, 2*(4), 425–444.

Masten, A. S., & Coatsworth, J. D. (1998). The development in competence in favorable and unfavorable environments. *American Psychologist, 53*(2), 205–220.

Matthews, W. (1999). Brief therapy: A problem-solving model of change. *The Counselor, 17*(4), 29–32.

McCann, I. L., & Pearlman, L. A. (1990). Vicarious traumatization: A framework for understanding the psychological effects of working with victims. *Journal of Traumatic Stress, 3,* 131–149.

McElwain, N., Cox, M., Burchinal, M., & Macfie, J. (2003). Differentiating among insecure mother–infant attachment classifications: A focus on child–friend interaction and exploration during solitary play at 36 months. *Attachment and Human Development, 5*(2), 136–164.

Mendez, J., Fantuzzo, J., & Cicchetti, D. (2002). Profiles of social competence among low-income African American preschool children. *Child Development, 73,* 1085–1100.

Mezzacappa, E., Kindlon, D., & Earls, F. (2001). Child abuse and performance task assessments of executive functions in boys. *Journal of Child Psychology and Psychiatry, 42*(8), 1041–1048.

Miller, A. L., Rathus, J. H., & Linchan, M. M. (2006). *Dialectical behavior therapy with suicidal adolescents.* New York: Guilford Press.

Min, M., Farkas, K., Minnes, S., & Singer, L. (2007). Impact of childhood abuse and neglect on substance abuse and psychological distress in adulthood. *Journal of Traumatic Stress, 20,* 833–844.

Mischel, W., Shoda, Y., & Rodriguez, M. L. (1989). Delay of gratification in children. *Science, 244,* 933–938.

Navalta, C., Polcari, A., Webster, D., Boghossian, A., & Teicher, M. (2006). Effects of childhood sexual abuse on neuropsychological and cognitive function in college women. *Journal of Neuropsychiatry and Clinical Neurosciences, 18,* 45–53.

Noll, J., Trickett, P., Harris, W., & Putnam, F. (2009). The cumulative burden borne by offspring whose mothers were sexually abused as children: Descriptive results from a multigenerational study. *Journal of Interpersonal Violence, 24*(3), 424–449.

Ogawa, J., Sroufe, A., Weinfield, N., Carlson, E., & Egeland, B. (1997). Development and the fragmented self: Longitudinal study of dissociative symptomatology in a nonclinical sample. *Development and Psychopathology, 9*(4), 855–879.

Ostby, Y., Tamnes, C. K., Fjell, A. M., Westlye, L. T., Due-Tonnessen, P., & Walhovd, K. B. (2009). Heterogeneity in subcortical brain development: A structural magnetic resonance imaging study of brain maturation from 8 to 30 years. *Journal of Neuroscience, 29,* 11772–11782.

Pearlman, L., & Saakvitne, K. (1995). *Trauma and the therapist: Counter-transference and vicarious traumatisation in psychotherapy with incest survivors.* New York: Norton.

Perry, B. D., Pollard, R. A., Blakley, T. L., Baker, W. L., & Vigilante, D. (1995). Childhood trauma, the neurobiology of adaptation, and "use-dependent" development of the brain: How "states" become "traits." *Infant Mental Health Journal, 16*(4), 271–291.

Piaget, J. (2003). Part 1: Cognitive development in children: Development and Learning. *Journal of Research in Science Teaching, 40,* S8–S18.

Piaget, J. (2008). Intellectual evolution from adolescence to adulthood. *Human Development, 51*(1), 40–47.

Piaget, J., Garcia, R., Davidson, P. M., & Easley, J. (1991). *Toward a logic of meanings.* Hillsdale, NJ: Erlbaum.

Piaget, J., & Inhelder, R. (1991). The construction of reality. In J. Oates & R. Sheldon (Eds.), *Cognitive development in infancy* (pp. 165–169). East Sussex, UK: Erlbaum.

Putnam, F. W. (1997). *Dissociation in children and adolescents: A developmental perspective.* New York: Guilford Press.

Pynoos, R., Steinberg, A., & Wraith, R. (1995). A developmental model of childhood traumatic stress. In D. Cicchetti & D. Cohen (Eds.), *Manual of developmental psychopathology: Vol. 2. Risk, disorder, and adaptation* (pp. 72–95). New York: Wiley.

Resnick, M., Bearman, P., Blum, R. W., Bauman, K., Harris, K., Jones, J., et al. (1997). Protecting adolescents from harm: Findings from the National Longitudinal Study on Adolescent Health. *Journal of the American Medical Association, 278,* 823–832.

Reviere, S., & Bakeman, R. (2001). The effects of early trauma on autobiographical memory and schematic self-representation. *Applied Cognitive Psychology, 15*(7), S89–S100.

Rogers, C. (1951). *Client-centered therapy: Its current practice, implications, and theory.* Boston: Houghton Mifflin.

Rothbart, M. K., Ahadi, S. A., & Evans, D. E. (2000). Temperament and personality: Origins and outcomes. *Journal of Personality and Social Psychology, 78,* 122–135.

Runyon, M., & Kenny, M. (2002). Relationship of attributional style, depression, and posttrauma distress among children who suffered physical or sexual abuse. *Child Maltreatment, 7,* 254–264.

Saakvitne, K., Gamble, S., Pearlman, L., & Lev, B. (2000). *Risking connection: A training curriculum for working with survivors of child abuse.* Baltimore: Sidran Institute Press.

Scheeringa, M. S., & Zeanah, C. H. (2001). A relational perspective on PTSD in early childhood. *Journal of Traumatic Stress, 14,* 799–815.

Schore, A. (2001a). The effects of early relational trauma on right brain development, affect regulation, and infant mental health development. *Infant Mental Health Journal, 22,* 201–269.

Schore, A. (2001b). Effects of a secure attachment on right brain development, affect regulation, and infant mental health. *Infant Mental Health Journal, 22,* 7–66.

Shapiro, F. (1995). *Eye movement desensitization and reprocessing (EMDR): Basic principles, protocols, and procedures.* New York: Guilford Press.

Shields, A., Ryan, R., & Cicchetti, D. (2001). Narrative representations of caregivers and emotion dysregulation as predictors of maltreated children's rejection by peers. *Developmental Psychology, 37,* 321–337.

Shoda, Y., Mischel, W., & Peake, P. K. (1990). Predicting adolescent cognitive and self-regulatory competencies from preschool delay of gratification: Identifying diagnostic conditions. *Developmental Psychology, 26*(6), 978–986.

Shonk, S. M., & Cicchetti, D. (2001). Maltreatment, competency deficits, and risk for academic and behavioral maladjustment. *Developmental Psychology, 37,* 3–17.

Simpson, J. A., Collins, W. A., Tran, S., & Haydon, K. C. (2007). Attachment and the experience and expression of emotions in romantic relationships: A developmental perspective. *Journal of Personality and Social Psychology, 92,* 355–367.

Smith, J., & Prior, M. (1995). Temperament and stress resilience in school-age children: A within-families study. *Journal of the American Academy of Child and Adolescent Psychiatry, 34,* 168–179.

Solomon, S. D., & Davidson, J. R. T. (1997). Trauma: Prevalence, impairment, service use, and cost. *Journal of Clinical Psychiatry, 58*(Suppl. 9), 5–11.

Spinazzola, J., Blaustein, M., & van der Kolk, B. (2005). Posttraumatic stress disorder treatment outcome research: The study of unrepresentative samples. *Journal of Traumatic Stress, 18*(5), 425–436.

Spiraling Hearts. (n.d.). *Yoga Bingo.* Available at *www.spiralinghearts.com.*

Stamm, B. H. (Ed.). (1999). *Secondary traumatic stress: Self-care issues for clinicians, researchers, and educators* (2nd ed.). Baltimore: Sidran Institute Press.

Streeck-Fischer, A., & van der Kolk, B. (2000). Down will come baby, cradle and all: Diagnostic and therapeutic implications of chronic trauma on child development. *Australian and New Zealand Journal of Psychiatry, 34,* 903–918.

Tamnes, C. K., Ostby, Y., Fjell, A. M., Westlye, L. T., Due-Tonnessen, P., & Walhovd, K. B. (2009). Brain maturation in adolescence and young adulthood: Regional age-related changes in cortical thickness and white matter volume and microstructure. *Cerebral Cortex.*

Terr, L. (1990). *Too scared to cry: Psychic trauma in childhood.* New York: HarperCollins.

Tinker, R. H., & Wilson, S. A. (1999). Through the eyes of a child: EMDR with children. New York: Norton.

Toth, S., & Cicchetti, D. (1996). Patterns of relatedness, depressive symptomatology, and perceived competence in maltreated children. *Journal of Consulting and Clinical Psychology, 64*(1), 32–41.

Tronick, E. (2007). *The neurobehavioral and social–emotional development of infants and children.* New York: Norton.

Urban, J., Carlson, E., Egeland, B., & Sroufe, A. (1991). Patterns of individual adaptation across childhood. *Development and Psychopathology, 3,* 445–460.

van der Kolk, B. (2005). Developmental trauma disorder: Toward a rational diagnosis for children with complex trauma histories. *Psychiatric Annals, 35*(5), 401–408.

van der Kolk, B., Roth, S., Pelcovitz, D., & Mandel, F. S. (1994). *Disorders of extreme stress: Results from the DSM-IV field trial for PTSD*. Unpublished manuscript.

van IJzendoorn, M. H. (1995). Adult attachment representations, parental responsiveness and infant attachment: A meta-analysis on the predictive validity of the Adult Attachment Interview. *Psychological Bulletin, 117,* 387–403.

Vondra, J., Barnett, D., & Cicchetti, D. (1989). Perceived and actual competence among maltreated and comparison school children. *Development and Psychopathology, 1,* 237–255.

Vondra, J., Barnett, D., & Cicchetti, D. (1990). Self-concept, motivation, and competence among preschoolers from maltreating and comparison families. *Child Abuse and Neglect, 14,* 525–540.

Wakschlag, L., & Hans, S. (1999). Relation of maternal responsiveness during infancy to the development of behavior problems in high-risk youths. *Developmental Psychology, 35,* 569–579.

Webb, N. B. (Ed.). (2007). *Play therapy with children in crisis: Individual, group, and family treatment* (3rd ed.). New York: Guilford Press.

Werker, J. F., & Tees, R. C. (1984). Cross-language speech perception: Evidence for perceptual reorganization during the first year of life. *Infant Behavior and Development, 7,* 49–63.

Werner, E. E., & Smith, R. S. (1980). An epidemiologic perspective on some antecedents and consequences of childhood mental health problems and learning disabilities. *Annual Progress in Child Psychiatry and Child Development,* pp. 133–147.

Werner, E. E., & Smith, R. S. (2001). *Journeys from childhood to midlife: Risk, resilience, and recovery.* Ithaca, NY: Cornell University Press.

Wolff, A., & Ratner, P. (1999). Stress, social support, and sense of coherence. *Western Journal of Nursing Research, 21*(2), 182–197.

Wyman, P. A., Cowen, E. L., Work, W. C., Hoyt-Meyers, L., Magnus, K. B., & Fagen, D. B. (1999). Caregiving and developmental factors differentiating young at-risk urban children showing resilient versus stress-affected outcomes: A replication and extension. *Child Development, 70,* 645–659.

Wyman, P. A., Cowen, E. L., Work, W. C., & Parker, G. R. (1991). Developmental and family milieu correlates of resilience in urban children who have experienced major life-stress. *American Journal of Community Psychology, 19,* 405–426.

Zelazo, P. D. (2001). Self-reflection and the development of consciously controlled processing. In P. Mitchell & K. J. Riggs (Eds.), *Children's reasoning and the mind* (pp. 169–189). London: Psychology Press.

Index